It Wasn't Pretty, Folks, but Didn't We Have Fun?

It Wasn't Pretty, Folks, but Didn't We Have Fun?

Esquire in the Sixties

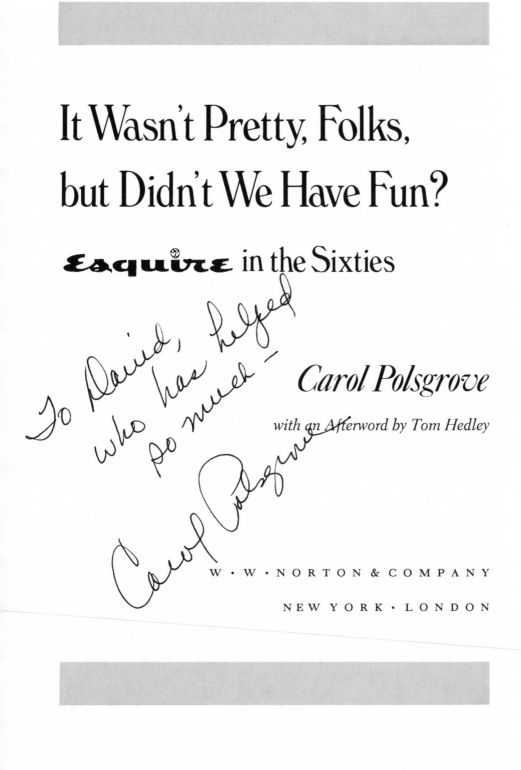

Carol Polsgrove

with an Afterword by Tom Hedley

To David, who has helped so much —

Carol Polsgrove

W · W · NORTON & COMPANY

NEW YORK · LONDON

FIRST EDITION

The text of this book is composed in Avanta with the display set in Typositor Windsor and Caslon. Composition and manufacturing are by The Haddon Craftsmen, Inc. Book design by Marjorie J. Flock.

Library of Congress Cataloging-in-Publication Data

Polsgrove, Carol.
    It wasn't pretty, folks, but didn't we have fun?: Esquire in the
sixties / by Carol Polsgrove.
      p.   cm.
    Includes bibliographical references and index.
    1. Esquire (New York: N.Y.)   I. Title.
PN4900.E8P65   1995
051—dc20   95-5457

ISBN 0-393-03792-4

W. W. Norton & Company, Inc., 500 Fifth Avenue, New York, N.Y. 10110
W. W. Norton & Company Ltd., 10 Coptic Street, London WC1A 1PU

1 2 3 4 5 6 7 8 9 0

To the memory of Edward R. Hagemann
1921–1994

Teacher and Scholar

Contents

Preface

I WAS FIFTEEN when John F. Kennedy was elected president and
the sixties began. I was in college when he faced off against
Khrushchev over Russian missiles in Cuba. I was in an English
literature class when he was killed in Dallas. I was visiting in West
Africa in the summer of 1964 when the Gulf of Tonkin resolution freed
President Lyndon Johnson to fight the Vietnam War. I was at work for
Associated Press the night the news came over the wire from Memphis
that Martin Luther King had been shot. When I heard Robert Kennedy
had been shot in California, I was ironing, and I felt, clutching my iron, as
if I were on a raft, adrift in a stormy sea.

Curiously, given the prominence of public events in my own life in the
sixties, when I first happened upon the material that turned into this book
I saw it outside the context of time. I had been writing an essay on Gay
Talese's magazine work in the 1960s, and I had wondered how Talese's
relationship with his editors at *Esquire* had affected his pieces, those artful
Esquire profiles he collected in *Fame and Obscurity*. I knew Harold Hayes
had been editor of *Esquire* in the 1960s—a legendary editor, one of the
great ones, like Harold Ross of *The New Yorker*. Had Hayes worked with
Talese? And might I be able to find correspondence between them? I
called *Esquire* magazine and asked where Hayes's old files might be.

That was how I learned that after Hayes's death, boxes of his correspondence and office memoranda had been deposited, at his request, in
the Z. Smith Reynolds Library at Wake Forest University, his alma mater
and my own. I was intrigued. I had been a magazine editor, and I was still
writing for magazines. I knew how powerfully the editor-writer relationship can shape the work of the writer. *Esquire* had given the sixties some

of the decade's finest writing, from Talese, Tom Wolfe, Norman Mailer, Michael Herr, and many others. Hayes's *Esquire* had been a magazine set apart, where reporters were writing a whole new kind of journalism, or so it seemed to us then. When I discovered Hayes had left a paper trail of his work—a map of his relationships with writers—I was elated.

In June 1991, I made my way through the files—letter after letter to and from writers: Talese, Wolfe, Mailer, Herr; James Baldwin, Garry Wills, John Sack, Richard Rovere. . . . There were writers I knew and writers I didn't know. There were office memoranda, letters home, even a few journal entries. There was an unfinished manuscript for a book on magazine editing. There was a lot—yet as I neared the end of my survey, I had an unsettled feeling, as if this were a puzzle and at least half the pieces were not on the table.

In one file I had come across an address for Hayes's old college friend Bob Sherrill, who had gone to work with him at *Esquire.* Was Sherrill still living in Durham, North Carolina? He was, and, before I left North Carolina, I drove over to meet him in his little house, and he pulled out his old *Esquire*s for us to look at together: big magazines, oversized, like *Life,* with those weird George Lois covers. As we rambled around in the past, the world of *Esquire* in the sixties took on a reality it had not had during my days of reading the papers.

I looked up other *Esquire* editors—and writers, art directors, photographers, most of them still in Manhattan, still carrying on the business of making culture: movies, books, magazines, television. Like all of us, they have forgotten much. They see the past through the veil of the years that have followed. But when they re-created conversations from thirty years ago, I could hear the voices, the scrape of chairs.

Robert Benton took me back to the late 1950s, when he was *Esquire*'s art director and New York was "a place filled with promise." David Newman, the *Esquire* editor who teamed up with Benton to write the movie *Bonnie and Clyde,* took me to *Esquire* parties of the early sixties, when writers drank too much and fought over women. John Berendt took me—along with Terry Southern, Jean Genet, and William Burroughs, three of the wildest literary men of the time—to the 1968 Democratic Convention. I looked up others and, one by one, they added their memories to the store.

Meanwhile, I was also reading my way through the magazine—sometimes, wonderfully, not in the bound library volumes but in my own copies, rescued from an attic of a bookstore in Greensboro, North Carolina. Eventually, I saw what I should have seen from the start: that I could not look at the creative world of *Esquire* apart from its time. This was not a puzzle but a story, the story of *Esquire*'s people passing through the sixties, when America was transformed in ways we have not yet fully fathomed.

For many of us who lived through that time, history pressed closely on our lives. For the men and women who created the monthly issues of *Esquire,* tracking history was their job. Most magazines try to catch their times on the wing, in one way or another, but because *Esquire* redefined itself in the late fifties as an avant-garde magazine, it tried harder than most. *Esquire* did its part to break up the monochrome of fifties culture in the early sixties, ranging widely across the scene, acquiring an attitude: an irreverent, skeptical edge—a cross between the *Harvard Lampoon* and H. L. Mencken's *American Mercury,* with the eclectic, iconoclastic spirit of the decade's turn—the spirit behind Joseph Heller's *Catch-22* and Thomas Pynchon's *V.*

How would that attitude weather the storms of the later sixties? What would *Esquire* do with the Vietnam War, the riots in the cities, the demonstrations on college campuses? *Esquire* negotiated the turn, publishing powerful reports by John Sack and Michael Herr on Vietnam. In the wake of summer riots, Garry Wills toured the ruins of American cities.

So vibrant was the journalism at *Esquire* that it inspired experimentation elsewhere. There began to be talk of a "New Journalism." Hayes himself turned away from the concept, contending that New Journalism was not new at all. He was right, in a way, but wrong too, because magazine journalism did renew itself in the sixties, before it went down for the count. With television competing for advertisers, big general-interest magazines—*Life, Look,* the *Saturday Evening Post*—were on the ropes. But other magazines were giving America some of the best journalism it had ever had: *The New Yorker,* the *New York Review of Books, New York, Ramparts,* Willie Morris's *Harper's,* and, toward the end of the sixties, *Rolling Stone.* Later on, some of their editors would say *Esquire* had opened the door.

Even now, the exuberance of the sixties *Esquire* seems unsurpassed. Today's magazines, by contrast, seem editorial starvelings, pale and thin, however swollen they are with advertisements. *Esquire* was a big, unruly book, its contents unbound by formulaic notions of what belonged there.

Esquire mixed on-the-scene reports with Diane Arbus photographs, un-worshipful profiles with charts of power in America, guides to campus protest with movie reviews by Dwight Macdonald, fiction by Raymond Carver, and surreal paintings by Jean-Paul Goude. In some respects a conventional man, as an editor Harold Hayes had few inhibitions. He would put just about anything into the magazine if *he* thought it belonged there. Tom Wolfe never got over the *Esquire* photo spread he remembered spotting in the early seventies: "portrait after portrait of chicken feet, in high resolution, double-size, triple-size . . . chicken feet!" he wrote in 1973. When he talked with me twenty years later, he was still bemused.

Hayes explained the free-for-all as a legacy of Arnold Gingrich, *Esquire*'s founding editor, who thought a good magazine was like a three-ring circus. The *Esquire* of the sixties owed plenty to Gingrich, who had already made *Esquire* a great magazine once, when he started it in the thirties and published Ernest Hemingway and F. Scott Fitzgerald. But as publisher, Gingrich mattered most to Hayes as a buffer between Hayes and company management. Even when *Esquire* prospered under Hayes's guidance, there were murmurs of discontent on the business side: Couldn't there be more service features, fewer controversial covers? Couldn't the editors take fashion more seriously?

Hayes did not care what reader surveys said people wanted to see in his magazine; he would give them what they didn't expect to see. He was never interested in the girl stories or travel reports he had to put in to satisfy the advertising staff; all those service pages were simply space he had to fill so he could get to the good part. He did what he had to do, but he never forgot that he was a journalist whose job was to help readers make sense of their times, not by editorializing or hewing to some narrow line, but by making his magazine a forum for provocative views and detailed reports, for scenes freshly viewed and ideas newly expressed, in words, images—whatever it took.

Not everyone liked him; he could be charming, but he could be cold. Everyone feared him, one staff member told me; everyone was in love with him, said another. Survivors still divide themselves into camps, arguing who was the greater: Harold Hayes or Clay Felker, who had competed with him for the job of *Esquire*'s editor and went on to create his own unique magazine, *New York*. Hayes—and his decisions—could stir passionate response. After he ran William F. Buckley's and Gore Vidal's attacks on each other in 1969, Buckley sued *Esquire;* the suit ended his friendship with Hayes. Still, twenty-five years later Buckley wrote to me, "He was a very great editor. . . ."

But Hayes did not make *Esquire* alone and would not have wanted a claim made that he did; *Esquire* was a group enterprise. Hayes did not always understand the people he worked with; some had talents he did not have, yet he had a sixth sense for what they could do. His greatest gift as an editor may have been his ability to bring out the best in other people. Writers and editors were not instruments of his will; they were co-creators. He believed "in a magazine that unfolds the story of the people who work for it," according to Gordon Lish, who succeeded Bob Brown and Rust Hills as fiction editor. And so this is the story not only of Harold Hayes, but of all who made *Esquire* in the sixties one of the most intricate records of its time.

I want to thank those who spent hours talking with me, sometimes several times, sharing correspondence and telephone numbers. I have listed their names in the Sources section at the end of the book. I have not showed the manuscript to any of them, except for Tom Hedley, who graciously contributed an afterword on Hayes's life after *Esquire*. I thank them all for entrusting me with their stories; if errors they would have caught have slipped through, I apologize. I apologize, too, for turning them into characters, so much more partial and incomplete than they are in real life, and perhaps different in many ways than they were then, at the time of my story. Clay Felker has a thankless role in this book as foil to Harold Hayes; he is, in real life, the star of his own story. Henry Wolf, the art director who set a new standard and style at *Esquire*, walks off the stage almost as soon as my story begins. I particularly regret the unhappy role Abe Blinder must play; the last major survivor of *Esquire*'s earliest days, he guided the company for many years. His gift of *Esquire*'s papers to the University of Michigan helped make this book possible, and in our several conversations he responded generously to my questions. In our casual dealings, he lived up to Robert Benton's description of him as "a lovely, lovely man."

I regret that I could bring in only a small number of the many who made *Esquire* what it was. How did I decide which stories to tell? I was guided partly by Hayes's own selection of articles for *Smiling Through the Apocalypse: Esquire's History of the Sixties*. I was guided, too, by the comments of other *Esquire* editors and writers I talked with. *Esquire* was often the subject of comment by newspapers and other magazines during the sixties, and I scanned those accounts to see what in the magazine was drawing attention. Because I wanted to show what was going on behind the scenes, the availability of correspondence affected my choices. Finally, the events and changing zeitgeist of the sixties weighed heavily in my choices, as did the requirements of coherent narrative.

In addition to those who participated in the story, several others helped me determine the course it would take.

Edward R. Hagemann, an ex-Marine who guided me through the University of Louisville graduate school in the seventies, compiled the first index to *Esquire*'s serious literary work, published as an appendix to *The Armchair Esquire* (1958); Hagemann and Gingrich had actually met. I was pleased to be following in Ed Hagemann's footsteps, and I grieved when he died, before he could read my book, although not before he had given the first several chapters his scrupulous editorial attention and helped me to understand the significance of Arnold Gingrich's achievement, the importance of Gingrich's vision of what a magazine should be.

I might not be professionally interested in magazines at all if Erwin Knoll, editor of *The Progressive*, had not started publishing my pieces in the 1970s and, later, hired me as an editor. Because of our relationship over the years, I understand the importance and complexity of ongoing writer-editor relationships in the lives of magazines and writers. He died in November 1994, and I will miss him. Himself a reporter on the Washington scene during the sixties (and once, even, a contributor to *Esquire*), he had read an early draft of this book and told me what I had left out.

After I began work on the book, Julia Kagan, an editor with experience at the top of several New York magazines—*McCall's, Working Woman, Psychology Today*—joined the Indiana University faculty as a visiting professor and became for me a valuable source. She provided counsel and accommodations, and, when the manuscript was completed, she read it on deadline. From the beginning, George Juergens, a historian at Indiana University, told me my proper subject was not editorial creativity; it was culture-making in the sixties. My brother, William N. Claxon, Jr., a member of the English faculty at the University of South Carolina, Aiken, has a fine gift for narrative; I asked him to tell me where my storytelling went astray, and he did, honestly and precisely.

I owe thanks, too, to Joseph Rebello, a University of Kansas graduate student (now a reporter), who interviewed Harold Hayes twice not long before his death and wrote a master's thesis that introduced me to the drama of the late fifties at *Esquire.* He shared with me his appreciation of Hayes's *Esquire,* which he encountered first in his home country, India, and found compelling, even at that distance from the culture out of which it came. He was the first of several readers of the sixties *Esquire* I encountered in the course of writing this book; their memories, too, helped shape my sense of what was important, and added weight to my belief in the vitality of this magazine.

Harold Hayes's young cousin Hayes McNeill, my contemporary at Wake Forest, may have spoken for many when he wrote to Hayes, not long before Hayes's death, that *Esquire* had "colored and shaped an entire generation of us in a way very few American publications have ever done." After Harold Hayes's death, McNeill brought his papers to Wake Forest. I owe him great thanks for that, and also for the insights he has given me into Hayes himself.

I owe special appreciation to Hayes's widow, Judy Kessler, who gave me unconditional permission to quote from his professional papers at Wake Forest when I began the project.

Hayes's first wife, Susan, who shared his *Esquire* years, spoke willingly with me, as did his son, Tom Hayes. Hayes's sister-in-law, Thomasine Hayes, wife of Hayes's brother Jim, helped me see the young Hayes, as he was before he went to *Esquire.* Several members of the Wake Forest community were helpful, especially Bynum Shaw, my former journalism professor, who knew Hayes in college and also wrote for *Esquire.*

The curators and staffs of the collections I have worked with patiently produced box after box of documents, responded to photocopying requests, and sought out specific documents once I was no longer on the scene. I want to give special thanks to Sharon Snow, curator of the Rare Books and Manuscripts Department, Z. Smith Reynolds Library, Wake Forest University, and her assistant, Megan Mulder; Saundra Taylor, curator of manuscripts at the Lilly Library, Indiana University, which acquired Gordon Lish's papers while I was working on this book and Rust Hills's papers as the book went to press; Nancy Bartlett, reference archivist, and Francis X. Blouin, Jr., director, Bentley Historical Library, University of Michigan; Thomas W. Southall, a former curator at the Spencer Museum of Art, University of Kansas; and Charles Niles in Special Collections at the Mugar Memorial Library, Boston University.

Indiana University has supported this research with generous grants from the Research and University Graduate School and the Bureau of

Media Research of the School of Journalism, which also provided me with released time to write the book. My dean, Trevor Brown, has always been ready to smooth my way and offer counsel in difficult situations. I asked Ralph Holsinger, the School of Journalism's longtime expert on communications law, to read my manuscript for legal problems, and he graciously complied. Ran Wei, a Ph.D. student at the School of Journalism, analyzed *Esquire*'s circulation and revenue figures, charting their rise and fall over the period and comparing *Esquire*'s fortunes with those of other magazines. Three other students—Bill Lebzelter, Holly Ellender, and John Meunier—rendered research assistance. Two members of the secretarial staff, Heidi Wampler and Lauren Kinzer, fielded phone calls and faxes and helped in innumerable ways.

Several friends have provided ongoing advice, encouragement, and good examples: Becky O'Malley, Sandra Conn, Gerald and Del Coomer, Holly Stocking, Rosemary Daniell, and Suzanne Lipsett. My young daughter gave me secretarial assistance on several occasions, and patiently waited on others. I thank my mother, Emma Claxon, and my father, Neville Claxon, for sustaining me in many ways, for many years.

My agent, Doe Coover of Boston, has from the start been a smart, caring guide, who found for me exactly the right editor: Gerald Howard, who cut his eyeteeth on *Esquire* and, besides, has Harold Hayes's ability to find the soft spots and slippery places. I thank them both.

A word about the title: It is not a quotation. I wrote it myself, in the spirit of *Esquire.*

It Wasn't Pretty, Folks, but Didn't We Have Fun?

Part One

Suddenly it was 1960 and John Kennedy was there, and the wise, the intellectual and the taste-making people did him homage. They didn't think he was a father or Gramps. They liked him because he was tough, because he was all pro, because he was a man who knew what he wanted and grabbed it.

ROBERT BENTON AND DAVID NEWMAN, *Esquire*, JULY 1964

ONE

Open the Windows

*T*HEY WERE TWO of the most creative people in New York in
1959, but not many knew it, not even themselves: Harold Hayes,
an editor at *Esquire,* and Diane Arbus, a former fashion photographer. Arbus had only lately left a successful fashion photogra-
phy partnership with her husband, Alan Arbus; they shot covers for *Glam-
our* and *Seventeen* and spreads for *Vogue.* But Arbus was sick to death of
the work that she did: mostly styling the models—doing their hair, their
makeup, selecting accessories, props. She had done it for years, and now
she had quit, and was roaming the hidden places of New York, at all hours
of the day and night, looking for something: forbidden images, unrecorded truths about being human, the uncanny edge other photographers had missed. She photographed a female impersonator, a beggar who
called himself Moondog, an escape artist named Randi.

Who could have guessed Harold Hayes would understand what she
was doing? Hayes—a tall, lanky southerner, son of a Southern Baptist
minister—was fascinated by the mundane. He once proposed to a sales
company a device for lighting charcoal briquettes without aid of lighter
fluid, twigs, or piles of paper. He wrote detailed, indignant letters to dry
cleaners who shrunk his pants and to credit card companies that sent him
cards in the mail. He enjoyed life, gunning his motorcycle through the
late-night New York streets after a party. In a conversation, he listened
intently, laughed appreciatively. He gave the impression he really cared—
really wanted to know what people were doing and thinking.

Their curiosity drew them together, Arbus and Hayes. He found her
genuinely warm, her sense of humor marvelous. She was fresh, almost
naive. He barely seemed to notice the vast differences between them. She

was a petite Jewish child of Manhattan, daughter of a prosperous furrier. She had grown up in isolation and wealth—ensconced in darkened sumptuous apartments with her brother, Howard Nemerov, who became a poet and novelist. She could be gracious and kind, fey and unconventional, but she was often deeply depressed and withdrawn. Shy, she had had to work hard to overcome her reserve—to be able to go up to strangers. She could dress well—she would show up for lunch with Hayes in a well-cut linen suit. But she was often indifferent to her appearance; an *Esquire* writer who had planned to take her to lunch when she met him for an assignment abandoned the plan when he saw how she looked, as if she had slept in her clothes.

Life seemed never to offer Harold Hayes a challenge he could not meet, a defeat he could not get past. Diane Arbus struggled to discover on film depths no one else had, then died by her own hand.

He puzzled her.

Tell me about Harold, she once said to another editor.

He's hard, the editor replied.

Hayes *was* hard when he wanted to be, his anger flashing out. Arbus found him curt on occasion. Once when he had asked her to destroy or return a letter stating she was on assignment for *Esquire*, she observed that his letter had been "somewhat lacking in human warmth," just the sort of letter to write to the telephone company. She invited him to lunch anyway and signed her letter,

> Yours,
> Sincerely,
> Cordially,
> Cruelly,
> Frankly,
> Fondly,
> Diane.

Different as they were, Hayes was among the first to recognize Arbus's astonishing talent. He saw it in the first pictures she brought to *Esquire* in the late summer of 1959. She did not appear at *Esquire* unannounced. She lived across the street from the writer Thomas B. Morgan, one of *Esquire*'s most frequent contributors, and he had sent her to *Esquire*. And her brother had a story coming out in *Esquire* in September. But the pictures themselves were her true entree: "Her vision, her subject matter, her snapshot style, were perfect for *Esquire*, perfect for the times; she stripped away everything to the thing itself," Hayes told her biographer, Patricia Bosworth.

When Hayes asked Robert Benton, *Esquire*'s art director, to look at Arbus's photographs, Benton did not expect much. He knew Diane Arbus as a fashion photographer—that was all. He said to himself: "Harold has no visual sense but I like Harold and I'm going to be polite to this woman. I'll get out of this as tactfully as I can, without making an enemy of Harold or Diane." Then he saw these remarkable images, some of them drawn from visits to Hubert's Museum, a flea circus at 42nd and Broadway: Hezekiah Trambles, "The Jungle Creep"; Andrew Ratoucheff, the Russian midget. Her peculiar subjects intrigued him, but so did the way she approached them, getting close, yet remaining detached.

How could they get Arbus into the magazine? They had a special issue on New York coming up; they wanted to make it distinctively *Esquire's*—unpredictable and complex, like a broken mirror catching the city's light from various angles. They already had an opening piece by a young *New York Times* reporter, the son of an Italian immigrant tailor—Gay Talese. It was his first for the magazine, a sequence of odd New York scenes and facts. Novelist James Baldwin was writing a piece on Harlem; another fiction writer, John Cheever, was writing about leaving New York.

They had a thought: Arbus had shown in these pictures what she could do with the lowlife of New York. Suppose she were to stretch to the other extreme and photograph New York's high life? She had done Hezekiah Trambles; suppose she were to try Joan Crawford? Or she could photograph a *haut monde* salon and compare it to Beauty City, a twenty-four-hour hair salon on 47th Street and Broadway. And why didn't she try the city morgue?

Thus began a freewheeling photographic odyssey: Arbus spent four months trekking off to stockyards, a children's dance class, the Bowery, a pet funeral, a charity ball . . . the list went on and on. Hayes suggested subjects and wrote a stream of letters and bona-fides to get her into places she wanted to photograph. As her requests for help came thick and fast, Hayes began to think she needed more than an editor and a secretary behind her: she needed an army. He did his best, but even his efforts sometimes proved futile. The New York City Department of Correction tried to get *Esquire* to cough up a donation in return for the privilege of admitting Arbus to the Tombs. Hayes declined. In a polite letter, he wondered "if this is really a proper reason for your exclusion of us."

The attempt to get a picture of Joan Crawford was no more successful. Crawford had never heard of Arbus. Could she see samples of her work? Or couldn't that photographer who had photographed her for *Town & Country* be assigned instead? Arbus did not mind missing Crawford. She had been out peering into Rolls-Royces and strolling up Lexington Avenue, where, she wrote Benton, she saw a man lying with his fly open in front of a church; above him, a church sign declared, "Open for Meditation and Prayer."

In the end, six photographs composed "The Vertical Journey: Six Movements of a Moment within the Heart of the City." The six-page spread appeared in July 1960, in *Esquire*'s New York issue: "The Jungle Creep" paired with a soft-focus young socialite at a charity ball, a self-possessed midget in a topcoat opposite a sedate Daughter of the American Revolution in long pearls, and, finally, a bare-chested madman confronting the last shot—the upturned feet of a corpse, a large identification tag dangling from a big toe.

The sixties had started at *Esquire*.

Arnold Gingrich and Dave Smart, an energetic Chicago entrepreneur, had started *Esquire* in the depths of the depression, wryly, as a magazine for "the new leisure," filling its pages with contributions from Ernest Hemingway, John Dos Passos, Erskine Caldwell, F. Scott Fitzgerald, Dashiell Hammett, and cartoons and sketches by E. Simms Campbell, a black artist who had graduated from the Art Institute of Chicago but had had trouble getting his work across the color line at other magazines. The design of Gingrich's first issue in the autumn of 1933 was simple and clean, the advertisements clustered at front and back. The fashions did not dominate, but they were important; Gingrich and his partner Smart— his boss, really, but they seemed like partners—meant to sell *Esquire* in men's clothing stores. Only 5,000 of the 105,000 copies of the first issue went to newsstands, until the newsstands sold out in a matter of hours, and the distributor called for more. The plan went into reverse: 100,000 issues went onto the newsstands and sold out.

By the end of 1937, *Esquire*'s circulation climbed to 675,000, topping the success of the trade magazine that Smart had started before Gingrich came along, *Gentlemen's Quarterly*, and another magazine they had started together, *Apparel Arts*. *Esquire* was doing so well that they launched *Coronet*, which started out as a small-format art magazine; a

European art magazine named *Verve;* and *Ken,* a political magazine taking its title from an old word for knowledge (as in "beyond our ken"). Intending to run articles in *Ken* that the rest of the press was too cowardly to run, Gingrich found himself under attack from every side; the Catholic Church gave him an especially hard time after he published an article by a Los Angeles prostitute and a report on the Spanish Civil War that displeased church officials. By mid-1939, both *Esquire* and *Ken* were being boycotted by Catholics in 1,500 American cities and towns. *Ken* dropped by the wayside, but *Esquire* moved on.

World War II brought a change. Angling for bigger paper allotments from the War Production Board, Smart and Gingrich expanded the girl pages, offering the servicemen pinups on double-page spreads. In 1942 a Catholic postmaster general began proceedings to take away the magazine's second-class mailing privilege on moral grounds. *Esquire* argued its case up to the Supreme Court and won. By the end of the war Arnold Gingrich was tired of it all, and maybe, too, he and Smart had begun to wear on each other's nerves. By the age of forty, Gingrich told Smart, he had done a full lifetime of work. He was ready to retire. He moved to Switzerland, and he and Smart severed ties.

Without him, *Esquire* misplaced its editorial soul. Dave Smart was "a mercurial, impatient, difficult man," his right-hand man, Abe Blinder, would remember. He swallowed his editors up—called them every night to pour out ideas. The man he hired to edit *Esquire,* Frederic A. Birmingham, was a nice man, but compliant—not the best choice to restore *Esquire*'s panache after the war. The luxurious look and the literary tone vanished in a thicket of Westerns and detective stories. The design was garish, confused. Circulation stayed high—around 800,000 in the early fifties—but blue-chip advertisers, wary of *Esquire*'s naughty wartime reputation, stayed away.

Esquire had moved to New York in 1950, settling into the curved-corner *Look* Building at 488 Madison Avenue (*Esquire* was on the fourth floor, downstairs from *Look*). All around were signs of what *Esquire* was missing. New York was booming. Skyscrapers were going up, shining towers of glass and steel. One summer day in 1952, Gingrich, back in the United States and working upstairs from *Esquire* at a Cowles magazine called *Flair,* lunched at the Stork Club with Dave Smart, who painted a glorious future if Gingrich would only come back to *Esquire.* Together they could ride the great postwar boom. If Gingrich would just return,

Smart promised to keep out of editorial decisions. "I've learned that the hard way," he told Gingrich, "but I know it now. So when you come back, you'll find me completely changed. I'll just stick to the business side."

How could Gingrich resist? He was back on the job right away, this time as publisher. By a stroke of bad luck, Dave Smart, the company's founder and the most dynamic of the Smart brothers, died within three months. His brother Alfred had died earlier. Now the youngest Smart brother, John, was left to represent the Smart family, the major stock-holders. Abe Blinder, who had been there almost since the beginning, took the lead in guiding the company's fortunes, and Fritz Bamberger, an Austrian refugee and Schopenhauer scholar, tried to get things moving on the editorial side. But the company wasn't the same without Dave Smart's explosive energy.

By another stroke of bad luck, the year when Gingrich came back to *Esquire*, the Federal Communications Commission lifted a freeze on li-censes for television stations, and television took off. Advertising agencies leaped to take advantage of an audience that could turn out to be massive beyond belief. *Esquire* could not hope to keep up with television's soaring numbers, especially after *Esquire* abandoned the girlie market to *Playboy*, a new magazine created by a young man who had worked in *Esquire*'s promotion department in Chicago—Hugh Hefner. But *Esquire* could reach out for an audience of affluent young men—professionals, execu-tives—who could afford good suits and good liquor and occasional trips abroad.

Gingrich set to work. He fired *Esquire*'s old art director and elevated Henry Wolf, a talented young Austrian who restored *Esquire*'s elegance. He invited Paul Gallico, George Jean Nathan, and Aldous Huxley to write something for every issue. He brought back Helen Lawrenson, a glamor-ous, talented writer, former managing editor of *Vanity Fair*, who had written that famous 1936 piece for *Esquire*, "Latins Are Lousy Lovers." He tried dramatic moves, articles like "Californians Are Crazy" and "Let's Secede from Texas." But the transformation was slow. By 1956, Gingrich was willing to entertain the idea that he might need young editors to help him do the job.

"Dear Arnold," Laura Bergquist had written to Arnold Gingrich on September 23, 1954, "I don't often go out on a limb for somebody, but there is a young man who has been working on *Pageant*, named Harold

Hayes, and I think he has real capabilities. . . . He's a southern boy, literary, minister's son, good on ideas, has been working heavily with pictures and cartoons, writes well, has a good eye for material, and is—I'd say—in his late 20's. Engaging young man too." Would Arnold talk to him about working for *Esquire?* During the war, Bergquist had worked at *Coronet;* Gingrich, an affable man, was happy to see the southern boy she thought so well of.

Harold Hayes had been born in Elkin, North Carolina, then lived in Beckley, West Virginia, until he was eleven and his family moved to Winston-Salem, North Carolina. There, he wrote later, along Stratford Road "the lawns were kelly green, the homes stately and symmetrical, balanced on either end by sun parlors, surrounded by box shrubs and set back an acre from the street." In Winston-Salem Hayes encountered, for the first time, the very rich, the kind of people who might appear in a story by his favorite writer, F. Scott Fitzgerald—the Reynolds and Hanes families, who lent their family names to high schools, auditoriums, stadiums, parks. When the time came for college, he traveled across the state to Wake Forest, a small Southern Baptist school, then in the town of Wake Forest.

He left school at the tail end of World War II to serve in the navy and was stationed at Newberry, South Carolina, then at Great Lakes, Illinois. After the war, he went back to Wake Forest to finish up and start law school, which he found "tedious beyond redemption." After a semester of law, he fled to the English department after barely earning the lowest passing mark in his class. In a creative writing class, he learned he could write, and he started keeping a journal in an effort to develop the skeptical stance he thought he would need as a writer.

Hayes had grown up in dogmatic circumstances. When he went home for spring vacation, he quarreled with his father, who seemed more narrow-minded than ever. Hayes was happier back at school, where he had resurrected the student magazine. It was a "yeasty time," one of his fellow journalists remembered—those years after the war, when GIs filled Wake Forest and colleges across the country beyond their capacity. Hayes loved jazz—he played the trombone, and would sit on an overturned potato-chip can in *The Student* office, directing jazz from records he brought in. When he learned that Dizzy Gillespie would pass by Wake Forest on a southern tour, he went out to the highway, flagged down Gillespie's bus, and brought Gillespie back to campus for a jam session, which Hayes wrote about in the magazine. Hayes took his job seriously. He traveled to Raleigh for a conference put together by a student editor at Duke who brought in an editor from the New York *Daily News* and a layout team from *Life*. The Duke editor's name was Clay Felker, and Hayes was impressed.

The Student that Hayes edited that year earned the North Carolina Collegiate Press Association award for "best all-around" college magazine, but by the time the issue announcing the award came out, Hayes was gone. He had taken a job in Atlanta, Georgia, writing newsletters for the telephone company, and then he transferred to the United Press, where he rewrote newspaper wire copy for the night radio wire and covered the Georgia legislature. His old friend Bob Sherrill from Wake Forest also moved to Atlanta, and the two of them drove up to Lake Burton in Hayes's first car, a '36 Packard convertible that broke down on the way back.

In August 1950, with the Korean War on, Hayes, still vulnerable to the draft despite his earlier service in the navy, joined the Marines, probably, members of his family thought, because his older brother Jim had been a Marine. For the next two years, he trained as leader of a machine-gun platoon at Camp Lejeune, North Carolina, then as intelligence officer at Fort Riley, Kansas. The work was good preparation for journalism, he noted on the brink of his discharge as first lieutenant, in a personal statement giving his background for the magazine work he had decided to seek. As an intelligence officer his responsibility was "to collect, evaluate, interpret and disseminate all information concerning the enemy." Granted, he was not doing much writing, "but the thought process remains the same."

In an application form he filled out on July 27, 1952, for a position with Cowles Magazines in New York, Hayes declared he was six feet two and weighed 155 pounds. He carried $10,000 in life insurance. He was single. He was leaving the armed services because he had been discharged, he had left United Press because the draft was imminent, and he had left Southern Bell Telephone after eight months because he "disliked commercial writing." Recent reading included *The Caine Mutiny, The Far Side of Paradise, F. Scott Fitzgerald: The Man and His Work,* and *Life, Time, The New Yorker,* the *Herald Tribune Book Review,* and the *Saturday Review of Literature.* Asked to list hobbies, he put down "music, reading, golf, tennis." Asked to list amusements, he put down "women." Asked if he regularly attended a house of religious worship, he said, "No."

"What is your ambition in life?" asked the printed form. "Editing," he replied.

Under "Remarks: such as travel, public speaking experience, etc.?" he offered, "Manevers [*sic*] in Carribean [*sic*]."

He did not get a job at a Cowles publication; instead, on the strength of a critique of one issue, he got a job as assistant editor at the magazine *Pageant.* He was twenty-six years old. At *Pageant,* a small-format general-interest magazine—a low-budget *Reader's Digest*—he learned the magazine trade at a small magazine with limited means, under Harris Shevelson, who made the editors under him turn in one hundred ideas every two weeks. Hayes stayed at *Pageant* for a little more than two years. Then, when Shevelson brought in another editor to take over a project he was working on, he quit in a huff. That was when Laura Bergquist wrote Arnold Gingrich on Hayes's behalf.

Gingrich was not hiring just then, so he sent Hayes on to a friend scouting for editors for a small newsmagazine called *Tempo,* and he told Hayes to keep in touch. Soon, Hayes was developing a new magazine—*Picture Week*—for *Tempo*'s owner. Without much of a budget to draw on, he made do with southern chutzpah. When he wanted to use some award-winning photographers' pictures without paying the photographers, one of them, Ann Zane, protested. Watching him run in and out of the office, banging into drawers, she told him he was the most nervous, hysterical editor she'd ever met and if he went on in this way he wouldn't last long. When Hayes ran an article enumerating "The Worst of Everything," an idea he had borrowed from the *Harvard Lampoon,* the owner fired the entire editorial staff.

Once again, Laura Bergquist asked Gingrich to see Hayes and, once again, Gingrich agreed. Hayes, a man attractive to women, had married a Broadway actress, Susan Meredith, and she offered him a suggestion. "Harold, you should go about it like an actress would. You should have a scrapbook with your pieces." Hayes put together a portfolio of all the features he had developed at *Pageant* and *Picture Week,* and once again presented himself to Gingrich. "This time," as Gingrich wrote later in his memoir, *Nothing But People,* "I took him in like the morning paper, knowing that in a Southern liberal who was also a Marine reserve officer I had an extremely rare bird."

When Hayes arrived at *Esquire* in 1956, he found a magazine dangerously adrift. Gingrich had been back four years, and was exercising final editorial judgment, although Fred Birmingham was still editor. Birmingham would pick stories out of the heap that came in the mail and take them to Gingrich. Henry Wolf would bring Gingrich the layouts. Gingrich would agreeably okay what they proposed, and somehow the magazine would make its way through production. Hayes was surprised. At *Pageant* and *Picture Week,* editors had taken the lead. Trained by Shevelson, a veteran of *Coronet,* an *Esquire* company magazine, Hayes had not expected to find at *Esquire* such a low level of editorial initiative. Almost everything in the magazine, words and pictures, was the result of queries from outside: virtually nothing was staff generated. Hayes spent a week reading through the dusty unpublished and unpublishable manuscripts that had piled up and found only one he thought was any good.

He was surprised, too, by the crumbled wall between advertising and editorial. Advertising salesmen would dash into the editorial offices and grab manuscripts to show to advertisers. "You can't do that," Hayes said once. "Who says?" said the salesman. Gingrich was sympathetic to advertising because he had worked in advertising and because he knew very well that *Esquire* was meant to make a profit. He did not seem to mind long lunches with advertisers or the hours talking fashion with retailers. There was another reason, Hayes learned, that Gingrich was not likely to put a stop to advertising's encroachments: Gingrich operated by the principle of *"laissez-faire."* Gingrich did not like to say no. Whether or not Gingrich had always been so unassertive, Hayes could not know, but Hayes had the feeling he was losing interest in the magazine.

In no apparent hurry to put Hayes to work, Gingrich suggested he acquaint himself with the history of *Esquire.* Hayes had never really read the magazine. He had sneaked looks at it at a neighbor's house when he was a boy; as a college editor he had admired its production techniques. Now he settled down to read. He read back issues of the magazine. He read a memoir by a former editor, Meyer Levin, *In Search.* He read the proceedings in the post office case. Gingrich was impressed. "It was the first time I had ever seen anybody so much as open one of those three books, so big, so dull, so dense, so fully packed with words, words, words."

Hayes himself was not sure what he was supposed to do in his new job as Gingrich's assistant. He seemed overjoyed when Ann Zane, the photographer who had predicted a short career for him, heard he had moved up to *Esquire* and gave him a call. She had the impression he had been all alone in his new office, just waiting for the phone to ring. "Where are you?" he asked. She was calling from Schrafft's, practically next door. "Come on up," he said, and greeted her like a long-lost friend.

After Hayes's first week, Gingrich sensed his frustration and told him, "Christ, I suppose we must have scared the shit out of you with the way we work around here." Hayes felt he needed to reassure Gingrich, instead of the other way around. He liked Gingrich, who seemed affably open, his door seldom closed. When Gingrich returned calls he would identify himself to secretaries as "Mr. Gingrich," but at *Esquire* he was "Arnold" to everyone.

Affable as he might be, within Hayes's first year on the job, Gingrich fired the articles editor, the picture editor, and Fred Birmingham. A new managing editor, Leonard Wallace Robinson, left to take a job at *Collier's*, but before he left, he hired a fiction editor, L. Rust Hills, who had been teaching in Europe and editing a literary magazine called *Quixote.* Hills set to work soliciting serious fiction, such as Leslie Fiedler's "Nude Croquet," a venomous story about New York intellectuals; Arthur Miller's "The Misfits"; and Thomas Williams's "Goose Pond."

Before Fred Birmingham left, he told a young man named Ralph Ginzburg that he ought to try for his job. Ginzburg was director of circulation promotion at *Look,* upstairs, but he had been freelancing for *Esquire,* which had paid him an astonishing $2,000 for a piece he had done on library holdings of erotica. Ginzburg interviewed for the job and was hired—not by Gingrich, who seemed to him spineless and not especially talented, but by the Austrian refugee Fritz Bamberger, who seemed to be running the magazine. Ginzburg thought he was hired to replace Fred Birmingham as top editor. It would mean a pay cut, but he would get to do the editorial work he wanted to do. After Ginzburg had already quit his *Look* job, Bamberger broke the news. There had been a change of plans: two men would share the editorial power—Ralph Ginzburg and Clay Felker, lately of *Look*'s competitor, *Life.* Ginzburg was shocked and disappointed, but he had burned his bridges. He and Felker started work the same day, January 2, 1957.

When Felker came to work that first day, he stopped by Hayes's office to shake hands, and Hayes brought up the Duke conference. Although the two of them had not actually met there, Hayes had been impressed by Felker and was predisposed to like him. But Felker said something abrupt and walked on down the hall. It didn't take Hayes long to see Felker as an ambitious man galloping full tilt ahead.

What Felker remembered most clearly about the day he and Ginzburg started work was Gingrich gathering his editors together to say, "All right, I'm turning the magazine over to you. I will preside over it, but it's up to you to think up all the ideas and assign the writers and so on." Gingrich was capable of coming up with ideas, Felker thought, but he had made a deliberate retreat. He had learned a lesson when he dismissed Jack Kerouac's *On the Road* as "nothing but bop talk." His sensibility had been shaped by the depression; he knew it was time to turn the reins over to younger men with a better feel for the sensibility of the young, postwar generation, *Esquire*'s potential audience. Advertisers wanted readers between the ages of eighteen and thirty-four; the median age of *Esquire*'s readership was in the mid-forties. Felker was thirty-one, Hayes thirty, Ginzburg twenty-seven—the young Turks, Gingrich called them. Their job was to create a magazine that would appeal to young men. "It was almost like a mandate," recalled Sam Ferber, a young man rising on the business side. "Open the windows and let the world come in."

Each young editor had a different idea of how to go about that. Hayes saw Ginzburg as more salesman than journalist, and not classy either; he wore bow ties and kept an army canteen on his desk. Ginzburg would think of a title that would play well, especially on the cover, then find a writer or celebrity to write the piece. Sometimes his ideas would be long shots. Once he proposed asking famous people to write on virtues—de Gaulle, for example, would write about honor. Hayes and Felker both said, "Oh, shit, Ralph, how are you going to get de Gaulle to write anything?"

"Let de Gaulle do his own refusing," Gingrich said. De Gaulle didn't refuse, and the epigram went onto the list of Gingrich's repeatable sayings, along with, when someone dumb does something bright, "Even a stopped clock is right twice a day," and a string of others.

Felker, like Hayes, was more of a newsman than Ginzburg, but while Hayes had learned to be a journalist as a wire-service reporter in a southern statehouse, Felker had been working in *Life*'s Washington bureau, living in Georgetown and playing softball with Senator Jack Kennedy. At *Esquire,* Felker was always talking on the phone, brainstorming, going out to meet people who mattered, or flying off to distant places—Saint-Tropez, Paris—producing stories in the *Time-Life* mode: politics, cultural trends. He had a sixth sense for the coming thing. Once, passing the Paris cafe Deux Magots, he recognized the French intellectual Simone de Beauvoir sitting at one of the tables. He stopped to ask if she would write for

Esquire about Brigitte Bardot, who had just appeared nude in *And God Created Woman*—the world's most famous feminist on the world's most luscious woman—and she did. When Felker heard that *Harper's Bazaar* had turned down Truman Capote's novella, *Breakfast at Tiffany's,* he told Rust Hills to try to get hold of it. Capote had left for Greece, so Hills phoned American Express in Athens and asked how he could reach Capote. A minute or so later, a high-pitched voice came on, "This is Truman Capote." No, said Hills, thinking there was a misunderstanding, he was trying to *reach* Truman Capote. "This *is* Truman Capote," the voice insisted. It was, and *Esquire* would publish *Breakfast at Tiffany's.*

Years later, Ginzburg would say that Felker had the keenest early-warning antennae of anybody he had ever met. He was totally inefficient, Ginzburg thought, but he could spot emerging trends and talent like nobody else, and would do anything to get hot talent in harness. Hayes, on the other hand, seemed to Ginzburg to have no editorial talent at all; he couldn't see how these two men even worked in the same place. Ginzburg had started out thinking of Hayes as Gingrich's office boy, but he eventually saw him as a willful executive, without aesthetic taste, who would have been more at home in the steel business.

Hayes knew he was not nearly the man about town Felker was, and he worried about it. He would tell Ann Zane, "Clay gets around, he goes to all the right places. I don't do that." But Hayes was capable of circulating in any society, and he plied companions with endless questions: Where were the new acting groups? Who was the best director in town? He was passionately curious—a small-town boy in love with the big city. He was good at ideas—he could take subjects that had been kicking around in the media and come up with ways to make them seem fresh. He liked to stir things up—run pieces that would be provocative, controversial.

In no time at all, editorial meetings turned into shouting matches, as each editor tried to pull the magazine in a different direction. The arguments were so fierce that once the young editors tried meeting ahead of time to reconcile their differences before they joined Gingrich. They came so close to blows that they decided in future to fight it out with Gingrich present as referee. They were not simply quarrelsome. They were ambitious, and Fred Birmingham's old office sat vacant at the corner of an L-shaped hall. Martin Mayer, a former *Esquire* editor and now a regular contributor, strolled through one day and remarked, "What they should do is seal off that office in concrete. Then you guys could get some

work done." Hayes thought the opposite was true: the office was "a beautiful red apple suspended way up at the top of the tree"—and they all
knocked themselves out trying to get it. Under the force of their energy, a
new *Esquire* began to take shape: more serious, more substantial, more
political.

The chill of anti-communism still hung in the air in 1957, and Madison Avenue was as cool to communism as any street in America when
Hayes proposed a piece on the Communist *Daily Worker*. It seemed a lot
like a small-town newspaper in North Carolina, he thought. Why not have
Martin Mayer write about it in just that way, describing its circulation,
staff, and so on—an objective approach to a controversial topic. Let
Mayer approach this loaded subject as if it were not loaded at all. Mayer
did, and produced an article that was innocuous, even dull. Felker fought
against its publication right down to the wire, finally writing a six-page
memorandum warning that the article would permanently damage *Esquire*'s reputation with readers and advertisers. Ginzburg—who thought
Felker was a reactionary, with Hayes not too far behind—leaped to
Mayer's defense. He wrote his own memorandum to Gingrich. "I thought
that the kind of ugliness contained in this memo went out the window
soon after the discrediting of Senator McCarthy." He concluded with a
plea: "Let's, please, put an end to the office politics which caused this
whole business and let Clay understand that Henry, Harold, you and
I work 'with' him, not 'for' him. Life will become lots more bearable
for all of us and we can continue with the job of putting out a great new
Esquire. . . ."

The *Daily Worker* piece was not yet on the stands, in the August 1957
issue, when Hayes asked Richard Rovere, a *New Yorker* columnist, to
write a piece that would take up the cause of Ezra Pound, the poet who
had broadcast propaganda for Mussolini during World War II and was
now confined to a mental hospital. After the piece ran, support from
writers poured into the office: letters from John Dos Passos, Van Wyck
Brooks, Marianne Moore, Howard Nemerov, Mark Schorer, Norman
Mailer, Babette Deutsch, William Carlos Williams, and others. The letters and article became part of the legal petition that led to Pound's
release the next year.

No political writer in the country was more respected than Richard
Rovere, and it was good to have him writing for *Esquire*. Not only was he

a good writer, but he was a *New Yorker* writer, and his presence in *Esquire* would remind readers that *Esquire* too, before its girlie days, had been, like *The New Yorker,* a "smart magazine," a stylish mix of literary writing and cartoons. Rovere's connection to *The New Yorker* did create a problem: since he was *The New Yorker*'s writer on Washington, he did not feel he could write about political subjects for *Esquire.* Hayes found a way through that particular wicket: he proposed a piece on Senator Joseph McCarthy that would not be—well—quite political.

Hayes had been talking with Laura Bergquist, who had become a senior editor at *Look,* and she had passed on to him an observation about McCarthy that Robert Kennedy had made to her—a comment on the suddenness of McCarthy's collapse, once the Senate censured him and he found himself out of the limelight. Another writer she knew, John Cogley, took up the theme in a column in *Commonweal,* and Hayes approached him first to do a McCarthy article for *Esquire.* Cogley had said no because he was too clearly identified as an anti-McCarthyite. That was not a problem to Hayes, who thought only a writer with a reputation as anti-McCarthy could write the article he had in mind without opening himself to the charge of praising McCarthy. As Hayes explained the idea to Rovere (and he told Rovere he had asked Cogley first),

> I never knew anything but the public image of McCarthy, which, although it is a gratuitous comment in this context, I found as horrifying as most. But McCarthy *was* a phenomenon in our time, and these thoughtful remarks of Cogley, attempting to humanize him, I found both fascinating and dramatic.
>
> Would it be possible to do this, show the man as a person—in light of personality characteristics that few of his political enemies or friends considered—without pitying him? Or absolving him of the tremendous damage he did to this country? And would it be possible to trace, somewhat clinically, the last months of his life in order to show the drama of his disintegration?

What Hayes was asking of Rovere was not all that different from what he had asked of Mayer, when he assigned the *Daily Worker* piece, or of Rovere himself earlier, when he wrote about Ezra Pound: restore to cutout villains a rounded human reality. Over the next few years *Esquire* set Thomas B. Morgan on Roy Cohn, William F. Buckley, Jr., on Whittaker Chambers, Dan Wakefield on John Dos Passos, and Brock Brower on Alger Hiss. In taking on these controversial political figures, Hayes was not just motivated by the desire to attract attention, Brower thought. "He didn't think he was organizing the counterreformation or anything like that, but he felt this was the great subject area, and that we, writing about this, would make a difference. And it was important to do this to clean up the atmosphere, to stop what we looked upon at that time as verboten topics and the unexamined past."

But Felker had been right to detect danger in this direction: Even approached as human-interest stories, political topics could present risks, especially for a mainstream magazine like *Esquire,* which served a politically diverse readership. Hayes learned how rough the waters could be after the Rovere piece on McCarthy appeared in the August 1958 issue as "The Last Days of Joe McCarthy." Rovere portrayed McCarthy as a demagogue, but "an essentially frivolous one. The world took him seriously, as indeed it should have, but he never really took himself seriously. . . . He was a hell-raiser, a born troublemaker, a political racketeer, a con man who loved the game for its own sake."

The public response to his *Esquire* article surprised even Rovere, an experienced man. In the book he published on McCarthy the next year, he said,

Though I wrote of him a good deal while he lived and was formidable, and never wrote flatteringly, I first encountered the full wrath of the McCarthyites in 1958, when I published an account of the last days of his life and an estimate of his character for *Esquire.* Then the furies descended. I have half a file drawer full of suggestions that I walk into the Atlantic Ocean until my hat floats, that I ask God's forgiveness for my acts of desecration, that I buck for the next Stalin Prize, and so forth. While he lived, I never knew such vituperation. For some of it, the institutional part, I tend to make a heavy discount. The house organ of the American Legion sought to discredit my testimony by painting me as a hardened sinner; a church publication, *Our Sunday Visitor,* sought to discredit the forum, *Esquire,* in which my attempt at explanation appeared. But what impressed me was the volume of letters from terribly anguished men and women who would not stand idly by while McCarthy's name was dishonored. The letters were ugly, threatening, in many cases vile. Yet they bespoke a love for the man which, though it was doubtless a form of self-love, was not entirely without a power to be affecting. Three hundred subscriptions, or a lot, to *Esquire* were canceled, and this was a tribute.

Rovere thought the reaction was so intense because McCarthy, dead, had become even more beloved by his supporters, but the intensity may have been due to the article's publication in *Esquire.* Commentary like this might be expected of *The New Yorker.* But *Esquire,* the fashion magazine for men?

At one point in their argument over the *Daily Worker* article, Felker had said to Hayes, "The trouble with you is, you just don't *know.*" Felker's comment bit deep and was one reason Hayes applied in spring 1958 for a Nieman fellowship at Harvard, which brought professional journalists in for a year of study. He was sick of the fighting at the magazine and, besides, he needed more education to handle the kind of material he and the others were trying to get into *Esquire.* He had been educating himself in the ways of New York intellectual culture, reading magazines like *Commentary* and *Partisan Review;* both Felker and Hayes thought the editors of the smaller cultural magazines were setting examples a magazine like *Esquire* could follow. But Hayes knew he had a lot to learn. He had been an indifferent student at Wake Forest. He would warn students when he spoke there that the world outside the college was a competitive world in which, he told students, "winners usually win at *your* expense. Someone else's victory means your failure." He had been a C-average man, he confessed, and out there in the world, the C-average man competes with the A-plus man. "He must either run for his life, or settle for a C existence."

Harvard was Hayes's bid for remedial education. Writing on his behalf to the curator of the fellowships, Arnold Gingrich confessed to mixed feelings. Of all his editors Hayes would benefit most from the year at Harvard—an observation that could be read several ways. But Hayes was also the editor *Esquire* could least do without. Hayes was becoming, in Gingrich's mind, the "pitch pipe" in the *Esquire* choir. As he wrote later in his memoir, "Hayes seemed to have a keen weather eye for the mood changes that were beginning to develop across the country, and particularly among the young, in the late 1950s, and he was good at working up features that appealed to this spreading sense of skepticism, disbelief, and disenchantment." Hayes used the words "brash" and "irreverent," Gingrich observed, in an effort to "salt up the magazine's personality, give it a difference of posture that would set it smartly apart."

Still, Gingrich agreed to let him go, and Hayes enlisted the additional support of Richard Rovere, Dorothy Parker (who, at Hayes's request, was now reviewing books for *Esquire*), and John Fischer, editor of *Harper's* magazine, who had talked with Hayes about coming to work there. Hayes became the first magazine editor to get the fellowship. Gingrich not only gave him a nine-month leave of absence but also made up the difference between the modest Harvard stipend and his salary at *Esquire.*

Eager to begin, Hayes wrote to the registrar in June asking for reading lists for the courses he hoped to take, among them Paul Tillich's Religion and Society and John Kenneth Galbraith's Social Theory of Modern Enterprise. Once in Cambridge, he tried to sample as many courses in American intellectual history as he could fit in, just sitting in on some and actually doing the assignments in others, studying under Arthur Schlesinger, Jr., Crane Brinton, H. Stuart Hughes, and Oscar Handlin. In one exam he kept in his files, Hayes did not distinguish himself. On a test in Schlesinger's course, he earned a B+ on one question and a C+ on another. His grade for the exam was B−. Yet Hayes's courses in intellectual history encouraged him to think grandly—to spin off big ideas for writers, to play the role of sociologist and map the culture. Harvard gave him, too, a better feel for the changes American culture had gone through over time.

While he was there, Hayes kept his hand in at *Esquire*. He wrote a jazz column for several issues and corresponded with Gingrich, passing on comments by dignitaries who addressed the Nieman Fellows. Ralph McGill had given a moving account of southern editors who were trying to push the cause of integration while staying in touch with their readers. Edward R. Murrow had been "gloomy as hell" over what he saw as "the fastest rate of decline of a civilization in the history of the world." Eric Sevareid had been "extremely complimentary about *Esquire*—said it was the best magazine going, unafraid to print anything. I nodded gravely."

Other interesting people crossed his path at Cambridge. His college friend Walter Friedenberg sent along a young woman he had met in India, where she had been on a fellowship: Gloria Steinem. She and Friedenberg had talked of marriage, but here she was alone in Cambridge instead. Steinem would come over to the Hayeses' apartment, and sometimes, in the kitchen, try to teach Harold the time-step, but she was more Susan's friend than Harold's. Susan seemed to Steinem free and life-loving in a way that Harold was not. He seemed to Steinem inflexible and puritanical, and he talked about how much he loved being in the Marines. He was so different from Walter Friedenberg that she was surprised they were friends.

One spring week while he was at Harvard, Hayes traveled south to acquire the notes Elia Kazan and Archibald MacLeish had exchanged during production of MacLeish's play *J.B.* The idea of publishing the dialogue between them so intrigued him that he had been unable to concentrate on his studies—"the extension of Jeffersonianism as developed by John Taylor." A week before he had planned to go, he broke away and went down to Washington, D.C. When he arrived at the theater where the play was in rehearsal, Hayes took a seat near Kazan and waited for an opening. As he described what happened next to Gingrich, "He looked around at me once or twice but he seemed to be terribly involved, so I sat still like an ass and waited longer. Then I heard him say something about 'getting the police—some guy just wandered in and sat down.' "

When Hayes crossed the aisle and told Kazan who he was, Kazan greeted him like a long-lost brother.

"Harold Hayes? Harold Hayes? Really, you're Harold Hayes?" Kazan exclaimed. "I expected a much older man."

Kazan gave him the folder of correspondence and Hayes returned to his hotel room. He read for three hours through the attempt of these men "to define the spiritual position of modern man in dramatic terms," with here and there references to the Beat generation and rock and roll. To Hayes, the notes read "almost like an intellectual detective story, with MacLeish intellectualizing like Hell and Kazan beating drama out of him."

It is not hard to see why the *J.B.* correspondence interested Hayes. MacLeish was a poet who had written a philosophical verse play. Kazan was a director who had made his name staging emotional, melodramatic performances on stage and film: *A Streetcar Named Desire, On the Waterfront, East of Eden.* Their notes documented their collaborative attempt to do something like the *Esquire* editors were trying to do: make thought entertaining. In an age where a whole generation of young men had gone to college on the GI Bill, why not put out a magazine for an audience that cared about rock and roll and the spiritual position of modern man, an audience that had heard of French playwrights and existentialists, an educated audience weary of television and eager to taste the delights of the mind, the cultivations of spirit and sense—and have fun doing it, too?

Not long before Hayes had left for Harvard, Ginzburg had gotten himself fired. *Esquire* had never run his article on library holdings of erotic literature because, he understood, the advertising department had gotten its first advertising contract with General Motors, and Jerry Jontry, the advertising manager, did not think such an article would play well with the automobile industry. *Esquire* was, after all, trying to shed its image as a

girlie magazine—Gingrich had even dropped the centerfold. When Gingrich turned down Ginzburg's request for a raise on the ground that *Esquire* had paid $2,000 for an article that never ran, Ginzburg had asked for
the rights to his article, Gingrich had turned them over, and Ginzburg
expanded the article into a book, which he published and promoted on his
own.

The book made a quarter of a million dollars—more, he said later,
than the entire *Esquire* company made that year, a fact that left management "fit to be tied." He was careful not to mention *Esquire* in his
promotion of the book, and when he agreed to go on the Mike Wallace
show he did so on the condition that *Esquire* not be mentioned. But when
John Smart saw Ginzburg's upcoming appearance announced in the
paper, he called Ginzburg in and told him if he went on that show, he
would lose his job. Ginzburg had made the commitment to appear, and he
wasn't going to back out. He didn't mention *Esquire,* but he appeared on
the show, and the next morning Gingrich called him in and, shaking like a
leaf, fired him. Ginzburg was sorry to go; he had loved his job.

Henry Wolf also left, moving his talent over to *Harper's Bazaar,* and
Gingrich named one of the young art associates, Robert Benton, to take
his place. Benton was a slender, gentle man still in his twenties—small,
soulful, the kind of man women wanted to protect, the kind of man,
Hayes thought, his mother would call "a *nice* boy." He had arrived in
New York just a year before Hayes, traveling on a Continental Trailways
bus and, said Hayes—probably speaking of himself as well—"bearing the
terrible responsibility country boys have for preserving the city's sophistication against the vulgarities of people already here." He collaborated
with his roommate and fellow University of Texas graduate Harvey
Schmidt on *The In and Out Book,* and they made their debut in *Esquire*
in September 1957 with an "In and Out Primer," "written and lavishly
illustrated by Robert Benton and Harvey Schmidt" (the illustrations were
small childlike sketches).

Benton, to all appearances, should have been Out. He seemed per-
petually poor, wore army shirts, and drove an old Citroën that looked like a
Paris taxicab. For a while when he first came to New York he tried to be a
cartoonist. He roomed with a couple of cartoonists who were actually
making a living with their cartoons. Benton would hopefully make the
rounds every week of the magazines that bought cartoons. Sometimes a

magazine would pick out several to hold for a few days, then would send them back; nobody ever bought one of Benton's.

Finally, one day a cartoon editor called him in. "I'd like to talk to you," she said.

He said to himself, Oh, she's going to buy one—thank God.

"Have you ever thought of another line of work?" she asked.

But Benton had a talent that made him first-rate for *Esquire:* he enjoyed discovering people who could do some things better than he could. He could seek out collaborators who had something he lacked, and join his strength to theirs. He had another quality, too: he had a subtle, offbeat take on the times.

Benton, Felker, and Hills did very well without Hayes. In fact, Felker had the satisfying feeling he was running the magazine—and doing a good job of it. He brought to *Esquire* some of the Magnum photographers he had gotten to know at *Life:* Bruce Davidson, Burt Glinn. He discovered David Levine at a little art gallery and started him drawing caricatures for the columns at the front of the book. Hayes himself congratulated Felker on the April 1959 issue, which included (among other things) Richard H. Rovere on "Kennedy's Last Chance to Be President"; Tennessee Williams's play *Sweet Bird of Youth;* a words-and-sketches piece by Harvey Kurtzman, who had created *Mad* magazine; and, to top it all off, a photo spread on Saint-Tropez featuring filmmaker Roger Vadim, his wife sunbathing topless, and, in another picture with another man, his former wife Brigitte Bardot.

Before Hayes's year at Harvard was over, Felker had assigned a piece that became a kind of prototype for other articles to come—a profile of Sammy Davis, Jr., by a former *Esquire* editor, Thomas B. Morgan. Instead of grazing through a clip file and pouring out facts and anecdotes in a gray sludge, Morgan followed Davis around for ten nonstop days, and, still in a fictive mood from a novel he had just written, tried to give his story the drama and feel of fiction. Then he did the same thing on his next assignment, a no-holds-barred profile of television impresario David Susskind.

Felker had delivered such a good performance while Hayes was away that Gingrich may have imagined moving him into Birmingham's old office. If he imagined it, he kept it to himself. Much later in life Felker would say he was volatile in those years—"really passionate" about his ideas, maybe, he admitted, even more passionate than the ideas called for. Perhaps, he thought, Gingrich did not believe he was ready to run the magazine, and perhaps, he admitted, he wasn't. He did feel Gingrich recognized his ability, but he also noticed when Gingrich took Hayes to lunch.

As the time neared for Hayes's return to *Esquire* from Harvard, he came down in March to have lunch with Gingrich, who made him an offer.

"Well, see, I've got some wonderful news for you," Hayes recalled Gingrich telling him.

"What's that?" asked Hayes.

"*Coronet*'s having some problems and they really need a fireball over there."

"You know, I don't really want to work there," said Hayes.

"You're a Marine, you can take on any beachhead."

"Yeah, but I've already been on that beachhead at *Pageant.* I really don't want to work for that magazine."

Gingrich gave him a raise and Hayes came back to *Esquire.* Benton noticed in him a great change: He had a new sense of what a magazine and a magazine editor could be. "He stopped being a journalist," Benton recalled. "He started thinking of himself as an editor in the largest sense— in a very different way."

The Years with Ross, James Thurber's memoir of legendary *New Yorker* editor Harold Ross, came out that year, 1959, and Hayes read it with appreciation—and yet with a feeling, too, that Thurber had missed the mark. Thurber brought Ross to life for Hayes, but Thurber did not tell Hayes what he wanted to know about Ross, because Thurber had understood Ross only as a writer would understand him.

"It is not so much that Thurber missed the point of the editor's role; he never understood it," Hayes wrote several years later.

Through his magazine, an editor addresses his times. He sets out to do this within fairly well defined commercial limitations, all conditions for the play of his imagination; but this is why he does what he does and, most often, the reason he behaves the way he does. . . . He is not placed on earth to serve selflessly the artistic pretensions of his writers: he is here to get in touch with the reader. This, too, is difficult for a writer to understand. Thus, an editor like Ross who bleeds over his writer-children (or seems to), God Blessing Them and reminding them to wear their overshoes on rainy days, begins to take form as a writer's notion of what an editor ought to be like. From the editor's point of view, it is a massive misinterpretation to see Ross only in these terms, chasing commas, "who he?"-ing, and playing practical jokes on Alexander Woollcott.

How did he come to arrive at a satire magazine in those days (when *Vanity Fair* and *The American Mercury* were doing fine)? How did he find the money to get it going? How did he manage to get total editorial control away from his backers? If he was so inarticulate, how did he manage to persuade his backers to stay with him through two years of running in the red? How did he arrive at his plan of action for the magazine, his "formula" for presenting regular features on a regular basis?

Why was he so interested in being an editor in the first place? What did he want to accomplish with his magazine? And what, as the years went on, did he feel he accomplished?

Hayes's questions tumbled thick and fast until finally he said,

But most of all, this editor would like to know what he did in the heat of things, around 1938, say, when he was at his peak, and he had just closed a good issue—as good, at least, as he could make it—and had nothing very good for the next issue, but had to start planning anyway. What did he do, Thurber?

Dubious Achievements

*T*HE DARK ARENA (the novelist would later write) was like a church crowded at midnight. Twenty-seven minutes before, several thousand true believers had poured onto the floor and surged in the gallery, sending up such a vast wave of applause for Adlai Stevenson that those in charge gave up trying to shout it down and turned off the lights. The lights came on again and the convention went on with its business, nominating another candidate that mid-July evening in Los Angeles in 1960: John Fitzgerald Kennedy.

Stevenson's press secretary, Thomas B. Morgan, took careful notes. Clay Felker had asked him to produce an insider's account of the 1960 Democratic Convention for *Esquire*. The novelist Norman Mailer kept notes, too. Felker had asked *him* to write an account for *Esquire*. Elsewhere in the hall were other men who had written for *Esquire* or would write for *Esquire* in the near future, although they were not writing for *Esquire* on this occasion. Richard Rovere was there, reporting on the event for *The New Yorker*. Gore Vidal was there; so were John Kenneth Galbraith and Arthur Schlesinger, Jr. But Mailer and Morgan were the ones with the assignment to make sense of the event for *Esquire*. And each of the two thought he was the only one with the assignment.

Mailer's assignment had come about by chance. One night that spring, Felker had been seated with the novelist, whom he had not met before, at the Five Spot, the jazz club in the Bowery where Thelonious Monk and John Coltrane played to painters and writers and whoever else wanted to spend a few hours on the frontier of serious jazz. Mailer and his wife were bickering, and Felker, trying to change the subject, suggested that Mailer might write something political for *Esquire*. It was not such a far-fetched idea. "Like many another vain, empty, and bullying body of our time, I have been running for President these last ten years in the privacy of my mind," Mailer had announced, in the first sentence of *Advertisements for Myself.*

Besides, sending a novelist out as a reporter seemed a good way to get around *Esquire's* long lead time—surely Mailer would come up with something worth reading even three months after the fact, the soonest *Esquire* could get it into the magazine. That was an advantage of using novelists as reporters, an experiment Hayes had already tried, with mixed success, sending James Baldwin out to profile Swedish filmmaker Ingmar Bergman. *Commentary* editor Norman Podhoretz had only lately observed that novelists seemed to be doing their best work in magazine articles—usually articles for little magazines like *Commentary,* or *Dissent,* where Mailer had published. It wasn't a new idea, really—Gingrich himself had run reports on Spain and other places by Ernest Hemingway, and *Holiday* magazine had long used novelists as travel writers. But it felt new—a fresh way for *Esquire* to approach the contemporary scene, through the unique sensibilities fiction writers would bring to their work.

Esquire had already given Mailer himself a shot at reporting, when he wrote text to go with Bruce Davidson's photographs of Brooklyn teenagers. Yet Hayes opposed Felker's proposal to send him to the Democratic Convention, even though Hayes had been responsible for *Esquire's* first publication of Mailer's nonfiction, an excerpt from *Advertisements for Myself.* He voted against sending Mailer to the Democratic Convention because, at this point, he tended to vote against any Felker proposal. Felker got it through anyway and took Mailer in hand. He met him in Los Angeles and introduced him around, and then, after Mailer started writing, flew up to Provincetown to check on his progress. He found Mailer on track and working hard. He had even interviewed John Kennedy at Hyannis Port, and Kennedy had endeared himself to Mailer by saying he had read not *The Naked and the Dead,* the novel Mailer usually heard about, but a later novel, *The Deer Park.* Mailer knew Kennedy's aides might have prompted him to say that, but Mailer didn't mind.

When the piece came in, Hayes saw he had been wrong to oppose it. Mailer was forceful, unpredictable, and stretched the boundaries of *Esquire.* "For once let us try to think about a political convention without losing ourselves in housing projects of fact and issue," Mailer announced. He was less interested in fact and issue than in history, the grand currents underneath the political froth on the surface. What great historical waves lapped across Pershing Square, the Biltmore, the sports arena? This was political reporting in the grand style, less reporting, even, than prophecy: Mailer was the man outside the walls, calling judgment down on a nation that had lost its courage, and Kennedy was the man who might help the country find it. Arriving at Pershing Square, Kennedy was "the hero, the matinee idol, the movie star . . . the Democrats were going to nominate a man who, no matter how serious his political dedication might be, was indisputably and willy-nilly going to be seen as a great box-office actor, and the consequences of that were staggering and not at all easy to calculate."

There was more of Thomas Carlyle in this writing than of Ernest Hemingway, and Arnold Gingrich did not like it. "This isn't writing," Gingrich said. "It's just smearing anything on the page that comes into his head." He told Felker he would not even have run it, if he had not left space in the magazine for it. Felker never heard Gingrich express such contempt for an article as he did for this one. Gingrich kept all reference to it off the cover; he also changed the title from Mailer's "Superman Comes to the Supermarket" to "Superman Comes to the Supermart," which he thought sounded better. Hayes, meanwhile, suggested that Felker break up the interminable type with long subheadings in the style of an eighteenth-century novel.

Nobody told Mailer about the title change, but he found out when he received his check and saw the invoice, "Superman Comes to the Supermart." He called Felker, and Felker promised to change the title back. Writers did not usually dictate the titles of their own pieces, but from his first appearance in *Esquire*, Mailer had demanded extraordinary control over how his work was played. Felker was in a bind: Given Gingrich's hostility to the piece, he scarcely wanted to defy him over two alphabet letters. Nor did he want to tell Mailer that Gingrich did not like his article at all. At a party just before the magazine came out in mid-October, Felker confessed to Mailer that he had not restored his title. After the November issue appeared, Mailer wrote a furious letter to the editor announcing his intention not to write for *Esquire* again. He cited the title change, an erroneous statement in the "Backstage" column, *Esquire*'s use of a ten-year-old photograph in the "Backstage" column, and the small subheads. He concluded:

"Good-by now, rum friends, and best wishes. You got a good mag (like the pulp-heads say), you print nice stuff, but you gotta treat the hot writer right or you lose him like you just lost me."

Too bad: his appearance in *Esquire* had made a strong impression. Even Tom Morgan, disappointed when he learned *Esquire* would not need a story from him because it had Mailer, still saw the importance of what Mailer had done. Pete Hamill, then on the staff of the *New York Post*, would recall,

It went through journalism like a wave. Something changed. Everybody said, "Uh, oh. Here's another way to do it." Mailer had altered the form, and you said, "Okay. It's not the same, and you've got to deal with that." Everybody in the business, guys my age, were talking about it. Norman took political journalism beyond what the best guys—Mencken, Teddy White, Richard Rovere—had done. Rather than just a political sense there was a moral sense that came out of the piece.

Arthur Schlesinger, Jr., a member of the Kennedy circle, had written in the January 1960 *Esquire* of a new mood in America—a need "for a faith that what we are doing is deeply worthwhile—the kind of inspiration and lift we had for a while in the Thirties and again in World War II." Schlesinger pictured Americans "waiting for a trumpet to sound." Like Mailer and many other intellectuals, Schlesinger was weary of the consumer society, a nation preoccupied with buying and selling. But Schlesinger and Mailer had very different ideas about what might come next. Schlesinger saw the coming decade in utopian terms, as a time when America would turn its affluence to better use: better education, better missiles to fight communism.

Mailer had a different take on the character of the culture—passions stuffed down under the smooth surface, the emotional costs of suburban life and cold-war politics, the violence urban blacks faced daily. When Mailer looked ahead, he saw not career opportunity and better health care, not affluence more widely shared, but a possibility that passions and people held down so long would erupt in chaos. He saw ahead not utopia but apocalypse: "the approaching nightmare of history's oncoming night."

That fall, at the third of the *Esquire* literary symposia Rust Hills organized every year for college campuses, Philip Roth told an audience at Stanford, "The American writer in the middle of the twentieth century has his hands full in trying to understand, and then describe, and then make *credible* much of the American reality." At San Francisco State College, James Baldwin issued a call to action: "Now this country is going to be transformed. It will not be transformed by an act of God, but by all of us, by you and me." On the University of California campus at Berkeley, John Cheever, drinking what appeared to be water, slid under the table and had to be escorted off stage.

Americans were passing through "a period of self-doubt and anxiety of great magnitude," Hayes wrote in a plan for an issue devoted to sophistication. Intrigued by the numbers he found in a research report by the advertising agency Doyle Dane Bernbach—millions of Americans traveling abroad, 1,142 symphony orchestras—Hayes asked: How could *Esquire* present the complex phenomenon of American's new sophistication? Not as *Look, Life, Holiday, Sports Illustrated,* or *The New Yorker* might do— oversimply—but with "humor, irreverence, fashion, fine writing, controversy, topicality and surprise. . . . Throughout the issue, we will define our theme, praise it, blast it, ridicule it, revise it, qualify it—and finally, prove it beyond all doubt."

He would run a lead piece by Richard Rovere and an excerpt of Saul Bellow's *Herzog,* still in progress; he would set James Baldwin on expatriates, Gay Talese on *Vogue,* Dan Wakefield on women, Marya Mannes on men, and Alfred Hitchcock on violence. He sent photographer Pete Turner out to take pictures and when Turner, new to *Esquire,* protested, "Harold, I don't even know what the word 'sophistication' means," Hayes reassured him: "Pete, don't worry about it. I'll tell you the places I want you to photograph, you just do it in your style. Everything'll be fine."

Hayes could always imagine (it seemed to those who worked with him) how things would turn out; he could see an idea—visualize the magazine in advance. He could see how to put together a mix of very different pieces that would hold together and seem distinctively *Esquire.* The 1961 sophistication issue, a big July issue like the New York issue, gave him a chance to showcase the talent that Gingrich admired most in him: reflecting the mood of the culture in a unique *Esquire* way. While the issue was still in process, Gingrich took the step Hayes believed he had decided to take as far back as Hayes's return from Harvard a year and a half before: Gingrich named Hayes managing editor of *Esquire,* and Hayes moved into the vacant editor's office.

Clay Felker had lost, Harold Hayes had won. Quick as Felker was to pick up the scent of new trends, in the end Gingrich chose Hayes, the preacher's son, over Felker, the midwestern man about town. Of the two, Hayes was, in Gingrich's eyes, better at concepts, the man who could see the big picture of what the magazine was and could be. Gingrich seemed more at ease with Hayes, too; he seemed to like him as a man. He would, as time went on, speak affectionately of him, as Hayes would of him, although they had little in common other than *Esquire*—Gingrich the fly-fisherman, the man of impeccable tastes, Hayes the trombone-playing son of the red-clay South. Sam Ferber, advertising manager at the time, was still puzzling over the irony thirty years later. "Harold was one of the most unsophisticated people I've ever met, right out of Winston-Salem. I used to kid him, I'd say, 'I can't believe that you're the editor of the magazine.' He said, 'Sam, remember, how many great editors were the sons of preachers?' "

Later, Gingrich would write as if he had known, nearly from the start, that Hayes would be his choice; in what Hayes called his laissez-faire style, he had simply waited for the change to come of its own accord. If a friend of Hayes's from Atlanta days had not been rising through the ranks of the *Saturday Evening Post* and bringing Hayes offers, Hayes imagined Gingrich might have waited still longer. Having finally granted Hayes the title, Gingrich sat back and let Hayes figure out how to use it.

The situation was not easy. Felker tried to leave—he made a bid for a job at the *New York Herald Tribune,* which was undergoing a dramatic renovation; he expressed regret to the *Tribune*'s new editor, John Lee Denson, when Robert Manning was hired instead to remake the Sunday paper. He still hoped to be part of the revolution at the *Tribune.* Meanwhile, for several months he held a second job as managing editor of *Infinity* magazine, published by the American Society of Magazine Photographers.

While Felker explored his options elsewhere, he stayed on at *Esquire,* a defeated competitor, his office next door to Hayes's. Brock Brower, the young writer who had done a piece on Alger Hiss that Hayes particularly liked, had gotten a job as an associate editor, and he could sense the tension between the two men. Every Wednesday afternoon the editors would meet in Gingrich's office, with its window looking out on Madison Avenue. Gingrich would preside behind his desk, and Hills would look on as Felker and Hayes, one on the couch, one on a chair, faced off, arguing.

Once Felker came in with Burt Glinn photographs of Shirley Mac-Laine doing a parody of the old Varga Girl calendar, with MacLaine playing all the months, from January through December. Hayes exploded: This was the old *Esquire,* he said: just nonsense—a waste of twelve pages.

Not at all, Felker said. It was a marvelous send-up, it was Shirley Mac-
Laine. The argument went on, back and forth—should it be used at all?
for how many pages? Finally, Gingrich stepped in: they would use the
pictures somehow. David Newman, who had joined the staff as Rust
Hills's assistant, had an idea. The old Varga Girl calendars had run little
ditties next to the girl drawings. He would parody the ditties with parodies
of twelve serious poets.

Newman had come to *Esquire* fresh out of the University of Michigan, Arnold Gingrich's alma mater, bearing a master's degree in English, a
manuscript for a novel, and a recommendation from Malcolm Cowley,
who had taught a graduate writing seminar there. Although he was hired
to read fiction and other unsolicited manuscripts, right away the others
noticed his funny, ironic way with words—just what *Esquire* needed: they
had decided that the magazine had gotten *too* serious and needed lighten-
ing if *Esquire* was to draw in more readers and younger readers. None of
the editors was advanced in age, but Newman was the youngest, very
bright and energetic. He liked fooling around with words, writing a set of
captions, just for the fun of it, to go with pictures of people living the good
life in the Hamptons:

What I Did On My Summer Vacation
How the Fun People in the Fun Hamptons Have Fun.

Mr. and Mrs. Edward Stone sitting on chairs, outdoors.
Everybody likes to see everybody eating and drinking on the grass.
Ferrante and Teicher play pianos on the beach. Some kid is there, too.
Arthur Laurents gets some sun in his yard.
Joe Bosco has a chair he made on a dock. He's not sitting in it.
Philip Gramma working on some of his art stuff.
Jose Mecalles leans on his house, on the outside of it.
Hans Hemmerschmidt looks over a naked lady's shoulder.
Bruce Lippo sits down in front of his work.
Max Lerner reads a book.
Charles Addams likes to watch Joan Fontaine drawing a picture.
Also he likes to swim in the water.
John O'Hara has fun inside . . .
and outside.
Sometimes we all get together on the sand.
Sometimes we all get together on the lawn.
Sometimes we all get together in a house.
Time to fly home to old New York, but we'll be back next summer for some more
     fun.

The rest—Hayes, Felker, Benton—all liked his tone, wise-guy, smart-ass, very collegiate. This was a great age for humor magazines on college campuses, and Newman had been a humor magazine editor. Hayes himself liked the *Harvard Lampoon,* and he liked Harvey Kurtzman, the creator of *Mad,* a humor magazine for all ages. In no time Newman was working not just for Rust Hills, he was working for everyone. They would all come to him with pictures that needed captions, or ask him to write the little heads on the letters to the editor.

Benton, especially, found something in Newman that clicked, and Newman, in turn, keyed into what Hayes once described as Benton's "bittersweet, crazy-legged point of view," a tendency to let laughter creep in where you wouldn't expect it. When Hayes asked him once to try to define it, Benton said, "You remember that old story about the preacher in a tent revival asking the congregation to testify what the Lord has done for them. One by one, they come forward. 'The Lord saved my house from a tornado,' one man says. . . . 'The Lord brought rain to my thirsty crops,' and so on. Finally one man is left out there. He is a terribly crippled old farmer, so bent he can hardly move, and the preacher says, 'Now come on, my man, come forward and tell us what He's done for you.' The cripple hobbles up to the pulpit and says, 'Well, He damn near ruined me.' "

Benton's humor wasn't like Newman's, which moved along at a faster clip, Yankee style, but the differences between them just made teaming up even better. They could play to each other's strengths and make up for each other's weaknesses. Newman would go into Benton's office or Benton would go into Newman's, and they would come out together with an idea they would take to Hayes. Their office identities began to merge; they became Benton-and-Newman. Hayes began giving them pictures, stories, ideas: "Let's get your take on this," he would say. And they would come back with what soon became the voice of *Esquire:* a wise guy thumbing his nose at the world.

One day in the fall of 1961 Hayes called Benton and Newman into his office, which seemed to Newman always dimly lit. (Hayes liked to turn his lights off and use light from the window.) Hayes had a copy of the *Harvard Lampoon,* which every year awarded a prize for the worst actress and the worst actor and the worst movie. The prizes got a lot of publicity. Why couldn't *Esquire* do something like that but on a larger scale? Could Benton and Newman come up with something? He wanted that tone— that thing that they did.

They went off and came up with the first Dubious Achievement Awards, published in January 1962: several pages of candid photos with brief captions, like Norman Mailer: "White Man of the Year." They thought the awards up together, but Newman did most of the writing. Newman came up with one idea that would become a cultural cliché. Something unfortunate had happened to Richard Nixon, as something always did, and Newman had remembered a regular *Life* feature: a big photograph of some mysterious event—maybe three people staring at something in horror—and the title would read, "Why are these people frightened?" Then you would turn the page and find out. So all through the first Dubious Achievements they ran a little candid picture of Nixon with the caption, "Why is this man laughing?" It became a running gag from year to year, because there was always a reason to ask that about Nixon.

Like the "In and Out" features Benton had done earlier, the awards were mock sociology, status classification in fun. They demonstrated dramatically the truth of what became a maxim for Hayes: Old wine *could* be put in new bottles, old material made fresh if given fresh form. From then on, maps, lists, doctored photographs, diagrams, quizzes, illustrated guides spilled out of the magazine's pages. "From the raspberry to the hoax, in words and/or pictures . . . and occasionally with some loss of dignity, the idea was to suggest alternate possibilities to a monolithic view," Hayes wrote later, in an introduction to *Esquire* pieces from the sixties. More than any other single feature, the Dubious Achievement Awards—irreverent, sassy, and smart—set *Esquire* on its new course.

While Benton and Newman were shaping up a new identity for *Esquire,* Rust Hills was polishing up an old one, bringing in short stories by Bernard Malamud, James Purdy, Italo Calvino—serious writers who would give *Esquire* something more than the pulp fiction most other magazines published. It was not always easy for Hills to get what he wanted into the magazine: Gingrich seemed readier to block fiction than anything else. Once, Evan S. Connell sent Hills a short version of *Mrs. Bridge* and Hills proposed publishing it. Gingrich refused.

"It's bland as junket and totally offensive," Gingrich said.

"But Arnold, how can a thing be bland as junket and totally offensive?"

"I don't want to discuss it," said Gingrich.

Then there was the time Philip Roth submitted "Defender of the Faith," the first of his *Goodbye, Columbus* stories. Hills thought it was just great and wanted desperately to publish it. Gingrich said no. He showed the story to Abe Blinder and to Fritz Bamberger. They agreed—it was anti-Semitic. Hills was furious. The story was about anti-Semitism, but it was not anti-Semitic.

Roth's agent sent it to *The New Yorker,* which accepted the story. Hills told Bamberger, "Aha, *The New Yorker* took that story that you said was too rough for *Esquire.*"

"Wait'll they publish it," Bamberger replied. When the story came out in *The New Yorker,* there was a terrible firestorm, Hills recalled later, and ever after, Roth had to live down accusations of anti-Semitism. But Hills did get other Roth stories into the magazine.

Hills had Gingrich's full support in one area: the annual *Esquire* literary symposia, which generated excitement on the campuses where they were held and press attention elsewhere, as three or four big-name writers got together for two or three days and argued with each other about the writer's role in society. The symposia had gone without major incident until the fall of 1961, when trouble struck at *Esquire*'s fourth annual symposium, held at the University of Michigan, the alma mater of both Arnold Gingrich and David Newman.

The weekend started off smoothly enough with a pre-symposium speech by Gingrich at the Adcraft Club in nearby Detroit, the biggest ad club in America—an important part of the schedule, since *Esquire*'s publicity office liked to use the symposia to earn points with the advertising community, and the *Esquire* advertising staff was especially interested in wooing the car manufacturers. Once the sessions began, the speakers were fine—Gore Vidal, William Styron, Nelson Algren, and Vance Bourjaily— although the audiences were disappointing, their questions, Gingrich said later, "aimless meanderings." The real trouble came after-hours.

After the first evening's panel discussion, a young professor in the English department gave a party in his house. It was a small house, with a small living room, a small dining room containing a tall breakfront filled with china and crystal, a small back porch, and a small kitchen. The house was packed with more than 150 people that warm fall night—more crowded than any party Hills had ever seen. Liquor and beer flowed freely.

Hills, Gingrich, and Newman were there, along with the featured writers, faculty members, and writing students—writers on motorcycles,

Newman called them, good old boys, swigging beer and smoking ciga-
rettes. There was a lot of drinking, and little fights started breaking out—
pushing and shoving. When Rust Hills went down to the basement to get
ice, the crowd above sounded to him like a herd of elephants, rumbling
and shuffling. Newman sensed a testiness in the air: something seemed
bound to happen, something unpleasant. Deep into the evening, Hills was
standing by the front door talking with his host and Newman was in the
dining room when someone leaned against the breakfront. Almost in slow
motion, its upper half tilted forward, spilling the gray chinaware out onto
the floor in a great crash.

Newman and Hills helped pick up the pieces and dumped them into a
cardboard carton, and the party continued. Hills was sitting quietly in a
dining room chair near the breakfront, considering what had happened,
when his hostess, apparently explaining the crash, reached up and touched
the top part of the breakfront. Again the door swung open and more china
spilled out. The hostess, distraught, had to be led away.

At another party at a graduate student's house, Allan Seager, Gingrich's co-moderator—a Michigan professor who had been publishing fiction in *Esquire* for years—fell down the stairs and was so badly injured he
never fully recovered. After that happened, one of the *Esquire* writers
brought a young woman back to the Union, where the *Esquire* contingent
was staying, and, as a group stood around the lobby, her boyfriend, a young
writer, roared up on a motorcycle and, a minute later, came barreling
through the doors. He walked up to his girl, who was standing there with
the *Esquire* writer, and socked her—knocked her down, got on his motorcycle and drove off. Leslie and David Newman wondered if they would
ever be able to set foot on their old campus again.

A correspondent at Iowa passed on to Hills word of how the chairman
of the Michigan English department felt about the weekend. Recalling
the literary parties of the twenties, he thought *Esquire*'s weekend was "far
worse." In fact, said the correspondent, "his disgust and anger for *Esquire*
is not to be checked. I finally got him to allow that you and Styron were
acceptable gentlemen, but with the rest I could get nowhere."

As the dust was settling from the Michigan weekend, Hayes wrote
Gingrich a memorandum outlining office problems—a swollen inventory,
missed deadlines, poor cost control, and sloppy follow-up on features. He
had a specific complaint about Felker: Felker was leaving his production
work for Hayes and other staff members to do. (That was unlikely, Felker

said in 1993—taking care of production details was important to him; maybe he had been on a trip.) Hayes was willing to keep on picking up after Felker if he had to, he told Gingrich, but there was a better way: "I propose that you allow me to assume sufficient responsibility and authority to control all these problems."

He laid out the new regime in detail:

All story ideas would go through Hayes. He would have the power to reject any he thought were no good. Ideas he liked he would pass on to Gingrich, along with essential information, like the price. *Esquire* had been accepting too much mediocre material. Hayes would have the authority to make an assigning editor send a manuscript back to a writer for revision. If a piece could not be revised into shape, then Hayes would have the power to reject it. Only manuscripts he approved would move on to Gingrich. Hayes asked for similar powers over other terrain: house features, layouts.

He closed with a strong pitch that left Gingrich room to say no. He assured Gingrich he was willing to go on with things as they were. But if Gingrich wanted to try out this arrangement, Hayes wanted his "complete backing." He did not want to leave any room for anyone else to go around him to Gingrich.

I didn't learn a hell of a lot in the Marines but one thing I did learn with great conviction was: if you put one man in charge of three others you have to let that man do it his way, even if what he does is wrong. The minute you let one of the guys under him counter his order, his authority is forever and totally dissipated. If he continues to do wrong, you get rid of him and get someone else. This is a risk I am perfectly willing to take.

But this is *my* only reservation about this proposal. If you'd rather not tie yourself down to such a strong commitment at this time, I'd rather you didn't, too. But if you want to try it, I'm willing. And I assure you I will do everything possible to develop the staff (including Felker) rather than squelch it.

Gingrich agreed.

On November 13, Hayes wrote another memo to Gingrich, a more succinct setting forth of the new hierarchy. It began:

GENERAL POLICY:
I will assume total responsibility for the running of the editorial staff.

In this new era, the staff would be responsible to Hayes, and Hayes would be responsible to Gingrich. Everything that went to Gingrich from the staff would go through Hayes. Everything from Gingrich to the staff would go through Hayes. "If the magazine succeeds, I succeed. If the magazine fails, I fail."

One of Hayes's first items of business as *de facto* editor-in-chief was hiring new junior editors. To free Newman to work more with Benton, he needed to hire a new "first reader" to read unsolicited manuscripts. Brock Brower had left after just a few months, feeling he was a better writer than he was an editor; Hayes planned to hire a new editor who could come from either an art or an editorial background, so long as he was "an idea man who would make a distinct contribution to *both* the editorial and graphic look of the magazine."

Hayes talked with one candidate, Michael Herr, who was just finishing up undergraduate studies at Syracuse University. Herr had read *Esquire* since he was in junior high school, in the early 1950s, and it had seemed to him incredibly urbane and sophisticated. He took to Hayes the first time he met him, and he thought Hayes liked him, too. Herr did not know any southerners to speak of, and Hayes was distinctly southern—pleasant and attractive. Herr liked Hayes's laconic humor and he liked the upfront respect he felt Hayes had for him. Hayes was wonderfully dressed, and he filled his pipe with Revelation tobacco, a plebian tobacco, the kind coal miners or army men used. Hayes did not take advantage of Herr's nervousness, nor was he patronizing. He was, Herr thought, a "gent," a gentleman in the truest sense: someone who doesn't want to see other people uncomfortable.

Herr did not get the job. Hayes gave it instead to John Berendt, a clean-cut Harvard graduate who had gone to school with Herr in Syracuse when they were boys. The *Harvard Lampoon* had produced a parody of *Esquire* for *Mademoiselle* back in July, and Hayes had liked it. He found out Berendt was responsible, asked *him* to read the last six issues of *Esquire* and critique them, and come up with ten story ideas. Berendt was on staff by the end of December 1961, along with a new first reader to handle unsolicited manuscripts, Bob Brown, a refugee from Ph.D. studies in literature at Yale, who would put his literate stamp on the magazine in heads and house copy. Brown and Berendt seemed the sort of bright, savvy young men Hayes needed to put out a magazine designed for readers who wanted their stereotypes stretched, their tired ideas put to rest.

Take American women, for instance: Hayes wanted to do for them what he had done for sophistication, he told former secretary of state Dean Acheson, inviting him to contribute to the next July's issue on women: "We would like to try the same technique—knocking down old stereotypes and definitions and replacing them with a new and more accurate impression."

The *New York Times* had run articles about the problem educated women faced—their difficulties finding meaningful things to do—and Hayes had seen the articles, but he had also encountered the problem in a more personal way. His wife, Susan, her career as an actress abandoned, was spending her days back in their small Riverside apartment with their young son Tom, while Hayes brought home a briefcase bulging with manuscripts. Her friend from the Harvard year, Gloria Steinem, was now in New York, and Susan had helped her get a job with Harvey Kurtzman, who had gone from editing *Mad* to publishing his own magazine *Trump*. Steinem felt sympathetic toward Susan, who complained about being stuck in the kitchen while the men were out there, doing all the things women wanted to do. Steinem was dating Robert Benton, and one weekend she and Benton babysat for young Tom while Susan and Harold were away.

She and Benton also teamed up to produce a satiric guide to succeeding on campus for the September 1962 college issue, an idea *Esquire* borrowed from *Mademoiselle,* and for the same issue, she wrote a serious article on how contraceptives were changing sexual mores. Clay Felker assigned that one and then had made her rewrite it because, he told her, she had performed the incredible feat of making sex dull. Still, Steinem liked Felker as an editor. He would take a writer's idea and "make it grow." Hayes, on the other hand, seemed to her authoritarian: he wanted the writers to prove his ideas. Benton sometimes thought that Gloria Steinem was someone Hayes had a hard time hearing. She had had a big influence on Benton himself, and he thought her wise-guy, romantic cynicism crept into the new *Esquire* tone.

Not long after the college issue bearing Steinem's articles appeared on the newsstand, Arnold Gingrich announced to the staff that Clay Felker was leaving *Esquire* "to undertake a project of his own in the field of the economic news service. . . ." There was more to Felker's departure than that.

On May 31, 1962, *New York Post* columnist Earl Wilson had reported that comedian Mort Sahl "almost had a rumble with an *Esquire*

editor who asked him over to his table to meet some VIPS—then suddenly remembered an old battle and called him four- and five-letter
names. Sahl left abruptly but gracefully."

On June 4, a Beverly Hills lawyer named Richard Mark of Kopald and
Mark wrote to Gingrich and Hayes describing an incident that he said
occurred on May 29 at Basin Street East, where comedian Mort Sahl was
appearing. According to Mark, Felker was there with a group that included Senator and Mrs. Jacob Javits (friends of Felker's) and several
other prominent citizens, among them Paul Sann, executive editor of the
New York Post. Mark said Felker had invited Sahl to stop by the table
after the performance. Sahl did, and according to Mark's account, he
brought up a description of himself in *Esquire* as "the light that failed."
As Mark told the story, Sahl asked if someone at *Esquire* didn't like him,
and Felker said he didn't, then called Sahl names that the lawyer did not
want to repeat; then, according to Mark's letter, Felker threatened to
"bury" Sahl, through *Esquire.* At the start of the letter, Mark explained
that he was writing Gingrich and Hayes about the incident because *Esquire* had invited Sahl to offer comments *Esquire* could use to promote its
thirtieth-anniversary issue; at the end, he raised the possibility of further
action, presumably legal, a possibility ominously suggested by a heading at
the top of the letter: "RE: Sahl vs. Felker."

As Felker recalled the episode in 1994, he did remember approaching
Sahl, although he recalled the conversation taking place in Sahl's dressing
room, where Felker had gone to plead the case of a writer, Arthur Steuer.
Steuer was writing a series of *Esquire* articles on comedians and had
wanted to do Sahl, and, Felker recalled, Sahl had turned him down. Although Felker could not remember what he said to Sahl when Sahl
showed no inclination to change his mind, he thought he might have said
something like, "Listen, you prick, we're going to do the story anyway."
That was Felker's standard response to unwilling subjects, he said later: to
report around them. The threat to "bury" Sahl in *Esquire* would have
been uncharacteristic of him, Felker said in 1994, and his fellow *Esquire*
editor David Newman concurred—Felker was just not that kind of guy.

On June 11, a week after the date of Mark's letter, Gingrich responded, explaining that Felker had been out of the office, ill (he had strep).
Felker's return might be delayed, Gingrich explained. "Under the circumstances, I can only say that neither I nor any of the other editors ever have,
nor ever will, make *Esquire* the weapon of a personal vendetta."

On July 2, 1962, the lawyer Mark wrote again to Gingrich, reminding Gingrich that he was still waiting for an explanation of the incident. On July 16, 1962, Gingrich replied: Felker had written to Sahl, Gingrich said, and Gingrich was confident their differences had been worked out. Felker was on vacation from July 20 to August 13, and during that time Gingrich and Hayes met with Byron Dobell, an editor at Time-Life Books, to talk with him about coming to work for *Esquire* as Felker's replacement. On August 5, Dobell wrote Hayes a letter outlining his thoughts about *Esquire*. On August 24, Gingrich put out a memorandum to the staff announcing Felker's departure October 1.

When Dobell came to work—and he was on the job before the end of September—he moved into Felker's office, with Felker's dancing shoes still in the closet. Hayes told him that Felker had had a dispute with Sahl in a nightclub, and in 1994 Dobell recalled reading a letter about it, although he did not recall the details of the letter. The episode either was not generally known around the office, or was considered so inconsequential that few of the survivors remember anything about it. Felker himself discounts it as an immediate cause of his departure, which he believed was precipitated by another event: in a moment of anger, he had torn up an art assistant's layout; Gingrich would not tolerate such an act of disrespect to someone's creative work, and suggested it was time for Felker to leave. Whatever the individual incidents contributing to the timing of Felker's departure, he himself believed it was the natural result of his defeat by Hayes in the contest for the editorship of *Esquire*. He also had an idea for a publication he wanted to try, although it never came off and he wound up, eventually, running *New York* magazine.

There were those who missed Felker. Not long after Dobell came to *Esquire*, editorial associate Alice Glaser gave him a roman à clef she had written about the contest between Felker and Hayes. "I can't believe he was such a son of a bitch," Dobell said, when he had read the book. "The things he did—," he said, naming the character who seemed like the villain. "And to think Clay was like that."

"You're crazy," he recalled her saying. "That's Harold."

Dobell, who would later work with Felker at *New York* magazine, thought a lot of love for Felker had to go underground after he left.

Dobell was not much like Felker—he seemed to David Newman "a very different breed of cat . . . a very staid, more formal person." When he sent Hayes his thoughts on *Esquire* before he was hired, he had envisioned expansive picture-and-text pieces on lawyers, archaeologists, doctors—or bridges, skyscrapers, roads. He had favored *Esquire*'s less frivolous writers: Richard Rovere, Martin Mayer, Dan Wakefield. He was not, he confessed, a fan of Gay Talese.

But Dobell soon got into the swing of things. On October 9, 1962, taking a cue from friends working on Broadway, Byron Dobell proposed "a kind of Emperor's New Clothes profile on the vastly overinflated, super-glamourized reputation of Josh Logan." Idolized by actors and the angels who backed Broadway, protected by friends throughout the theater world, Logan had been responsible "for some of the most vulgar shows in Broadway history." Logan was hitting bottom this year with productions of the musicals *All-American* and *Mr. President:* "the first loaded with Logan's campy taste that runs to muscle-men and hyper-sexualized caricatures of women, the second loaded with god knows what according to the advance notes."

Why not assign Gay Talese, who was still on staff at the *New York Times* but writing regularly for *Esquire,* to shadow Logan during the premiere and opening night celebrations of *Mr. President,* an Irving Berlin creation? "If the show is as awful as predicted, Gay can then flash back into a reprise of Logan's career, influence and batting average. I know several people who could contribute some important insights into Logan's frightening drive to produce a 'hit' and his mechanical, cliché-ridden directorial techniques that have ruined half a dozen shows."

The *Times* unions went on strike on December 8, 1962, and Talese had plenty of time to settle down and watch Joshua Logan in rehearsals of Peter S. Feibleman's *Tiger Tiger Burning Bright,* which would open in January 1963. This was the kind of reporting Talese liked to do and seldom got to do as a newspaper reporter: just being there, observing, waiting for the climactic moment when the mask would drop and true character would reveal itself. Talese was less interested in exposing Logan's theatrical machinations—the line laid down by Dobell—than in portraying a man going down. He portrayed Logan as a man overwhelmed by his mother and insecure in his masculinity. The story built to the climax, as Logan crossed words with Claudia McNeil, the star, who reminded him of the Negro nurse of his plantation childhood, dominated by women.

"I've had enough of this today, Claudia."
"Yes, Mr. Logan."

"And stop Yes-Mr.-Logan-ing me."
"Yes, Mr. Logan."
"You're being a beast."
"Yes, Mr. Logan."
"Yes, Miss Beast."
"Yes, Mr. Logan."
"YES, MISS BEAST!"

Now McNeil was angered: "You . . . called . . . me . . . out . . . of . . . my . . . name," she said.

Logan turned to his co-producer. "I just don't know what to do with her. She's like some queen up there, or something . . ."

"YOU'RE THE QUEEN!" McNeil fired back.

A more conventional reporter might have kept that dialogue in his notebook; Talese put it into the story (although later, in his collected pieces, "queen" was changed to "empress"). *Esquire* titled the story "The Soft Psyche of Joshua Logan" and illustrated it with an Art Kane portrait in moody blue. Although Talese had kept himself out of the piece, the narration was so laden with judgment that *Esquire*'s lawyers feared a libel suit, despite Talese's insistence that every word in the piece was true. Talese finally called Logan, who was in Mexico, and read him the entire piece, and Logan confirmed it—which just showed, Hayes observed later, the rapport a good writer can have with his subject.

"The Soft Psyche of Joshua Logan" was a breakthrough piece for Gay Talese—he wrote it with a new confidence and control. From that point on, his profiles gave the *Esquire* attitude a new dimension. Looking back later on the *Esquire* of the early sixties, Tom Morgan, whose own profiles had set the stage, would say Hayes had been concerned about all the "self-creations and para-occasions" that were adding up to "a frightening denial of reality," as Daniel J. Boorstin had warned in his 1961 book, *The Image. Esquire* couldn't help but be part of the process—it was a commercial magazine filled with advertising and celebrity profiles. At least *Esquire* could expose the machinery behind the stage whenever it could.

Even *Esquire*'s more decorous writers got into the act, and they didn't stick to show business; there was plenty of posturing in the political world, too, and they went after it. Talk of "the establishment" had become fashionable—*Esquire* itself had run an article on the British establishment a couple of years back; C. Wright Mills had weighed in with a serious book-length analysis, *The Power Elite.* A conversation with Harvard economist John Kenneth Galbraith gave Richard Rovere the idea of

writing a parody of the genre. In a sober report on "The American Establishment," published in *Esquire* in May 1962, Rovere observed that some
states had virtually outlawed the establishment; in Indiana there was a
move for a law requiring the registration and fingerprinting of establishment agents. To make sure that readers understood the parallels to the
Red hunts of the fifties, the editors topped the article with a quote from
novelist Gore Vidal, whose *Esquire* column on "The Wrath of the Radical Right" had led Francis E. Walter, chair of the House Committee on
Un-American Activities, to cancel his *Esquire* subscription: "Not since J.
Edgar Hoover's *Masters of Deceit,*" proclaimed Vidal, "has there been
such an exposé of such startling impact. . . ."

Rovere had published the piece originally, in shorter form, for *The
American Scholar;* he was scarcely prepared for the reception it got when
he published it in *Esquire.* The piece drew notice from the *New York
Times,* the *Daily News,* and the *Chicago Tribune.* The scary part was how
many people thought Rovere was serious. In the *New York Post,* Milton
Viorst, writing about " 'The Establishment' and How It Grew," reported
that a John Birch Republican congressman from California, John Rouisse-
lot, had read the article into the *Congressional Record.* According to
Viorst, the Library of Congress even asked Rovere for his source material
when staff couldn't find the sources he cited.

Abe Blinder, president of the *Esquire* company, received a call from a
close friend saying the president of a national educational foundation had
told him at dinner that *Esquire* had done a disservice to its country.
Blinder hastened to assure his friend: The piece was satire, intended for a
sophisticated audience. His informant maintained that many readers had
taken it quite seriously. Hayes invited Rovere to write an article on the
subject of gullibility.

Rovere did not take him up on the invitation, but Rovere's friend John
Kenneth Galbraith, who had become Kennedy's ambassador to India,
kept the satiric ball rolling by offering his own social dissections in *Esquire*
under the pseudonym Mark Epernay, a name he got off a wine bottle. His
first piece offered a concept, "the McLandress Dimension," which measured the "intensity of the individual's identification with his own personality" by counting the minutes and seconds an individual could keep his
thoughts on something other than himself. The article reported the
McLandress Coefficient for Eleanor Roosevelt as two hours, Elizabeth
Taylor as three minutes, and Richard M. Nixon as three seconds. McLan-

dress theorized that lower ratings were an advantage for politicians.

After the piece was published in October 1962, a newspaper reporter from the *Boston Globe* called Hayes to say he had not been able to find either the institute or the doctor himself. Hayes had agreed not to blow Galbraith's cover, so he blamed a researcher for failing to identify the article as a hoax; it had come in as an unsolicited manuscript, Hayes told the reporter, who reported Hayes's response in his article. Jerry Jontry, *Esquire*'s advertising director, protested Hayes's response in a memo— eventually, he said, readers would not believe anything in *Esquire*.

Esquire had taken on a definite tone, the product not just of one or two minds—although Benton and Newman had sharpened its definition with the Dubious Achievement Awards—but of a group effort. They were like artists, Benton thought, drawing a horizon for a landscape in which they all worked. Some artists left more indelible marks than others— Diane Arbus, for instance, who proposed a photo story on eccentrics to be called "The Characters in a Fairy Tale for Grown Ups." Benton and Hayes liked the idea until they started getting calls, like the one from a distressed Bishop Ethel Credonzan of Jamaica, Queens, who wanted to know why *Esquire* had taken to publishing pictures of spiritual subjects. Hayes advised Arbus she could not take a picture of someone she meant to use as an "eccentric" if the subject did not know that was her purpose. Eventually *Esquire* decided against running the pictures, but Benton and Hayes both liked Arbus's work, which was distinctive without being pre- dictable, and her eerie images would find their way into the magazine on a regular basis, tinting its mood.

Like Arbus, Terry Southern, a Texan with his own eccentric sensibil- ity, passed through the offices and left a trail. The author of *The Magic Christian,* a cult book for young readers of David Newman's generation, Southern even worked at *Esquire* one summer when Rust Hills took off. Before Hills left, Southern came in to learn how to use Hills's card file, three-by-five index cards in wooden boxes that looked like shoe boxes. On the cards was listed every fiction writer anywhere, it seemed, and their agents, and publishers, and past publications. You could say, David New- man recalled, "Did you ever hear of a guy named Joe Smith?" And Hills would go to his file and pull out the card: "published in *Prairie Schooner* in 1949 a short story about a kid whose mother has epilepsy. He teaches at Ohio Wesleyan and his phone number is. . . ."

When Southern turned up to get acquainted with Hills's file system, he was wearing a dark blue suit with a hole in the knee the size of a quarter. Before he left for lunch at a fancy restaurant, Southern went to the art department and borrowed some blue-black ink, rolled up his pants, and colored his knee to match his pants. Once on the job, Southern worked quietly behind closed doors, preparing stories for publication and reading unsolicited manuscripts. Only after Hills returned did the truth come out: Southern, a man with a bizarre sense of humor, had singled out the worst writers he came across and had spent hours writing them long encouraging letters.

Southern wrote several pieces for *Esquire,* including "Twirling at Ole Miss," an account of a baton twirling contest for teen girls (with frequent asides on southern racism), and an interview with a man who claimed he would have gone on the Bay of Pigs invasion—if only he could have gotten out of Guatemala. Southern worked on the screenplay of *Dr. Strangelove,* the funniest movie ever made about the atomic bomb, and before the movie came out in 1964, Southern sent Newman the mock *Playboy* fold-out used in the movie. Would *Esquire* like to run it, along with text from "Strangelove"? "Or does Big Arne fear an open clash with coarse Hugh Heff?!?" he asked. It didn't run; *Esquire* passed up the chance, too, to run an article Southern wrote on the movie, despite Southern's accurate forecast that the movie was *"categorically* different from any film yet made and that it will probably have a stronger impact in America than has any single film, play, or book in our memory."

Black comedy, theater of the absurd: the stiff pretense of healthy-mindedness that ruled fifties mass culture had given way in the early sixties to a suspicion, hard to escape in a nuclear age, that the apparently sane were really crazed, and the apparently crazed deserved more respect. Joseph Heller's *Catch-22* came out in 1961; Ken Kesey's *One Flew Over the Cuckoo's Nest* in 1962. Lenny Bruce made people laugh darkly. *Esquire* ran a story by Gay Talese on a group of New Yorkers who had moved to Chico, California, to escape nuclear destruction, and another offering "nine places to hide" from the bomb. (The list prompted one reader, an unorthodox Indianapolis minister named Jim Jones, to move his family to Belo Horizonte, Brazil.)

Writers and editors could range across a broad expanse of subjects, so long as their pieces had what Hayes called "point of view" or, sometimes, "p.o.v." Hayes knew how to nudge writers and editors in just the right direction, getting into house copy that particular tone, irreverent, knowledgeable, never overly impressed with anything. He placed enormous emphasis on titles, copy blocks, captions. Editors had to get the attitude of *Esquire* across in these small pieces. He wanted the copy diamond perfect.

Newman would go into Hayes's office, and Hayes would be sitting there with his feet up on the desk.

"He'd say, 'Read this piece and give me a title for it'—or a subhead—and I'd come in with four of them. I'd put them on different pieces of paper, and he'd look at the first one and sort of smile like he knew what I was after, and then when he'd get to the third one, which I'd put in that spot because I was building toward it, he would laugh out loud, and say, 'That's it!' And he'd hand it to his secretary, and he'd say, 'Good work.' And you'd walk out and you'd feel wonderful. He was very quick to praise when he meant it.

"And when he was tough on you, it was always with the caveat that 'you're so good I can't believe you're giving me something that isn't up to your best standard.' So it was never scary and it was never mean."

Hayes presided over idea meetings every Wednesday, but there were other meetings—constant meetings—always stimulating. When someone was stuck on a problem Hayes would sometimes send around his secretary, Connie Wood, to fetch the others to solve it. There was an easy feel to the office—an openness to whatever came up. When Pete Turner told Hayes he had always wanted to do a picture story on railroads, Hayes said, "Great, do it." Turner got on a train at Grand Central Terminal and rode out to the Northwest, to Seattle, down to San Diego, across the Southwest to New Orleans, and then got off at Penn Station.

Coming back from an assignment, Turner would wait for Hayes to come down the corridor, the *tap-tap* of his brown suede shoes announcing his approach. "What you got, Pete?" he would say. "Let's see what you got." And if he liked it he would call in more editors, and pretty soon there would be a whole bunch of people having fun and talking. Hayes was never hip, Newman thought, but he knew the magazine should be hip and he should listen to hip people. What an exciting office it was, Connie Wood recalled—with all these young people like Benton, Newman, so terrific, smart, and Hayes bustling around, stirring things up.

But it was Rust Hills who brought Norman Mailer back to *Esquire*, adding volume and resonance to the magazine's new voice. About a year after Mailer left, Hayes and Hills had been riding home together in a cab, and had fallen to talking about Mailer's self-interview in *The Paris Review.*

Good stuff, they thought, and a real shame they had not gotten it. Hills said they ought to try to get Mailer back. Hayes argued that the magazine was more important than any single writer and, besides, look how Mailer had bad-mouthed them. A feeble point, Hills said. *"I* would never ask him back," Hayes retorted. Hills said he wouldn't mind, and so he did, promising, as Hayes recalled it later, "that the magazine would kiss Mailer's ass in Macy's window if that should be what it took to make amends."

Actually, the letter Hills wrote was more decorous, a model apology. He acknowledged *Esquire*'s carelessness in handling the convention story. "We ought to do things better, God knows we ought," he said. He had been shocked to find, when he got to *Esquire,* that sentences and titles were changed without the author's permission. He himself tried not to do that. But there were so few editors to do the job; as a result, the magazine was under-edited. In fact, he argued, that was its virtue. Many voices could be heard. "There is not the sameness, the all-the-stories-sound-alike quality that you get in a well edited magazine." If Mailer would come back to *Esquire,* he would give him an "absolutely firm, personal guarantee" that what Mailer wrote would appear as he approved it. If Gingrich insisted on changes Mailer would not approve, then the magazine would just not run the piece at all.

Mailer accepted the offer, and *Esquire* ran an apology that, as Hills said later, "made Mailer seem a little foolish for asking for an apology." Mailer came back to *Esquire* with a July 1962 article on Jacqueline Kennedy, then offered to write a monthly column for every issue for a year and a major feature every three months, in return for guaranteed fees.

Hayes talked the idea over with Hills, who set down his thoughts in a memorandum. The choice seemed to be either too much Mailer or no Mailer at all. "That much Mailer is undoubtedly more Mailer than we feel we want now, and we'd probably rather not have it—and it seems insane to spend that much [$700 per column] for something we'd rather not have," Hills argued. At the same time, it was better to have Mailer than not have him. The truth was, Hills said, with the possible exception of J. D. Salinger, Mailer was the only writer they would even think about making such a deal with. Mailer had a reputation as the most exciting writer around. Besides, there was a precedent in *Esquire*'s own history: In the thirties *Esquire* must have run almost that much by Hemingway, and it was not always his best writing. And Fitzgerald's Pat Hobby stories came in for criticism, but publishing them had been good for the magazine. Finally, Hills pointed out, the contract would run only a year.

Hayes once called Hills "a fidgety and charming man who always managed to see more sides than existed to any question." Hills concluded complexly:

"I vote reluctantly to go along with signing him up—reluctantly, because this much dough will surely cut into our funds for other writers to some extent, and because it is so much of one man's voice in the magazine. But although I vote yes reluctantly, I also vote strongly—that is, I feel very strongly that to sign him up is the better of the two alternatives."

Mailer wrote twelve columns in all, issuing diatribes against taped television and totalitarian architecture, plastic and housing projects, and commenting—belatedly, given *Esquire*'s long lead time—on passing events. He began "The Big Bite" in late 1962 with the deaths of Ernest Hemingway and Marilyn Monroe and moved on to the Cuban missile crisis—that October week "when the world stood like a playing card on edge." One month he wrote of the joy of keeping a quotations book and shared favorite quotations from an assortment of authors—Thoreau, Jack London, Hemingway. The next month he confessed he had made all the quotations up himself, proving that "readers who trust writers are often abused." He put some of his column material into a collection, *The Presidential Papers,* and when the collection came out he ran excerpts in his column, recycling passages that had appeared there just a few months before.

His column wore an improvised air, as if he were saying exactly what was on his mind in the day or so preceding the deadline—it was irreverent and fresh, and grand themes played through it: God and the Devil, totalitarianism and cancer, modern Americans' hatred of nature and fear of death. College students read *Esquire* to see what Norman Mailer was saying. He was a clear asset to the magazine. However difficult Hayes found him to deal with—and he did find him difficult—Hayes saw what he was doing for *Esquire.* He brought to the magazine a boldness Hayes liked.

"He had the audacity to address the President of the United States directly from our pages, thus we acquired the audacity. He spoke out boldly on politics, sex, architecture, literature, civil rights, cancer, anything that challenged his imagination, and many things did. Most of the time, when he shouted people listened; and to hear him, they had to read *Esquire.*"

Something was happening over at *Esquire*—George Lois could tell. Something focused, something smart. A Greek florist's son from the Kingsbridge section of the Bronx, Lois had spent a year at Doyle Dane Bernbach advertising agency, then had set up his own creative agency with two partners: Papert, Koenig, Lois. For Joseph E. Seagram & Sons, they came up with a series of print ads for Wolfschmidt, the company's vodka:

"You're some tomato," said a Wolfschmidt bottle, standing upright, to a red tomato. "We could make beautiful Bloody Marys together. I'm different from the other fellows."

"I like you Wolfschmidt," says the tomato. "You've got taste."

A week later, another ad followed:

"You sweet doll, I appreciate you," said the Wolfschmidt bottle, now lying prone, pointing to an orange. "I've got taste. I'll bring out your inner orange. I'll make you famous. Roll over here and kiss me."

"Who was that tomato I saw you with last week?" said the orange.

Years later, Lois recalled his first lunch with Hayes at the Four Seasons. He had been honored when Hayes asked him out, an idea Clay Felker had come up with before his departure. The minute Hayes and Lois sat down together, Lois was charmed by the man—the rumpled Mark Twain look, the hank of hair, the directness. Hayes got right to the heart of the matter. As Lois recalled the conversation, it went something like this:

"I've got a problem with the covers. It's always such an ordeal," Hayes began, and he was right: the sober covers, often heavy with type, did not match the spirit of the contents inside.

"Well, how do you do the covers now?"

"Everybody sits and talks and talks. They go away—they come back."

Lois knew right away what the problem was: too many minds were at work, they couldn't focus.

"Give it to one person," said Lois. "Find a graphic designer and say, 'Take a look at my issue and package it for me.' The cover should make a statement, tell readers not only what that issue is about but what *Esquire* is about. One cover would build on another, until people understood: this was a great magazine."

It *was* a great magazine, he told Hayes, and mentioned five or six terrific articles from recent issues. Hayes was doing an incredible job. He just needed someone to wrap the package.

"Well, who?" Hayes asked.

"Let me think about it," said Lois.

"How about you?" said Hayes.

"I run an agency," said Lois.

"Old buddy," said Hayes, brandishing his cigarillo, "do me one cover, just one cover. Show me—"

"Look," Lois replied, laying down a rule that would last for all his time at *Esquire,* "the only way I'd do a cover is if I do the cover and that's it. That's the cover. I ain't gonna argue and I ain't gonna talk and I ain't gonna have it compared to twenty other pieces of junk and I ain't gonna come over and discuss it."

"No, no, you can work just with me."

"Yeah, I'll work with you but I gotta tell you, and I don't wanna sound obnoxious, but I gotta have, like, control over it."

Hayes looked Lois in the eye—and it was a make-or-break moment. "Okay, do whatever you do. We'll run it."

"Okay," said Lois, "I'll do it."

A couple days later, Lois called him and asked, "When is your on-stand date? When does this thing get on the stand?" Hayes told him and Lois said, "Okay, terrific." Here was what he had in mind: About two weeks after the October 1962 issue went on the stand, Floyd Patterson, heavyweight champion of the world, conscientious, considerate, beloved, was going to take on a challenger, Sonny Liston, a fighter who had come up from the meanest streets, a man with the Mob at his shoulder. This was a fight everyone was talking about. Norman Mailer was going to cover it for *Esquire;* James Baldwin would be there, too, and so would Gay Talese, both writing for other publications. Lois had seen an advance piece on the fight in the lineup for the issue, and he wanted the cover to reflect that piece but he also wanted to do something more brash.

"I want to call the fight on the cover," he told Hayes.

"You want to *what?*"

"We'll get a guy who looks like Patterson—his build. We'll get the color trunks he's gonna wear, I hope, and we'll show him in the middle of the ring, left for dead. They've had the fight—he's left for dead."

Hayes understood. Though Lois loved boxing, he was going to say something unkind about it on the cover of *Esquire,* something derogatory: If you win they take you out to the show, but if you lose they leave you for dead.

Lois called up Cus D'Amato, Patterson's manager, and told him he wanted to know what color trunks Patterson was going to wear, but he couldn't tell him why he wanted to know. So D'Amato wouldn't tell him what color trunks Patterson was going to wear. Lois had photographer Harold Krieger shoot his Patterson stand-in both in black Everlast trunks and in white Everlast trunks. They shot the pictures in the abandoned St. Nicholas Arena on West 66th Street: a dark figure, face up, out, in the center of the square ring, flanked by empty seats.

Lois showed Hayes two covers, one with white trunks, one with black. Hayes loved them. They flipped a coin to decide which trunks they would go with—the trunks they were betting Patterson would wear. Black won.

Lois told *Esquire*'s publicity office to say the *Esquire* issue coming out was predicting a knockout—a wipeout of Patterson. Gingrich didn't like it. He started off his Publisher's Page for the issue by making his position clear: "Since this issue will achieve currency barely a fortnight before the Patterson-Liston title fight, we thought we'd better take advantage of this last chance to tell you that we don't agree with its cover." Lois's point was fine—the loneliness of a boxer's defeat. What Gingrich did not like about the cover was its prophetic note: he preferred "to believe that Liston can be stopped, and that Patterson is the one that can do it."

He was wrong and Lois was right. Patterson wore black and Patterson lost. He went down (as Norman Mailer reported a few months later in *Esquire*) two minutes, six seconds into the first round. After that first Lois cover appeared, Patterson face up on the mat, the lighting eerie, subdued, Hayes got on the phone:

"George, we got people calling here. People hate what you did, people love what you did. Oh my God, I love it."

"Terrific," Lois said.

"George," said Hayes, "you've got to do some more. George, do a couple more."

After that, he did *Esquire*'s covers every issue, giving everyone—readers, writers, editors, advertisers—a monthly reminder of what they could expect from *Esquire:* the unexpected.

Was everyone at *Esquire* happy with the new provocative *Esquire*? They were not. Back when Hayes was planning the issue on sophistication, he had tried to convince the advertising sales staff that they could sell the idea of a sophisticated magazine for sophisticated readers. General magazines might be dying, but *Esquire* would be a general magazine with a difference: aimed at "the best informed and most curious people in America." The sales staff was not persuaded. *Esquire* readers might be sophisticated, but that did not mean advertisers were. If the salespeople tried to explain the sophistication of *Esquire*'s editorial policy, one salesman said, the average advertiser would simply not know what they meant.

In spring 1962, the advertising department's unease over the new direction had flared into open revolt. On April 23, 1962, the department's top executives, Jerry Jontry and Sam Ferber, had fired off an eight-page memo to Arnold Gingrich laying out a lengthy critique of editorial handling of fashion pages, which Hayes and Benton tried to give the flair of the rest of the magazine, for instance sending Pete Turner off to photograph President Kennedy for a special report: "The Monogram on this Man's Shirt is J.F.K.," which led the January 1962 issue as an editorial feature. Getting that spread had involved some subterfuge—a pretense of photographing the man, not his clothes; on the scene, Turner had had a tough time explaining to Kennedy why he was leaning over to get a shot of Kennedy's shoes.

The resulting spread had as much charm as a fashion feature could have, but what about that piece David Newman had come up with for April—"Deadly 7 Dressers"—pictures of celebrities who wore dumpy suits and shorts too short for them, accompanied by text that sounded suspiciously like parody? The advertising staff could not help detecting a whiff of disrespect for fashion in the editorial air. For Jerry Jontry and Sam Ferber the fashion spread *Esquire* ran every month—eight pages or so— was a crucial draw for advertisements for men's clothing, which, along with whiskey, was an advertising staple for *Esquire*. Unlike the old days, when *Esquire* began, *Esquire* had a bunch of competitors for the clothing ads: *Gentlemen's Quarterly, True, Playboy, Sports Illustrated, Argosy.* These were competitive times.

And what was the editorial response?

By their own admission [wrote Jontry and Ferber], most of the *Esquire editorial and art departments* would be happy if we could do away with the fashion pages ALTOGETHER and devote this space to something else *more interesting to them.* Their own personal appearance, by and large, indicates their complete lack of interest or understanding of fashion. They never attend an *Esquire* fashion show, trend clinic, or color clinic. They never call on a store or visit the market, or even talk to a reader about fashion. Yet when our fashion department brings

the full report and lays it at their feet they suddenly become experts in something they haven't the slightest interest [in], or what is worse, the slightest understanding [of]. . . .

Look at how Hayes had overruled *Esquire*'s fashion experts, Oscar
Schoeffler and Chip Tolbert, and devoted five pages to the "stretch suit,"
in the interest of "making a clever acrobatic picture story." And what
about that spread on white buckskin shoes? Nobody was wearing white
buckskin shoes; the shoe manufacturers and stores were still laughing.

Jontry and Ferber laid out their demands. They wanted Schoeffler to
have veto power over a spread before it went to Gingrich. They wanted a
more uniform format. They wanted *Esquire*'s advertisers to be featured in
the fashion pages (with credit, of course). They wanted the fashion pages
to show a range of styles. "We love publishing independence as much as
anyone, but let's face it—we are fighting for our lives in the men's apparel
business. . . ."

It was the start of an ongoing tug-of-war over the fashion pages, as
Hayes struggled to make them part of the magazine—and at the same
time resented their very presence. Hayes described *Esquire* years later as
"an immensely commercial magazine that was constrained by all sorts of
silly, stupid, in-house laws" that required him to run spreads that would
lure advertisers: eight pages of fashion every issue, with credits; a page on
liquor; a spread on gifts; two hi-fi pieces a year; a car feature each June; a
demure girl story. When he sat down to plan an issue, he had to begin by
blocking out twenty pages of editorial copy for this stuff before he could
get down to serious business. That still left far more pages to devote to
other things than most magazines would have in the years to come, but
Hayes felt the indignity. "Abe, please don't turn this magazine into a
catalogue," he pled once with Blinder. "I'll do whatever's necessary to
make money," Blinder replied.

Hayes felt, too, the constraint of having Fritz Bamberger looking over
his shoulder to make sure he didn't run something that would lose Detroit.
Even after Bamberger took a position at Hebrew Union College, he read
manuscripts for potential problems of libel and taste—anything that
might offend readers or advertisers. His objections did not carry absolute
weight, but Hayes could not dismiss them out of hand. Management had
a legitimate interest in the commercial consequences of what the editors
did.

The company's financial situation was better in the early sixties than it had been in the early fifties when Gingrich returned, but it was still dicey, prompting Gingrich in April 1961 to warn Dwight Macdonald, *Esquire's* unruly movie columnist, not to invite unnecessary attacks: "The current recession has made all magazine people, circulation as well as advertising, much more sensitive to pressures from all sides." By 1962 Blinder had killed off *Coronet.* He was also taking steps to make the company less vulnerable to the whims of publishing: he had begun a process of diversification, so that the company's fortunes would not depend on its magazines alone. In mid-1962, a market research report on *Esquire's* readers offered glimmers of hope. The income of new subscribers (whose median age was 42.2 years) was up, and 70 percent were reported engaged in executive, professional, or managerial occupations. But the number of advertising pages dropped 4 percent in 1962; the company itself (although not the magazine) posted a small loss. Management made no bones in-house about the magazine's precarious position. Robert Benton would recall the management line: "Listen, circulation is going down, if it continues going down we're going to fire you. And if we fire you and it goes down, we're going to sell the magazine."

It was a tricky time, and Hayes kept his eyes on the newsstand sales— the magazine's best barometer of its changing fortunes. When a harshly critical piece on Attorney General Robert Kennedy—"The Best Man 1968"—sent newsstand sales soaring in March 1963, Hayes was jubilant. He wrote its author, Gore Vidal, "Well you were right—the newsstand sale is up and still climbing—conceivably to the highest mark we've reached in the past two or three years (excluding the big December issues)." Besides that, Vidal's attack had been featured by wire services, network radio, *U.S. News and World Report, Time,* and *Newsweek.* Hayes knew he needed successes like that. Byron Dobell remembers him saying, "If the circulation goes down three months in a row, we're out of here."

THREE

Red Hot Center

FOR WEEKS during the winter of 1962–63, a cardboard and rubber-cement concoction blocked the doorway of Rust Hills's office: situated on it were the names of agents, book reviewers, magazines, book publishers, academic critics—the brokers of literary power in New York.

"I guess everyone knows that everyone in America reads," Hills explained to Hayes in a memorandum, "but less commonly realized is the fact that everyone writes. I don't mean 'it seems sometimes to me that nearly everyone wants to write'—I mean: *everyone* writes."

With the appropriate promotion efforts (for instance, a press release to writers' magazines, columnists and book-page editors, and 1,254 teachers of creative writing on a list in his office), *Esquire* ought to be able to sell an issue the next July that would tell all those writers

what the good writers are doing and what the bad ones are up to; how the successful writer lives and how the unsuccessful writer lives; who are the agents with power and judgement, who are the "literary" book publishers and magazine editors and who are the critics that count—and how all of these forces interact with one another. The reader should get examples of the good current work and learn what to expect in the future. He should also be given an amount of malicious and satirical comment on the bad writing and the literary politicking. In general, I think he should be given a comprehensive but not dull picture of what's up, what's REALLY the situation, in the world of writing.

Hayes bought the idea, and the staff went to work. Robert Benton and David Newman found a couple of writers willing to act out their lives for a photo piece: screenwriter George Axelrod, who wrote and was rich, and a Beat "writer" named John Filler, who refrained from writing and was poor. Carl Fischer gathered together twenties literary survivors in front of his camera. Terry Southern wrote about Mickey Spillane. Rust Hills invited Vladimir Nabokov, Flannery O'Connor, and several other novelists to send in excerpts of works-in-progress. Norman Mailer cast his eye over a field of contemporaries and thought up mean things to say about their newest novels. William Styron's *Set This House on Fire* was a "bad maggoty novel" and Styron himself (who appeared elsewhere in the issue talking to James Jones) "a fat spoiled rich boy"; James Baldwin's *Another Country* was "powerful" but "abominably written"; John Updike had the instincts of a novelist but served up "mud pies in prose."

Esquire's lawyer objected: Some of Mailer's comments did not appear to be "fair comment," allowable under libel law, since Mailer admitted he was personally involved with Styron and acknowledged, too, his "spite" and pleasure when Styron failed. Mailer ought to make his criticism more impersonal. To ask Mailer not to be personal was to ask Mailer not to be Mailer; Mailer merely admitted his animus ("On record are the opinions of a partisan") and went on.

Meanwhile, Gay Talese was out interviewing *The Paris Review* crowd, George Plimpton and his friends, the social center of New York literary life. Talese heard many stories about their life in Paris, some on the record and some not. In Paris the crowd had been poseurs, rich young men who pretended to be poor. "There was something very *manqué* about them," said Patsy Matthiessen, Peter's then-wife. James Baldwin observed that "they were more interested in kicks and hashish" than he was. Back in New York, they were Peter Pans, trying to escape "the inevitability of being thirty-six," drifting in and out of Plimpton's apartment, rubbing shoulders with James Jones, William Styron, Jean vanden Heuvel, Lillian Hellman, call girls, "a junkie or two," "a retired bunny from the Playboy Club," and other knowns and unknowns, several of whom were also in the *Esquire* crowd. One night earlier that year, Jacqueline Kennedy appeared, wandering gracefully through the party, and Talese put her into the story.

Based entirely on interviews, the piece presented one challenge after another to the *Esquire* fact-checker, who noted at the beginning of her report, "We have used our discretion in checking information relating to the personal lives of individuals discussed in this article. In many cases it was necessary to check lightly in order to maintain the good will of the persons contacted." The report proceeded, confirmations and corrections of spelling mixed with less certain remarks:

Mrs. (Matthiessen) Goldberg [Peter Matthiessen's former wife, Patsy] was
extremely reluctant to talk about the information she had given our author in
personal interview; . . . .

Author tells us that he is a personal friend of Mr. Humes. He assures us that
all information concerning Humes is accurate and that we should not attempt to
investigate further the stories told about him. . . .

We are sorry to say that we accidentally read this word to Mr. Matthiessen in
reviewing with him the information contained in this passage. He feels that the
use of the word *condescendingly* here puts him in a bad light. . . .

We would like to state, for the record, that in regard to information included
about Alexander Trocchi, we were not able to trace his history through the court
records. . . .

Talese did some fact-checking of his own, reading a couple of sections
of the manuscript to Harold Humes, one of the key figures in it. Humes
was dismayed by the tenor of what he heard. The mythology that had
grown up around the expatriates was "a grotesque and dangerous lie."
Talese had not questioned the lie; instead, he had asked Humes "to agree
that the shape of the fifties was banged out of the matrix of the twenties."
The truth was that those years in Paris, for many of the expatriates, were
"a time of fear and misery." There was something else Talese needed to
face: "that if there is such a thing as 'the Paris Review Crowd,' then you,
old bean, certainly exist at the heart of it. . . ."

Eleanor Perenyi had the formidable job of writing about Edmund
Wilson, America's most august literary journalist, who was not, at first,
inclined to cooperate. When Perenyi asked him for an interview, Wilson
pronounced himself "annoyed with *Esquire* for publishing a malicious
statement about me in that Mary McCarthy article," a piece by Brock
Brower in the issue on women the previous July. He declined to do anything for *Esquire.*

It is difficult to know which statement Wilson objected to; Brower
quoted several unkind remarks by Mary McCarthy. He could have minded
McCarthy's testimony at her divorce trial that, as she told the judge, "he
got up from the sofa and took a terrible swing and hit me in the face and
all over." Or perhaps he simply minded her remark that the former husband in *A Charmed Life,* one of her books, couldn't be Edmund Wilson
because the character is a successful playwright and "everybody knows
that Edmund never had a successful play in his life!"

At any rate, Wilson was not pleased, and what could have been a coup
for Perenyi was looking doubtful. She asked Hayes, with some hesitation,

if he would consider—"I guess there's no other word for it—an apology?"
She passed along Wilson's address.

Hayes replied, "I'm damned if I'll apologize to Edmund Wilson. What
we did to him is no worse than *The New Yorker* has done to many more
notable men of the past and that certainly hasn't stopped him from writing for *The New Yorker*. We apologized to Norman last July and I'm
convinced more than ever that that was a mistake." He told her he still
wanted the piece if she wanted to do it.

Perenyi wrote back, acknowledging that the note she had suggested he
write was the kind "I guess no man can really write to another." She would
try proceeding with the piece, although she wouldn't get far if Wilson's
friends would not talk with her. "It is an undoubted fact that while nobody minds talking about Mary McCarthy, who is widely loathed—not by
me—Edmund is a different matter," she said.

"I didn't mean to seem mad at you," Hayes replied. "I spent half an
hour trying to write the old bastard but could find no way to keep us all
from sounding like worms. Then I got mad at him."

The lull was temporary, and what happened next demonstrated a side
of Hayes that earned him a reputation as a tough guy with writers. After
Perenyi turned in the piece and revised it (Wilson did give her an interview after all), Hayes told her she would need to cut about eight manuscript pages—space was tight. Perenyi was upset. Hadn't Hayes told her
when she first turned the piece in that it seemed short? And why was her
deadline so early (February 1)? If it had been later, the editors would have
known better what length they wanted.

Hayes snapped back: "You wrote it long, and it didn't justify the
length. You were given the deadline of February 1st, because that was the
deadline I wanted to give you, and deadlines, as you ought to know, are an
editor's business to set and a writer's business to refuse if he or she can't
make them." He went on down a line of accusations until finally he said,
"You have raised hell with so many people here they are coming to feel
you are part of management. And you say you are not difficult to work
with! Please let me know when you're going to get *really* tough."

She replied: "I can only say that I hope you won't (to paraphrase your
letter) let me know when you're any more annoyed than 'somewhat.' I
doubt if I could take it."

Hayes backed down, restored much of the cut material without going
into why, "since any more developments in the Wilson Affair would prob-

ably give us both nervous breakdowns," and said, finally, "I like the piece. Honest."

There was one figure on the literary scene who was far away, but Hayes was determined to have him in the issue: the Beat poet Allen Ginsberg, who had moved with Peter Orlovsky to India. Hayes asked several editors if they would go; nobody wanted to make the trip until, finally, editorial associate Alice Glaser agreed. Hayes trusted Glaser—a graduate of Radcliffe, she was very bright; she was also devoted to the magazine. While Gay Talese saw her as shy, another writer, Dan Wakefield, found her friendly. He always remembered the night they had dinner together and it was snowing, and they thought up a board game for writers—"Stockholm." They drew cards that moved them forward or backward around a board—cards like "get an agent, take three moves forward" or "bad review in the *Times,* take three moves back." The winner won the Nobel Prize for literature and got to give an acceptance speech.

Off to India, Glaser, prone to anxiety even at home in New York, flew to Benares, then took a rickshaw across town in the direction of the Ganges. She found Ginsberg and Orlovsky on the third floor of a sweltering tenement in a Hindu section of town. They had adapted nicely to their surroundings, which offered apartments for $2 a month and plentiful marijuana. Dressed in loose robes, their hair untamed, they even looked right.

In fact, behind the peaceful scene a melodrama was unfolding. The police were watching Ginsberg and Orlovsky: they had begun to wonder why these Americans were staying so long in India and, besides that, mingling with the lower classes as they did. Perhaps they were CIA? Ginsberg had ruffled the feathers of a professor at Benares Hindu University when he gave a reading there, and a copy of Ginsberg's *Howl,* with passages underlined, ended up in the hands of the local police. Suspicion mounted when *Esquire*'s photographer, Pete Turner, arrived before Glaser and drew official attention: this was not the kind of publicity India wanted—beatniks doing who knows what.

"Drugs, my God," Turner recalled, "they had more drugs within a block or two: they took me to the store—it was beautiful, they must have had three hundred bins of different colors and powders and whatnot, and ganja this and ganja that, different colors of ganja—you know, pot— psychedelic God knows what, they'd chew it or smoke it or whatever. But those guys were in heaven. You could go there and that was like a corner tobacco store. They had everything you could imagine, and they said, 'You oughta try some of this.' I said, 'Okay.' I took a puff of this stuff and I couldn't believe it—it was enough to make you want to jump out of your skin. I did not enjoy it at all, and this Indian fellow says, 'Oh, you're having a bad trip? You have to chew on a lime. I get you some lime.'

"So he gets the limes and I'm chewing on them and he was right, it went right away. Apparently the citric acid in lemons and limes neutralizes a lot of whatever it is in pot—or ganja—that gets you wrecked."

Turner took Ginsberg's photograph as he stood, waist deep, in the river in front of a cluster of curly-horned cows.

By the time Glaser arrived, a man from the Criminal Investigation Department was hanging around the poets' neighborhood and had told their landlord that he would get in trouble for letting them have a room. The day after Glaser got there—she stayed a week—they learned their request for a visa had been denied. None of this fuss got into the story, except obliquely, in a quote from Ginsberg's journal—a "jolly" policeman asking, "Why do you want to stay here in India so long?" Although Glaser's high heels prevented her from accompanying Ginsberg and Orlovsky on their walks, the visit sounded, on the whole, pleasantly upbeat. Ginsberg lay comfortably on the floor of their room, blowing out sweet smoke, and Orlovsky offered Glaser tea, which she declined, having taken stock of the hairs and flies clinging to the dishes in view.

The hardest part was still to come. Back home in New York, Glaser had to write the article. Glaser was a skilled, graceful writer, who brought her own personal flair to titles and other house copy, including "Backstage," the column about each issue's contents. But when she came back from India, she blocked. That, at least, was what art assistant Jill Goldstein thought happened. True, Glaser was also ill, feverish, in bed. But, Goldstein believed, Glaser's confidence was faltering; this piece was not only a chance to prove herself as a writer—the magazine really needed it. The cover illustration featured an impassive Ginsberg with a pretty young woman who says, over a drift of cigarette smoke:

> Mr. Mailer is here.
> Mr. Albee is here.
> Mr. Styron is here.
> Mr. Jones is here.
> Mr. Nabokov is here.

> But who would have
> dreamt you would
> come all the way
> from the Ganges to be
> at our little party,
> Mr. Ginsberg.

Ginsberg had to get into the magazine.

Goldstein advised Hayes to send someone over to help her. Gay Talese
was fast becoming a pinch-hitter for Hayes. Once James Baldwin had
been assigned to write text to go with Tom Keogh's sketches of Harlem at
night, and he turned in a polemic instead. Hayes called Talese: Baldwin's
mad, he said, and won't rewrite. "Come up and look at these pictures."
Talese did not know anything about Harlem at night, but he booked
himself into a Harlem hotel and asked a fellow reporter at the *Times* who
did know Harlem to take him around to some bars after-hours. He had to
write the piece fast, and he was not a fast writer, but for Hayes, he tried to
be. After the piece ran, in September 1962, Hayes said, "It's not your best
piece," and Talese made up his mind. Fuck you, Harold, he said to himself. From then on he would set the agenda.

But when Hayes asked Talese to help Glaser with the Ginsberg story,
Talese went to her bedside. He had her tell him all she had seen and
heard. He did not even look at her notes. Then he wrote the story—mostly
Glaser asking questions, with the poets responding, all apparently in one
session. The scene was mellow, relaxed. At the end of it the two poets fell
asleep; Glaser kissed them and left. The piece ran under her byline.

When the issue came out, attention was paid. A young southerner,
Willie Morris, who had just come to work for *Harper's* magazine, studied
Rowland B. Wilson's drawing of *The Paris Review* crowd that accompa-
nied Talese's piece and wondered: "Would I ever be part of all that?"

The people who were a part of it weren't all that happy to be a part of
it in *Esquire*. George Plimpton called Talese in a state of mind Talese
described as "hysterical." He told Talese (by Talese's account) that his
Paris Review article had ruined him and his chances for a career as ambassador, and it had upset Jackie Kennedy besides. He was afraid the references to junkies and call girls would show up in *Newsweek* and *Time*.
Talese did not think that would happen, but when Plimpton insisted it
would, Talese called *Newsweek* and talked to several staff members; he

told one of them he had heard Mrs. Kennedy was upset. That night at a party, Plimpton told Talese he had misunderstood—she was not upset after all and Plimpton was distressed that Talese had told *Newsweek* she was.

Neither *Time* nor *Newsweek* reported on "Looking for Hemingway," although, Plimpton wrote Talese, *Time* did circulate a memo pointing out the references to drugs and call girls, and *Newsweek* actually prepared a story on the piece—"a dilly"—but the piece was killed. Plimpton was relieved when the piece stayed within the pages of *Esquire* and did not leak out into what he called "the public press." He had been concerned about "an excessive reek of narcotics in the piece."

But Plimpton still was not happy. In a long letter from Italy—twelve and a half pages double-spaced—he pointed out a series of inaccuracies that took him seven double-spaced pages to describe: they had not posed as paupers, the French did not despise them, they did not edit the magazine between turns at pinball, he did not have parties "any night of the week," and so on.

He went on: "You told me at great length your theory that there is a key to every story, a cornerstone that holds up the edifice of character, and frankly I'm very suspicious of this, and the sort of interpretive journalism that can result. . . . and in the case of the *Review,* a composite group, varied, from different backgrounds, violent differences—one cannot responsibly boil all this down . . . and say with any hope of justification that we were looking for Hemingway. . . ."

What Talese had done, Plimpton said in another, shorter letter, "after all those hours, all those interviews, was to get it wrong. . . ."

Talese returned a three-and-a-half-page, single-spaced response to Plimpton's twelve-and-a-half-page double-spaced letter: The errors Plimpton pointed out were trivial, he said; Plimpton was nitpicking. Besides, different sources had told him different things. As for getting The Crowd wrong, all Talese was doing was writing about The Crowd from *his* point of view. ". . . I thought I captured the true flavor, the truth of spirit and mood, as I see the PR Crowd; it was a painting, I told you, not a photograph, and since you did not like the painting, you are naturally entitled to throw eggs at my painting. . . ."

Plimpton wrote back: "A mistake is a mistake. . . ." He answered Talese on a few other points, then said, "Anyway, let's cut this short. You believe your portrait is accurate and true, funny and witty, etc., and nothing I say is going to dampen your appreciation. . . ." The next day he backpedaled, half-apologizing. "It is important to feel very strongly about one's work, to defend it with tenacity."

Rust Hills's power chart, "The Structure of the American Literary Establishment," drew fire from a wider field. Hills had put the final version of the chart together one night in a studio with a designer who could send type out and get it back in an hour. They had organized the names in columns of small type—editors, agents, writers, magazines, publishers, college writing programs—under headings: "The Poetry Situation," "Campuses," "Book Publishers," "Ivory Tower."

A splash of red spilled like ink over the lists: "The Hot Center"—*The Partisan Review* and *The Paris Review* and all of their writers; Random House and Farrar, Straus and their writers; and the Russell and Volkening literary agency and its writers. At the center of the hot center was Russell and Volkening's Candida Donadio, a young New York Italian with a sexy telephone voice ("like a purr," John Berendt thought).

Donadio had begun her career in the mid-fifties, about the time Hills and Hayes had started work at *Esquire.* By the early sixties, she was sniffing out the most exciting writers: Thomas Pynchon, author of *V.,* and Joseph Heller, who wrote *Catch-22.* There was something spiritual about Donadio—even psychic. Some said she could read authors' minds, or believed that she could. John Berendt recalled hearing about something she said to Pynchon when he called her one day. "Don't squash them," she said. She could picture him in his kitchen, and she pictured a line of ants going in formation up to the window. She knew what Pynchon was thinking.

More to the point, she had a sense of mission about being an agent. Valerie Elliott, a young woman who worked for her in the later sixties, remembered, "Her one concern seemed to be to act in the right way. She didn't seem to be doing things for money, or glory—it just all seemed to be that she wanted to act in the right way for the people that she loved. She usually took to people instantly or not at all. . . . Everything she seemed to do was so that the world would get on, and that people would get on, and that books would be placed. She always said—books had a life in the world. It was always putting things in the world that should be there."

Donadio and Hayes had formed a working friendship. He had invited her to his office almost as soon as he started working for *Esquire*—he wanted to know whom she was representing, what they were doing. They talked often on the phone. He would tell her ideas he had for stories, and she would suggest writers. He would take her to movie screenings, and he got her to buy a mink coat at Alexander's so she could go directly from work to parties, cocktails, dinner.

"You'd look good," he'd say. "It's good for you to know how the rich live."

He was, she thought, "damn bossy." He would say, "C.D., I want you to tell her this and this." And she would say, "Why do you have to interrupt me? I already told her. Why don't you stop writing scripts for me?"

He was kind, but he did have force: he wanted things his way.

She enjoyed being out with him. He never seemed to be shy; he had a sense of his professional and his personal worth. He was attractive, and, though his wardrobe was not huge, he wore clothes of good quality. He loved being in the thick of things. He had social grace. One day he called her and said, "Arnold wants you to come in—how about four o'clock?" She arrived at the office, nervous—she was very young and very shy, and there was Arnold Gingrich looking very prominent: nice rich voice, gentlemanly, smart. And he said, "I just want to take a look at you—this young woman who's creating such a stir."

Nobody could reasonably object to Donadio's central place on the power chart, but they *could* object to their own place on it or to the fact that they were on it at all. Hills had not meant anyone to take his power chart literally, especially those blotches of categorizing color. He did not mean, for instance, to make a distinction between John Steinbeck, a Viking author who escaped the reach of "The Hot Center," and Evan S. Connell, Jr., another Viking author whose name was half under the red. But some of the writers (not Steinbeck, but others) did take the chart literally, and minded not being red hot. Willie Morris could not help observing that *Harper's* appeared just above the category "Squaresville." Others were deeply offended by their placement or lack of placement in the columns under the blobs of color. One who did make the red category, Burton Raffel, confessed he felt "shame, and then anger." He knew another writer who felt similarly smeared: being categorized so commercially "made him feel 'slimy'." Some critical readers thought the chart further established the establishment. Thirty years later, looking over the chart again, Hills said, "I always thought this was pretty funny. But I think people thought that it enhanced the establishmentarian nature of the literary world—that it somehow endorsed it, when in a way it's mocking it, and certainly it's mocking everybody who's in Squaresville."

The *New York Times Book Review* editors belonged in Squaresville, along with their book reviewer Orville Prescott. "If Orville Prescott in the *Times* reviews a book unfavorably, most of the people on this chart will probably think a little better of it," Hills explained in his introduction. The *Book Review* had its revenge in an August 4 critique by Mark Harris, who did not let the fact that he'd published in *Esquire* stop him from complaining. The establishment chart would strengthen budding writers' misconception that you had to know somebody to be published, Harris said. The writer should write and not worry about the power structure of publishing. Rust Hills responded in a letter eventually published on September 29, delayed while Hayes negotiated with the *Times'* Sunday editor, Lester Markel, over how long Hills's reply could be. Harris was confusing writing with publishing, Hills said. "Of course Faulkner worked in Mississippi and Frost in Vermont—but where did they send their manuscripts, Iowa City?"

Critic Theodore Solotaroff, an editor at *Commentary,* was somewhat more generous than Harris had been. Writing later about all the fuss over the literary issue, "a relatively notorious spread," Solotaroff said it was easy to put *Esquire* down for trivializing the literary world, but the literary situation was pretty much as *Esquire* had shown it to be. Hills had identified "a new and very fluid marketplace." The older centers of literary life—lively journals like *The Partisan Review* and the *Kenyon Review*— had once provided a community of thought independent from mass society, but they had lost vitality. They had been displaced by "the entrepreneurs who have set up shop where Madison Avenue runs into Greenwich Village." *Esquire* had picked up on "the shrinkage of extremes between the serious and the trivial, between hard thought and easy attitudinizing, between originality and novelty, relevance and chic, distinction and celebrity." In truth, Solotaroff said, although *Esquire* had refrained from saying so, *"Esquire* is itself 'the red hot center' of our literary vacuum."

Despite the attention the issue stirred up, it did not do well on the newsstand: it was the only issue that year to sell fewer copies on the newsstand than the year before, a fact that Abe Blinder, the company president, pointed out to John Smart, the chairman of the board, who pointed out to Blinder that it was good for the company to produce such an issue. Yes, Gingrich agreed, the low newsstand sales appeared to be a setback, but the low sales shouldn't scuttle future special July issues, which were a useful way to build the magazine's character. After all, the issue had been taken seriously in the *New York Times,* the *New York Herald Tribune,* and *Publisher's Weekly;* attention had been paid.

To celebrate the issue, the magazine held a party in its party room, Exhibit Hall, where the advertising people met clients for lunches and the staff held Christmas or birthday parties. Every writer in New York was there, it seemed—just standing around drinking and talking. And suddenly, somebody said, "Oh my God. Oh shit."

They all turned around and there was a man in a jumpsuit—Leo D'Lion, identified in a caption of the literary issue as an "actor and chess hustler"—and he was going around the room waving his arm like a magician casting a spell on people. It was a kind of dance, but it seemed threatening. While everyone tried to ignore him, he wove his way around individuals, who tried to be cool. He was black, and nobody wanted any kind of racial unpleasantness, so they would just force a chuckle and turn away. But he got more and more in their faces, and their smiles froze. Suddenly he started unzipping his zipper. Inch by inch he peeled off his jumpsuit. And there he was: a naked man, dancing around the room.

Some people laughed, a lot averted their eyes. Byron Dobell said, Better call the police, and he did. Jill Goldstein simply said to the naked man, "This is silly, why don't you put on your clothes?" And he did.

One writer who was *not* at the party for the literary issue (or on the chart) had watched what was going on at *Esquire* with something like envy. Tom Wolfe was a feature writer at the *New York Herald Tribune,* and he kept an eye on his competition, which included Gay Talese over at the *New York Times*—and now at *Esquire,* too. Wolfe was a man with a scholarly bent (he had a Ph.D. in American Studies from Yale), and he admired the way Talese could write a magazine article, all based on facts, and have it come out sounding like a short story, like that opening to the Joe Louis profile, with Louis's wife meeting him at the airport:

"Joe," she said, "where's your tie?"
"Aw, sweetie," he said, shrugging, "I stayed out all night in New York and didn't have time—"

The month after the literary issue, Tom Wolfe got his big chance at *Esquire.* Dobell had already tried him out on a tipping guide to New York

City, and Hayes hadn't liked it. Then Wolfe had come up with the idea of going to California to write about customized cars. After some debate (since Hayes wasn't crazy about what he had done so far), *Esquire* paid his way. Then, for months, he hadn't turned in a story. Dobell had called, Wolfe had stalled. In August, a traveling exhibit of customized cars—cars redesigned, reshaped for the sheer fun of it—had come to New Jersey. Hayes thought the next issue could use a good image, so he asked photographer Ben Someroff to take a big studio portrait of one of the weirdest cars, and Hayes put it in the lineup for the next issue. Now *Esquire* needed text, and needed it quickly. *Esquire* would have just two weeks to prepare the photograph and accompanying text for the engraver in Chicago.

Hayes told Dobell to call Wolfe and explain that *Esquire* had to have his story. The loss of $350 in expenses *Esquire* had paid for Wolfe's trip to the coast had ballooned by another thousand on the photograph. Give him a deadline, said Hayes: the Friday before the Monday the photograph would be sent to the engraver. Wolfe said he would try. On Friday Wolfe sent the word: the piece just wouldn't come. Hayes called his automotive editor, Diane Bartley, and asked if she could turn a reporter's notes into something usable on custom cars. He would get her the notes by Monday.

Type out your notes, Dobell told Wolfe, and *Esquire* would have someone else write the story. That night Wolfe began typing.

"Dear Byron," he began, and started telling about the customized car show, just as he saw it, putting everything in, typing away lickety split. By midnight the memorandum was twenty pages long and he was still typing. He had started around 8 P.M. About 2 A.M. he turned on rock-and-roll music from WABC and sped on. He finished up about 6:15 A.M.

Dobell took the "Dear Byron" off the top of the forty-nine-page manuscript, took out some of the Salingerisms—phrases from *Catcher in the Rye*—and *Esquire* had a story on customized cars. To Hayes, here was an example of how a relationship between a writer and an editor can bring forth something a writer might not have produced alone. When Wolfe wrote "Dear Byron"—when he began to tell his story to Byron Dobell—at that moment Wolfe broke away from the straitjacket of standard magazine form and style. "From this decision, and at that very instant," Hayes wrote later, "came the first words of an extraordinary new voice—italics, ellipses, exclamation marks, shifting tenses, arcane references, every bit of freight and baggage he had collected out of his past, from newspaper beats back through postgraduate studies in art history at Yale."

Compared to some of Wolfe's later pieces, the customized car piece was actually pretty tame. What made it different from most magazine and newspaper pieces was that it was so natural—as Hayes said, just as if he were telling something to somebody.

"The first good look I had at customized cars was at an event called a 'Teen fair,' held in Burbank, a suburb of Los Angeles beyond Hollywood," he began. "This was a wild place to be taking a look at art objects— eventually, I should say, you have to reach the conclusion that these cus- tomized cars *are* art objects, at least if you use the standards applied in a civilized society. But I will get to that in a moment."

Fascination with teen culture wasn't new, but enthusiasm for it was; and Wolfe had managed at one and the same time to convey the fun of it all *and* ridicule the stuffy art world that would deny that customized cars could be art. It was the kind of double perspective that delighted *Esquire* editors, and Hayes, who had had his doubts about Wolfe, happily sched- uled the piece for publication in the November issue. David Newman wrote a title that caught the flavor of Wolfe's later voice almost better than the piece itself did: "There goes (VAROOM! VAROOM!) that Kandy Kolored (THPHHHHHH) tangerine-flake streamline baby (RAH- GHHHH!) around the bend (BRUMMMMMMMMMMMMMM- MM . . . . . .''

A question arose about Wolfe's byline. There was another, more fa- mous Thomas Wolfe, a writer from North Carolina who wrote long Whit- manesque novels. A writer destined for fame should not be confused with another writer. Suppose they added a middle initial? They could if they liked. His middle name was Kennerly. They bylined the piece "Thomas K. Wolfe."

Hayes himself came up with Wolfe's next assignment. Hayes had heard that Cassius Clay, contender for Sonny Liston's title, would be in town to make a recording, and Hayes arranged through the record com- pany to talk with Clay. *Esquire* would like to do a cover story on him, Hayes told Clay. How much would *Esquire* pay? Clay asked Hayes. Noth- ing, Hayes replied. "We don't work that way; we don't buy stories. We consider it an honor to be on the cover of *Esquire.*"

It didn't seem that much of an honor to Clay. So then Hayes said, "Well, okay, we'll make an exception, because it's you. We really wanta do this story. I'll give you $150—but you have to let our man be with you for five days. I'll pay you $50 on Monday, $50 on Wednesday, and $50 on Friday."

Clay thought it over. His backers didn't give him much spending money when he came to New York so that he wouldn't spend it on hangers-on. A hundred fifty dollars was a hundred fifty dollars. He agreed. He kept his side of the bargain, letting Wolfe follow him around. On Tuesday, after a recording session, they got in the car full of people and Clay looked out the window.

"You know it's a beautiful day, I'd like to walk," he said. "Tom," he said, "why don't we walk back to the hotel?" They got out and were walking along, and suddenly Clay put his arm around Wolfe's shoulders and said, "What day is this?"

"Tuesday," said Wolfe.

"It feels like Wednesday," said Clay.

Wolfe gave him his Wednesday money; Clay stuck to his bargain, and Wolfe wrote a story about Cassius Clay in New York, a Talese-style piece, showing a man in his world. Because it was unaccompanied by a color illustration, it was published in October, the month before "Kandy Kolored" appeared. Wolfe was rapidly becoming a regular.

Wolfe's next piece, on Las Vegas, had a sharper edge. He ridiculed "the old babes" who played the slot machines and he paid visits to the Clark County Courthouse and the County Hospital psychiatric ward to view the casualties. A legal adviser vetting the piece suggested that given the negative cast of the article, one of the subjects of the photographs that ran with it might claim libel by association, although the claim would probably not fly in court. There was in "LAS VEGAS (What?) LAS VEGAS (Can't hear you! Too noisy) *LAS VEGAS!!!!*" less joy of discovery than there had been in "Kandy Kolored," but Helen Lawrenson, *Esquire* contributor and one of Gingrich's pen-pals, was crazy about it anyway. She wrote Gingrich, "He is so great, that guy, that I am practically paralyzed into permanent writing impotence every time I think of him. . . ." David Newman would remember the opening for years: "Hernia, hernia, hernia, hernia, hernia, hernia, hernia, hernia. . . ."

Not long after Wolfe discovered his voice at *Esquire*, Hayes hired a new editor, Bob Sherrill,* his old friend from Wake Forest College. A North Carolina mountain man, Sherrill talked like Tom Wolfe wrote, his

---

*Not to be confused with the other Robert Sherrill, author of *The Last Kennedy* and other books and a writer for *Esquire*.

words skittering around in an energetic collage. He was a man alive to the world—antennae out, picking up strange vibrations. If there was a censoring mechanism anywhere in Sherrill, it operated weakly: he seemed utterly open. He had the journalist's obsession: to find out things that hadn't been told and tell them, not just tell them but *tell* them—grab the listener by the lapels and tell the story.

One day he and Wolfe and Hayes were sitting in Hayes's dim office talking about story ideas. What about dirt-track racers? Sherrill suggested. Wolfe had done customized cars as folk art. Why not dirt-track racing as folk sport? Wolfe didn't seem all that interested in North Carolina mountain guys who raced Fords and Chevrolets around dirt tracks. Sherrill began naming some of the drivers, and when he got to Junior Johnson, Wolfe's interest picked up. Was that his real name? Junior? Junior Johnson?

In the spring of 1964, Wolfe went down to Wilkes County, North Carolina, the ancestral home of the Hayes family, to meet Junior Johnson and watch him race. Junior was a burly man who had made a reputation as a whiskey runner, outdriving federal agents around mountain roads, before he made his name as a racer. He had a big following, and they watched curiously as Wolfe, a southerner, too, although not their kind of southerner, stood around in a green tweed suit (he favored white suits but he was trying to look casual), baking in the hot southern spring sun. Wolfe made several trips to North Carolina because he could never stay long; he had to get back to his job at the *New York Herald Tribune*.

Still no story appeared.

Finally, Hayes called him up. "Tom, when are we going to get that piece?"

"Harold, I'm working on it very hard."

"You've told us that before. This is *not right.*"

Not that it was unprofessional, or not fair to *Esquire,* or that he wouldn't get paid. "This is *not right.*" Wolfe was crushed, and worked day and night to get the piece finished: "The Last American Hero Is Junior Johnson. *Yes!*"

It was one of his best—Wolfe floated comfortably along, dropping into hill country accents with no big to-do, falling back into his own repertoire of voices that ranged from rhapsody to sociological chat to straight-talking journalist, just telling a story. Again finding artistry in an unlikely place, he never balanced better on the line between enthusiasm and ridicule. Reading "Junior," reporters in North Carolina who had watched Wolfe come in and snatch the story right out from under them were amazed: "What does this guy know? What are all these sentences?" Remembering how they felt, one of them, John Baskin, a young newspaper reporter who had watched Wolfe work around the pit crew, said, "I just got quiet and started figuring out how to do it."

By the time *Esquire* published "Junior Johnson" in March 1965, Wolfe was writing more often for Clay Felker at *New York,* the Sunday magazine of the *New York Herald Tribune,* where Wolfe was a staff writer. Hayes did not give him up easily; once when Wolfe owed both Hayes and Felker a story, Hayes sent him a cable relaxing his *New York* deadline and signed the cable with Felker's name. But Hayes had to concede, eventually, that Wolfe was more *New York*'s than *Esquire*'s.

Roaming New York for Felker, Wolfe served up dizzying pastiches, verbal versions of abstract expressionist art—questions, exclamations, foreign phrases, an explosion of details: a knockout in a world where most journalists wrote in lockstep. To those standing by, it might have seemed as if, under the pressure of circumstance, Wolfe had burst forth self-created, like Venus appearing out of the sea. In fact, the style developed as Wolfe went along, and he took what he needed wherever he found it—from comics, commercials, disc jockeys, J. D. Salinger, but mostly (he himself has said) from Ben Hecht and from Boris Pilnyak, Yevgeny Zamyatin, and Andre Sobol, Russian writers he had discovered in the library at Yale. Writing fiction between 1917 and 1927, when the revolution was young, the Russians had shown Wolfe how to glide across a social field, gathering telling details, pouring them all out in a rush:

"In the nunnery," wrote Pilnyak in *The Naked Year,* "in the morning, in the *Execcom* (where, too, there were balsams at the window),—in the *Execcom,* there gathered, sign of the times, leather men in leather tunics, (bolsheviks!) everyone a standard leathern man, each of them hefty, and hair in curly ringlets sticking out on his neck from under a forage cap. . . ."

Wolfe had been struck by the "bizarre combination: the rawness of the material of the revolution, written with this very mannered, very literary French technique," derived from French symbolism. He thought these guys were wonderful, and he kept reading them after he left Yale, until finally the time came to use what he had learned from them: documenting his own revolution, a theatricalization of American life that made Wolfe's words spin.

Bangs mane bouffant beehives Beatle caps butter faces brush-on lashes decal eyes puffy sweaters French thrust bras flailing leather blue jeans stretch pants jeans honeydew bottoms eclair shanks elf boots ballerinas knight slippers, hundreds of them, these flaming little buds, bobbing and screaming, rocketing around inside the Academy of Music Theater underneath that vast old mouldering cherub dome up there—aren't they super-marvelous!

"Aren't they super-marvelous!" says Baby Jane. . . .

He wrote that later for *New York,* but he had figured out how to do it over at *Esquire. Esquire,* in turn, had gained something from Tom Wolfe, who cast his hyperactive eye across American culture and found it dazzling. What was all this, this American *stuff,* and what did it mean? A writer like Wolfe changes a magazine, Hayes wrote later. He sets a new standard—stirs competition among writers and editors. Something happens at such a magazine, Hayes said: "A personality has begun to form."

FOUR

Around the Bend

*I*N THE FALL OF 1963, as Tom Wolfe made his debut in *Esquire*, circulation reached an all-time high, approaching 900,000, and the *New York Times* advertising columnist Peter Bart granted *Esquire* a place among America's leading cultural magazines—*The Reporter, Harper's, Atlantic Monthly, Saturday Review, Commentary*, and *The Nation*. To Jerry Jontry, *Esquire*'s advertising director, this was cause for alarm. If America was experiencing a "cultural explosion," Bart had said, you couldn't tell it from the circulations of these leading cultural magazines. Oddly, his own numbers, offered toward the end of the column, belied his skepticism: in most cases, circulation had actually risen.

But the damage was done. Jontry started hearing reports that advertisers would not want to use *Esquire* because Bart's column gave them the impression *Esquire* was slipping. In a worried memorandum to Arnold Gingrich, Harold Hayes, Abe Blinder, and John Smart, Jontry pointed out that all the other magazines mentioned were small magazines, not known for their success in advertising. It was fine for *Esquire* to be seen as a specialized magazine, but if it was going to be seen as a literate magazine, it had better be seen as a *"popular* literate magazine."

Gingrich replied in a terse, one-paragraph memo sent to everyone who had gotten Jontry's memo: "Jerry is magnifying the bad and minimizing the good in this column. The 'specialized' is not differentiated from the 'literate' in the column itself—only in Rev. Jontry's sermon on the subject."

Jontry did not give up; he was wrestling with a real image problem. A few weeks later, in a memorandum dated October 1, 1963, he told Gingrich that to non-readers, *Esquire* was a cross between a "Grandfatherly

Playboy" and a "cultural magazine." Although he himself, personally, liked the new magazine—it was "gutsy, stimulating"—he was having trouble summing it up for his ad salesmen.

If Gingrich, Blinder, and Smart had doubts about where Hayes was taking *Esquire,* they suppressed them. The very day Jontry wrote that memo, October 1, the company bestowed on Harold Hayes the title of editor of *Esquire.*

In a memorandum defining his new power, Hayes proposed to Gingrich that he and Gingrich have a mutual veto. Gingrich could say no to whatever Hayes wanted to put in the magazine and Hayes could say no to whatever Gingrich wanted to put in.

"Sure. Sounds good," Gingrich wrote on the corner of the memorandum.

"While the man didn't have it in him to say no," Hayes said later, "I certainly did, and from that time on *Esquire* became more my magazine than his."

Gingrich did not retire completely from editorial duty. He kept on reading manuscripts and scribbling a few words of praise or criticism on little pieces of paper attached to the corners. He had a particularly sharp eye for obscene words, and he did not mind saying when he could not appreciate a piece, or just did not understand it. When he found some copy William Burroughs had written incomprehensible, he attached a hopeful note: "Maybe if it just runs, gutterlike, between captioned pictures, it will pass by unnoticed, like so much dummy type." Sometimes he used his "Publisher's Page" to kvetch, leaving the appealing impression that at *Esquire* even the powers that be had the right to think their own thoughts.

Once a month Hayes made a formal presentation of the upcoming issue to Gingrich, Blinder, and the men in charge of advertising—Jontry and Sam Ferber—with an open phone line to salesmen in California. The idea was to fill the advertising staff in on the contents so they could sell advertising, but the meeting also gave management a chance to keep tabs on Hayes. Hayes was always nervous about the presentation. He would go over it in advance with Byron Dobell, now managing editor, to make sure it was rehearsed and under control, and he tried not to couch anything in controversial terms.

As a rule, Dobell recalled, management did not mount major challenges to editorial decisions, although, over the years, several pieces were blocked, one of them not long after Hayes was made editor: a piece on sexual behavior at Bard College. *Esquire* had announced the piece as forthcoming, and a Bard alumnus, who was also a public relations and advertising man, spotted the announcement and raised questions about it in a letter to Blinder, Gingrich, Hayes, Jontry, Smart, and Walter Karp (the author of the article). He sent a copy of his letter to the president of Bard and to the president of the Bard–St. Stephens Alumni Association.

As Dobell recalled the incident, Hayes came to him with management's concerns, and Dobell went over the piece carefully and satisfied himself that it was fair. Hayes suggested asking the novelist Ralph Ellison, whom he knew and who taught at Bard, to read the piece. As Dobell recalled, Ellison returned a judgment that led Hayes to kill the piece, a decision that cost *Esquire* a chance to break ground on a new social phenomenon—the loosening of sexual mores on college campuses. To Dobell, the decision was wrong, and an embarrassment to the magazine.

The episode was unusual; management did not routinely intervene in editorial affairs. Blinder and Smart might raise questions, even objections, but deferentially, as if they acknowledged the principle of editorial independence and were attempting to sway by persuasion. As a rule, they relied on Arnold Gingrich—and Fritz Bamberger, still the arbiter of taste—to protect company interests. To the editorial staff, seldom privy to higher-level debates, Gingrich sometimes appeared to be part of the scenery—a sleepy older man, playing his violin in the early morning hours, not paying much attention to what was going on. In fact, aside from courting advertisers in endless letters and lunches, Gingrich played a significant role: he was a buffer between Blinder and Smart and their new editor, Harold Hayes.

Hayes proved right away that editorial independence could carry a big price tag. For the December issue coming up, George Lois had complied with an advertising staff request to produce a Santa Claus cover. He had flown to Las Vegas with Carl Fischer, the photographer who did most of the covers, and, with the help of Joe Louis, he had gotten the new, mean heavyweight champion, Sonny Liston, to pose—wearing a Santa Claus hat. As the shooting proceeded, Liston looked progressively meaner. Finally, Liston suddenly flung off the Santa cap and announced, "Had me enough of this motherfuckin' crap." Louis brought him back for the final shot, but if he had been mean-looking to start out with, now, Lois thought, he looked *really* mean.

When the cover came into the office, Hayes showed it around, as he always did—flashing it by the advertising director, advertising promotion manager, circulation director, circulation manager, publisher, president, and chairman of the board. It was still late summer and the climate outside and in, Hayes would recall, was sticky.

"Jesus *Christ,* Hayes, you call *that* Christmasy?" said the circulation manager. "What the hell are you trying to *do* to us?"

It *is* Christmasy, Hayes maintained. Look at the Santa Claus hat. But nobody saw the wit, Hayes wrote later, "in the magazine's mockery of its own commercial intent." Jerry Jontry was recovering from an appendectomy at New York Hospital when the cover came in. He called Hayes to ask if *Esquire* couldn't wait until Saks Fifth Avenue installed black Santa Clauses before putting a black Santa on the cover of *Esquire.* At least Hayes could identify Liston by printing his name on the cover. Then it would be a cover about a world champion, not a cover about a black Santa Claus. Hayes actually did raise the question with Lois—not telling him it was Jontry's idea—just asking: "Do you think we should identify him on the cover?"

"No, this is a black man, Santa Claus," Lois said. "He just so happens to be Sonny Liston."

So there Liston was, eyes peering out from under a lopsided Santa Claus hat. "The cover is, at first glance, simple and pleasant," *Newsweek* reported in a full-page story about *Esquire* on December 16. "Then it turns savage. It is the face, uncaptioned but unmistakable, of the heavyweight champion of the world, Sonny Liston. He is glaring. . . ."

Lois's Santa Liston cover became one of the most controversial in the history of American magazines. "It's hard to understand today," Lois remembered, "but the idea of a black man as Santa Claus pissed off half the country." Outraged letters poured into the *Esquire* office. Gingrich tried to explain that the idea was to turn the "meanest man in the world"—a Scrooge—into Santa Claus. *Esquire* had not been trying to make a racial comment; in fact, he wrote one reader, *Esquire* was neutral on the question of race, and he cited several articles to prove his point, including one in the upcoming January issue—"The Segs": "the candid and unqualified views of the five most influential segregationists in the south today."

Gingrich didn't point out the transparent object of their long monologues: to let them hang themselves with their own words, an achievement enhanced by the sinister Carl Fischer photographs that accompanied the text. Fischer excelled at putting an editorial spin on his portraits, and it was usually unflattering. In the case of "The Segs"—and it was one of the few times Hayes gave him specific instructions—Hayes had told him not to use a wide-angle lens to distort the faces; he did not want the segregationists accusing *Esquire* of deliberate unfairness. Fischer had cheated: he had recopied the pictures on his enlarger to get more texture in the skin and coarsen the images. The result was distinctly unflattering, and Gingrich, who often displayed ingenuity when he replied to angry readers, had to stretch to offer "The Segs" as evidence of *Esquire*'s neutrality on race.

Years later, in a 1981 article in *Adweek,* Hayes tried to explain the tumultuous response to the Liston Santa Claus cover.

Sonny Liston was a bad black who beat up good blacks, like Floyd Patterson; there was no telling what he might do to a white man. In 1963, when this was the sort of possibility that preyed on white men's minds everywhere, George Lois's Christmasy cover was something more than an inducement for readers to buy Dad extra shaving soap. In the national climate of 1963, thick with racial fear, Lois's angry icon insisted on several things: the split in our culture was showing; the notion of racial equality was a bad joke; the felicitations of this season—goodwill to all men, etc.—carried irony more than sentiment.

What nobody seemed to notice, advertising manager Sam Ferber said later, was the relationship of the cover to the lead piece of the issue—a five-page spread of news photos, each on a separate page with a Bible verse underneath in ironic counterpoint: Communist soldiers retrieving the body of an East German shot trying to scale the Berlin Wall; a Buddhist monk who had set himself on fire; New York policemen dragging away a black protester—"a page out of the Bible and a page out of reality today."

The cover won an award from the International Federation of the Periodical Press as the Finest Front Cover of a men's magazine in 1963. An art history professor called it "one of the greatest social statements of the plastic arts since Picasso's *Guernica.*" The Liston cover cost *Esquire* at least $750,000 in pulled advertising, not in that issue, which advertisers had no warning was on its way, but in future issues. That was the number both Hayes and advertising director Jerry Jontry used for the record, but Sam Ferber, advertising manager under Jontry, figured the loss was even greater: some of the defectors stayed out a long time—one of them, a leading shirtmaker, for ten years. It was a loss the magazine could ill afford, then or later, Jontry would tell Hayes almost twenty years later.

At the time, management was "pretty forebearing," Hayes would say, looking back. George Lois kept on designing *Esquire* covers, and Hayes was not fired. The thought of firing Hayes never occurred to Blinder, Gingrich, or Smart, advertising manager Sam Ferber believed. "They thought Harold was brilliant, and he was, and he was."

Just days after the Sonny Liston issue went on the stands in mid-November, Sam Ferber presented a five-year plan at a turbulent management meeting where all the department heads were presenting five-year plans. The magazine would need to make a decision, he said: either make the commitment to being a mass magazine and increase circulation or make a commitment to being a quality magazine and cut circulation to yield high-quality demographics. Although Ferber wanted to cut back on cut-rate subscriptions that did not net high-income readers, he said building circulation was the only way to reach a management goal of bringing in $11 million in advertising, up significantly from the $8.3 million the magazine would report at the end of the year. To build circulation, the editors would need to back off from the emphasis on the hip and the esoteric and attend more cheerfully to service features. They needed more girl stories and fewer "kookie" covers.

The morning meeting was ending, the arguments suspended for lunch, when someone came in with the news: President Kennedy had been shot.

Rust Hills, in his office, was on the phone with Norman Mailer. "I can't really concentrate on this," he told Mailer, "because word's come in that Kennedy's been shot in Dallas."

"It was in the cards," Mailer said.

The meeting on *Esquire*'s future was never resumed.

Two pieces already scheduled for upcoming issues were canceled—a forecast of the 1964 election by Gore Vidal and an article on Arthur Schlesinger, Jr., by Thomas Morgan. A sampler of the British magazine *Private Eye* had to undergo changes. January 1964's Dubious Achievements issue was ready on press, and all the editors could do was blank out some of the faces in copies that had not yet been run; it was too late to take Johnson and Kennedy out of the lineups on the cover.

In the days after the assassination, Hayes was preoccupied with the metamorphosis Kennedy underwent in the public mind: the wry, candid private man—the skeptical man Hayes himself could find attractive—had disappeared in a cloud of pomp. "My mind is still boggling from the switch that seemed somehow to career through the nation—sweeping along formerly disabused intellectuals, leaders of the Negro Protest, Southerners, West Coasters and everyone else," Hayes wrote to Tom Wicker of the *New York Times.* "What interests me is not the fact that all these people were capable of being so deeply moved (and even changed) in the face of a national tragedy, but that they all came to see the man—in the most human terms—as a different sort of man altogether."

As Hayes had once asked Richard Rovere to present the human side of Joe McCarthy, he now asked Wicker to write about "Kennedy without tears."

Wicker wrote back on December 22, 1963. Yes, he was interested, if Hayes would write a longer letter, saying more about what he had in mind. Wicker also expressed gratitude for a piece *Esquire* had run on David Halberstam, the *New York Times* reporter who had been taking a beating for his coverage of the war in Vietnam. "I want you to know all Dave Halberstam's friends appreciate that good piece in your current issue. Dave is a great man and has taken a licking from the likes of Joe Alsop. It shouldn't happen to a dog."

That piece on Halberstam, by George J. W. Goodman, represented *Esquire*'s first serious notice of the war. "The war in Vietnam is a small one," Goodman noted, "but it is the only one around at the moment. . . ."

Later, *Esquire* editors and writers would look back at Kennedy's assassination as a turning point, a bend in the road. His presidency had released new energies, Hayes would write at the end of the sixties. Everyone wanted "to be like Jack—young, rich, powerful and attractive." Then came the assassination, like a spark setting off the energies he had collected around him, "traumatizing the country more than any event in recent memory."

Yet even before Kennedy's death, Robert Benton and David Newman had felt a great shift in the culture, a shift that Jack and Jackie Kennedy were part of but that was much larger than either. Benton and Newman had been watching European films—Ingmar Bergman's and Federico Fellini's, but especially the French New Wave films of Jean-Luc Godard and François Truffaut. As they looked at American culture through the filter of the French New Wave, they saw toughness gone soft—fifties cool in its decadent stage. They gathered examples, organized them into categories, and produced a big photo-and-text spread for the next July issue: "The New Sentimentality." Its favorite couples were Mr. and Mrs. John F. Kennedy and Jean-Paul Belmondo and Jean Seberg of *Breathless.* John Kennedy was "the pro" and Jacqueline Kennedy was "the pro's wife." Belmondo was "cool and tough, but soft in the center. He was destroyed because he let love carry him away." Jean Seberg "was fragile, but hard."

Failure was all right, but success was better. The world was absurd; better go through it disguised. Don't have friends, have accomplices. Do fall in love, but don't expect it to last. Don't carry the torch. Bounce back. Read Robert Lowell, the poet who understands "the order of chaos." Contemplate Marilyn Monroe: "Look what can happen to you when you screw up your life." Consider Humphrey Bogart, who "says that a man can both care and not give a damn."

Despite its title, "The New Sentimentality" did not so much announce something new as mark the end of something old: the cynicism of the fifties, which had turned out to be as vulnerable to romance as had the pieties of an earlier time. "The New Sentimentality" became for Hayes a landmark piece, a midpoint in what he thought of as the descent of the sixties. He began to talk about giving Benton more time to team up with Newman on other features—even switching Benton from art direction to special projects, house features that could strengthen the personality of the magazine.

Benton believed Hayes had something in mind other than using his talents the best way and strengthening *Esquire;* Benton began to feel maybe he ought to be looking for a new way to make a living. The tone he had tried to give *Esquire* as art director—a wry, dry wit—was, he thought, "static" to Hayes. Hayes's idea of irreverent wit was Harvey Kurtzman. Benton liked Kurtzman, but Kurtzman was not his idea of irreverent wit.

Jill Goldstein had been working with Benton as art assistant, and she was aware of tension between him and Hayes, although she was not sure whether the differences between them were specific—differences over particular features—or broader than that: ideological differences, or maybe simply the differences between a word person and an art person. Benton was wonderful, she thought, amazingly talented, but he was not particularly articulate. Two or three times he asked her to type up a note to Hayes for him, maybe, she thought, because he figured he might not be able to get his ideas across face-to-face, especially if he got angry.

Considering his uncertain position, Benton had wondered what he would do if he left *Esquire.* He did not think another magazine or advertising agency would hire him—he was too quirky, offbeat. He had a friend who had sold a movie treatment to Doris Day for $25,000. With $25,000 and what *Esquire* would pay him for special projects, he could make do until he could figure out his next move. The trouble was that he did not think he could write. But Newman could.

By this time, Benton and Newman were best friends; eventually they would move into the same apartment house together, push their kids side by side in their strollers. Already, they talked all the time, sifting their experience for ideas for the magazine. In the morning when they came to the office, they'd tell a secretary they were going out to talk about ideas, and they'd have breakfast at Schrafft's. Sometimes Diane Arbus would join them and they'd talk about great subjects for her to photograph— Mae West, Blaze Starr—but usually they'd go alone.

By coincidence, they'd both read a book by John Toland, *The Dillinger Days.* The book mentioned Bonnie Parker and Clyde Barrow, who robbed banks during the depression. When Benton was growing up in east Texas, his father had told him about going to Bonnie's and Clyde's funeral, and he had heard other stories about them. Benton started telling Newman the stories, and something about Bonnie and Clyde reached out and spoke to them.

Earlier, they had gone to see François Truffaut's movie about a woman and two men who loved her, *Jules and Jim,* released in 1961. Benton and Gloria Steinem had split up and Benton was deeply unhappy. "I went to see *Jules and Jim,* and for me it was not about Catherine, it was about survival, all I cared about was survival, and I somehow saw it eight times in the next two months, and you can't watch a movie eight times without beginning to see certain structural elements." Benton and Newman began to imagine a French-American movie based on the Bonnie and Clyde story: *Jules and Jim* and *Shoot the Piano Player* rolled into one. They found a young fledgling producer who put up a little money, and they took a two-week break from *Esquire.* They went to east Texas, found Bonnie's and Clyde's graves, met one of the sheriffs in on the final ambush of the outlaws, and interviewed people with stories to tell. They steeped themselves in fact and mythology and came back to *Esquire* to write a movie. They would sit in one of their offices at *Esquire,* or go down to Schrafft's, or to the hamburger hamlet around the corner, and talk about it.

By the time they were ready to write the outline, toward the end of

1963, Benton had left the job as art director and was working on special projects, on contract; he was coming in only a day or so a week. Newman called in sick, and they worked on the outline in Benton's apartment. At one point, Peter Bogdanovich, an *Esquire* writer who was doing the monograph for a Museum of Modern Art retrospective on Hitchcock, called to ask if they'd like to come over and watch a Hitchcock film. They stopped working on *Bonnie and Clyde* and went over to the museum, then went back to writing *Bonnie and Clyde.*

"That more than any other picture that we ever did was formed by *Esquire,*" Benton recalled. "It came out of that magazine world notion of immediacy—working for a magazine teaches you to pay attention at a very visceral level. . . . We put everything we knew into that movie about relationships—what we felt were relationships at that point in our lives. We brought the same thing to discussion of the script that you would bring to that weekly meeting about story ideas. And I think one of the things that gives the movie a sense of impact—if it still has it—is that it comes out of that sense of urgency that working on a magazine gives you."

Benton and Newman did not have any idea what a movie treatment really was—they wrote a script without dialogue and asked a staff member at the French film office if she would pass it on to Truffaut. She knew them because they were always asking her for stills of French stars— Jeanne Moreau or Jean-Paul Belmondo—to use in *Esquire.* When visiting directors had come along, she would even introduce them to Benton and Newman, but she could not forward their treatment, she said, because if she did that for them, everybody else would want her to do it for them. They pleaded. She agreed to read what they had written. She read it and said she would make an exception. She got the treatment to Truffaut, who told Warren Beatty about it, Beatty bought it and starred in it, and Arthur Penn directed it.

Bonnie and Clyde would be released in 1967 and would turn out to be one of the most successful and discussed American movies of the 1960s. By 1967, American real life had turned undeniably violent and Bonnie and Clyde seemed to mirror the times: romping across the American land-scape like teenagers on a joyride, tough-guy romantics, spinning a vision of life as "somebody," choosing to die in a hailstorm of bullets rather than give up their idea of themselves. Yet the film had been written out of an earlier time, the age of the New Sentimentality, the mood of *Esquire* in the early sixties, as America went around the bend.

Esquire itself was in a state of transition. To replace Benton as art director, Hayes called Sam Antupit, who had worked for Henry Wolf at *Harper's Bazaar* and *Show* and had given a durable and distinctive design to the *New York Review of Books,* a new magazine for intellectuals.

"I'd like you to start in two weeks," Hayes said.

"I don't know, it's going to take me at least two weeks to think it over. I'm not sure—"

"What do you mean?" Hayes replied.

Antupit had never met Hayes, but he had heard about him, and almost everything he had heard about Hayes wasn't good, especially from designers. A bull in a china closet—that was Antupit's advance impression of Hayes, and it was confirmed when he actually met him. What was this guy from North Carolina doing, telling the rest of the country what New York was all about? The bravado of the man intrigued him; he took the job.

Hayes told Antupit right off that he hated art directors, and Antupit had the idea Hayes might not even want to give him the title of art director. Antupit was firm about it: he would have the title or he wouldn't have the job. Okay, Hayes said.

"That's the way it was with Harold," Antupit remembered. "You'd build suspense three days, trying to think up a good defense for your position, and then you'd present it to him, and he would tilt his head, put his feet up, look out the window, puff on his cigar, or something that would distract you, and then he would say—," his voice lighting up, "Yeah!"

In Antupit's hands, *Esquire* began immediately to look different. The graphics editor who had handled layout for a few issues after Benton left had been using a different typeface for the title of each article in the "sandwich"—the section in the middle of the magazine where each feature ran for several pages without interruption by ads. Much as he loved type, Antupit wanted readers to open *Esquire* at any page and know it was *Esquire.* He put all the heads in Baskerville and used type size for variety, doing as much as he could with as little as possible. He did it that way not only because he respected type, but also because Hayes was always changing heads at the last minute: "That should be 'A,' not 'The,'" he would say, and a complex typographic structure would crumble. Antupit made other changes as well. David Levine had been drawing minuscule caricatures for the columns at the front of the magazine; Antupit gave him more space to spread out his talent—full pages, sometimes—and eventually added full-page satiric art by Burt Silverman and Edward Sorel. Something all but vanished, too, under Antupit: the full-page cartoons that had been part of *Esquire* for thirty years but didn't seem as good as the rest of the magazine.

George Lois went on doing the covers, and Antupit liked that arrangement just fine. There was a lot less whining from editors than there would have been if there had been monthly in-house battles over whose stories would be cover stories. Everyone knew Lois was making the call, picking the cover story from the list of contents Hayes gave him every month. Everyone knew that the article he chose was not necessarily the best or the most important in the issue; it was the article that made the best cover. Sometimes editors did complain that Lois was giving the article an interpretation the writer or editors had not meant it to have. They might have a point, Antupit thought, but it seemed to him that Lois never actually misinterpreted an article, never sensationalized.

Antupit enjoyed life at *Esquire*—enjoyed using unlikely photographers for the fashion pages and turning cocktail spreads into luminous still lifes. He enjoyed, too, finding talented illustrators for the fiction. Antupit did sometimes cross swords with Byron Dobell, who had had a strong background as a picture editor, first at *Pageant,* then at Time-Life. Once Antupit called Dobell "a beady-eyed idiot," and Hayes made him apologize.

What for? Antupit asked.

"You go in and apologize to that man," Hayes said. "There's no reason to say that."

There were times when Hayes's and Antupit's own relationship went awfully wrong, usually, Antupit thought, when Hayes didn't have an idea and didn't know what he wanted. For a good while, an idea floated around for a picture story on John F. Kennedy's Boston. Finally Hayes collected a lot of pictures and turned them over to Antupit. Because Hayes had a writer coming in to look at the layouts, then write the piece, Antupit was working under deadline. He worked on the layouts for several days, and they were awful, because there was no idea there.

"JFK's Boston—" Who knew what JFK's Boston was? Not Harold Hayes, not Sam Antupit. Finally, it was six or seven in the evening, on a Friday, and Hayes said, "I guess you're going to have to stay tonight until it's finished."

"No, I'm not. My kids are in a school play, and I'm going to see that play. And I've worked enough on this stupid article. I'll do it over the weekend or I'll finish it on Monday, but I'm not staying."

"You'll finish it tonight," Hayes said. "And just remember: There is no justice."

"No," Antupit replied, "but there's always revenge." And he left the office. On Monday, he came in and said, "Okay, I'm going to finish this up today."

"No," said Hayes, "we're not doing that article. That's not an idea."

Despite the occasional tension, Antupit liked what he was doing, and he revised his estimation of Hayes. After thirty more years in publishing, he would say, "I have never worked for a brighter editor, ever. I've been in too many places since then, and someone will say, 'Well, aren't I the best editor you ever worked with?' I just tell 'em, 'You're in one of Harold Hayes's shoes.' "

One day that spring of 1964, Hayes told Jill Goldstein he really needed to add another staff member, an associate editor. He was losing Newman, who was going on contract with Benton to do special projects for *Esquire* and other magazines. Hayes may have been prompted, too, by something more than the need to keep the numbers stable. On March 9, he put out a memo that suggested restlessness with the staff he had.

Coming from a murkier background than the rest of you, I am astonished you all work so well together. I have known some good editors in my day and most of them were mean. All of you are nice folks, and not only that, you are wittier, hipper and generally better informed than I am, which is the way it should be.

Now, given brains, talent and sunny dispositions, why doesn't *Esquire* get better and better each month?

He laid out for them his theory of the active editor:

A passive, inert, dull magazine *(Show, Harper's, The Nation, Life)* is usually made up of editors who sit around and wait for writers to send them queries, or pictures, or finished pieces upon which they can react and thus fulfill themselves ("I like this lots and think we ought to publish. . . ."). Some of these editors write well but the peripheral talents of editors seldom keep such magazines from being passive, inert and dull. Magazine editing is not just the act of choosing, it is an act of assertion. Magazine editors who do nothing but read manuscripts and/or write copy blocks, no matter how well they perform these chores, are *only* performing chores, the same chores that exist at other magazines. Important chores to be sure, but not all *that* important.

Lively, dynamic, interesting magazines (*The Saturday Evening Post, New Statesman, Encounter, The Realist,* now *Playboy,* alas) are made up usually of editors who *give* something to their magazines. The process, as I understand it, usually goes like this: "If I had this magazine and it were all mine, what would I like to see it do?"

Esquire had alternated between being a passive magazine and being a lively magazine. At the start, in the thirties, Arnold had done everything and because he was an "active, curious, intelligent editor" *Esquire* had been good. Then in the mid-forties when he left, it had turned passive, the product as much of freelance writers as of the editors.

In recent years now known down the hall as the big change, the editors acted the only way they knew how to bring the magazine back to life. They started asking themselves what the magazine *ought* to be doing. Controlled from within by editors who assigned ideas they were enthusiastic about to writers they were also enthusiastic about—(whether or not the writer was enthusiastic about *Esquire*) the magazine became more effective than when it was controlled from the outside by standard, favored, competent but uninspired regular writers—the operating policy known to good editors as "opening the mail". . . .

As I say, all this ought to be fairly obvious. If it is, I am astonished and dismayed at how little you all seem to care. About four months ago, I asked each of you to turn in 10 ideas each Friday (child's play for committed editors). Byron requested the deadline day be shifted to Monday and then, later, the number reduced to five. On this dark March the ninth, I received my weekly packet: Six from Sherrill (the only editor who consistently produces ideas without being asked), two pass-along queries by a writer from Byron, one pass-along query by a writer from John—the lowest point in a situation that's been deteriorating over the past six weeks. . . .

We're facing the August line-up now, and there's absolutely nothing in the house. I can't tell you how miserable all this makes me feel.
HH.

The memo may have been merely motivational, but Bob Sherrill thought Hayes was frequently assailed by the conviction that there was somebody better out there—editors, art directors with more imagination than the ones he was working with. And Sherrill felt, too, that Hayes was always looking for an editor who would be *his* man: in tune with his own editorial instincts.

Byron Dobell had proved to be a solid managing editor, who tried to keep the staff from falling apart when Hayes, as Dobell recalled, was being "particularly horrible." To Hayes, *Esquire* seemed to be the Holy Grail; Dobell would come along and say, "Look, folks, it's just a magazine." He got Hayes to trim the weekly ideas requirement from ten to five to keep the staff from going crazy, and when an editor could come up with just three ideas, Dobell would say, "Write two stupid ones." Pleasant, unprepossessing, Dobell brought to *Esquire* his Time-Life experience in orderly process. Every Friday afternoon, after the staff gathered for drinks in Hayes's office—modest occasions, nothing wild—Dobell and Hayes would walk up Park Avenue together for drinks on their own, and talk over the week at the office. Still, Hayes was restless, looking for new talent to enrich the mix at the magazine.

Don Erickson, a Rhodes scholar and experienced editor, worked at *Cyanimid,* a trade magazine, and lived in the same building as Goldstein; they talked about *Esquire* all the time. Dobell had met him and had been impressed; at Dobell's request, Erickson wrote down some thoughts on *Esquire:*

I still dote on *The New Yorker*—oh, not the fiction much, or the Talk of the Town very often, or the short humorous pieces. But the longer reporters' pieces and the annals of this and that. I like nothing better than to settle down and give myself up to what I know will be a superb research and organizational job, flowing along from one section to another with an ease that makes your skin crawl (pleasurably). But this isn't what I mean by magazine excitement. This is definitive stuff. This is The Word, not the brilliant passing word. *The New Yorker* has got itself raised to the empyrean. It comes to you, somehow, encased.

Well, *Esquire* is the only other magazine I dote on, and I think I like it because it is fallible. It breathes like the people who put it together, some issues up higher than others; it's uneven, unexpected, surprising. It assumes nothing (as *The New Yorker* does) and attempts to make the reader feel that the merest ephemera it treats of is monumental. It labors to make the reader interested (good for it, it's competing on earthly terms), but it has the grace to realize that this month's monuments will quickly give way to next month's. The new *Esquire* seems wonderfully important. But it throws away easily.

And that's excellent. The whole point of a magazine is that you throw it out—unlike a book. It hasn't shot its entire wad. One holds a moment of time caught glitteringly for an instant within the soft covers. And there'll be another next issue (a pox, here, on those hard-cover coffee table magazines—magazines that aren't). You have managed to strike a balance between the intense drumbeat buildup and a don't care relaxation which results, for me, in exactly the feeling a magazine ought to give its readers.

They say Inigo Jones designed his masques for the court of James I and said that they "created heaven on earth for one night—therein (the one-night bit) lies their supreme enchantment." Well, something like that is the sense of excitement that *Esquire* is able to convey.

How would he strengthen the magazine, were he editor? He would retain the contributions the magazine made to literature as a "responsible publisher"—its publication of fiction by Norman Mailer and John Cheever, plays by Tennessee Williams, letters from F. Scott Fitzgerald. But he didn't know how he could be of much help there. "I don't know any great writers," he confessed. He did think he could improve the service features in the magazine. He thought *Esquire* had found an "admirable tone" for its service features, the tone of a scout at an Oxford college, who explains to young men "what to do and how." But in the features that used pictures, *Esquire* was trying too hard for cleverness—apologizing, it seemed, for instructing its readers. *Gentlemen's Quarterly* handled fashion better than *Esquire* because, Erickson said, "that editor really *believes* men should be better dressed—or so he manages to convey."

There were other things about *Esquire* that he did not like: the pictures, which were too often studio illustrations instead of photojournalism. (Hayes did prefer illustrations with strong ideas behind them.) He had not been moved by *Esquire* pictures since Bruce Davidson's pictures on juvenile delinquents in June 1960. And the text that went with the pictures did not seem to him to have "that lovely air of inevitability that makes both picture and words seem wedded to the page." He had the feeling the caption writer was "in a swivet to make it fit and make it clever." He thought the captions for girl features and fashion had a "forced cleverness." The cartoons were "often lousy," the travel notes "endless." The only one he had liked recently was a piece on Scotland by Howard Fast.

He would keep *Esquire* in "the eternal sophomore mode"—"the key to what you are and should keep on being." The sophomore year was the year when you understood "what it all meant." Whatever happened, you related to "an Important Truth." Then you grew up and saw there was no central truth, or stopped caring, and then along would come *Esquire* and rekindle that old excitement. Everywhere in an *Esquire* story, no matter how superficial the subject, there seemed to be a paragraph on "What it All Means." He liked that, and he would see that his writers kept on seeing each subject as part of a bigger whole.

As much as he liked the sophomoric quality of *Esquire,* he thought there was room for the don—"the man of letters in his booklined study," like John Updike in a review he had read elsewhere. "A delicious, soft, secure piece of writing: a man toying with words. I read this in a steel and formica cafeteria, but during the reading I was surrounded by panelled walls, decanters of sherry, and dogs on the hearth rug."

Erickson started work at *Esquire* within three weeks of that letter. Hayes must not have hesitated much over hiring him, but Arnold Gingrich apparently did have reservations. Hayes called Goldstein into his office and said Gingrich was not sure about Erickson. Hayes said to her, as she recalled, "Well, do you think this fellow is—has the right attitude? A.G. seemed to feel there was something—hmm—" Hayes paused, searching for the word, and came up with something like "a little off-base."

"Do you know anything about his personal life?" Hayes asked Goldstein.

She knew what Hayes was getting at and suspected it was true—she did not know for sure, but she guessed that Erickson was gay.

Well, she replied, she and Erickson lived in the same building; they socialized and were friends. "He's made a couple of passes at me," she said. It was true, but she knew, too, that he meant nothing by them.

Her answer seemed to satisfy Hayes, who, according to his old friend Bob Sherrill, was not a man to be troubled by anyone's homosexuality. Gingrich, himself a ladies' man, probably had no deep personal prejudices either, but he had always been concerned that a men's fashion magazine might appear to be a "primer for fops." Once when Gore Vidal wrote a column about Washington police beating up homosexuals outside the YMCA, Gingrich cut the line that specifically identified them as homosexuals. "We have enough trouble with *Playboy* already," Gingrich had said.

But Gingrich approved hiring Erickson and, on the job, Erickson proved to be the soul of discretion. Some years later, when Hayes was having dinner with an editor, Gordon Lish, Lish asked Hayes about Erickson's sexuality.

"None of your fucking business. And I don't know anyway," Hayes replied.

Hayes was easing into the groove of being editor at *Esquire.* During the week, he came home with a satchel bulging with manuscripts and settled down to read, sometimes with a drink, although he was not a heavy drinker (he came to prefer breakfast with writers at the Plaza to debilitating martini lunches). On the weekends, sometimes, he drove with his family to Stone Ridge, New York, where they had bought a country home, but when he stayed in town he would go into the office on Saturday, sometimes taking along his son Tom, who would find a calculating machine to play with.

Hayes worked hard, but his work did not wholly consume him. He had taken tennis lessons several years before and had become a dedicated player. He would play in the morning before he came in to work; he would play at lunchtime, on courts all over the city. Sometimes he would bring home tennis partners at the end of the day to play on courts near his apartment. Tennis was a way for him to release his aggression, his wife Susan thought: Take *that,* he could say to himself, smashing the ball back.

She was less aware, then, of another form of release for Hayes: the extramarital affairs he was weaving through his complex life. Later on, when she knew more about them, Susan spoke of the sexual ambience at *Esquire,* which, despite its broadening horizons, still focused on a man's "prowess, his intellectual interests, and his inner feelings, and the men's inner feelings were always generated from this quality men have that God gave them, that it was ready to go at any moment: it didn't take much, a few drinks, a few fine words, a pretty face, a lifted skirt—and that was kind of the undercurrent about the magazine. It was a men's magazine. . . ." Susan knew women were attracted to Hayes; she did not know the extent of his amorous activity. He kept his life in compartments, maintaining relationships—with his wife and children, parents, lovers, friends—on terms he found acceptable.

Friends found him warm, always welcoming, a man capable of enormous enjoyment, especially of anything creative—music, the theater. He and Susan had become friends with Ann Zane Shanks and her second husband, television producer Bob Shanks, whom she had married after her first husband died, and they would all four go to clubs in the Village to listen to jazz. Bob Shanks always felt better for being with Hayes, who was so full of joy and optimism, curious about everything, open to the world. Hayes took a long view of life—people erred, people failed, but the grand design went on. Later on, when they went through a difficult experience together, Hayes gave Shanks a copy of Rudyard Kipling's poem "If," and Shanks thought the poem was important to Hayes:

> If you can keep your head when all about you
> Are losing theirs and blaming it on you. . . .

Despite Hayes's extramarital activities, Bob Shanks felt Hayes had never abandoned his upbringing as a minister's son; he had brought with him from North Carolina a set of values that gave his life a moral center. A dutiful son, Hayes maintained his ties to home, returning for a long visit at Christmas, writing friendly letters to his mother and father, and other members of the family. He was especially close to his brother Jim.

In late May 1964, Hayes reported to Jim that things were looking up—the good-looking blond on the May cover had helped. The Kennedy issue was just out—the issue containing Tom Wicker's article, "Kennedy without Tears." Not everyone liked the cover, a photograph of Kennedy's face with a hand wiping away a tear that had fallen there. The *New York Herald Tribune* reported that designers were wondering, "Has Esquire magazine leaped off the bridge of good taste?" The cover problem wasn't getting any easier, Hayes wrote to his brother—in fact, nothing was getting easier at the magazine; but he did not seem to mind—life was good.

In late July, he wrote his parents that the August issue featuring the baseball establishment chart was selling well, and the late-summer riots in Harlem and the Bedford-Stuyvesant section of Brooklyn were a safe distance away from his apartment on Riverside Drive.

In September, he wrote a friend on the West Coast that he had gotten a Honda motorcycle, which he rode to work. He could get from his Riverside apartment to the garage near the office in twelve minutes. His office walls needed painting and the fluorescent lights were burned out, but he had wealth, fame, and the admiration of celebrities.

Well, not quite. Hayes's stock with one celebrity, never especially high, had fallen.

For the first eight months of 1964, *Esquire* had been running a strange, violent novel by Norman Mailer in serial form: *An American Dream*, a satiric picaresque tale that Tom Wolfe thought was modeled on Dostoyevsky's *Crime and Punishment.* Mailer was writing the novel as it was being published, as a test of his skill and a way, too, of making sure he wrote it quickly—he had several children and former wives to support. The story began in the January issue with the line (written and set in type before the assassination) "I met Jack Kennedy in 1946. . . ." The assassination had given the opening a peculiar context, but a more pressing problem surfaced with the second installment, when Rojack went downstairs to his wife's maid's room.

For all its pretty pinups of saucy girls in the past, *Esquire* had never been the kind of skin magazine that actually served up sex. Arnold Gingrich was not, personally, a prude, but he did not like the trend toward openness in publishing all those "clinical details." He had said so just recently in the publisher's column he wrote about a piece Anthony Lewis had done for *Esquire* on sex and the Supreme Court, which had lowered the legal bar to sexual frankness in literature. Not that Gingrich favored censorship—oh no—but that did not mean he wanted obscenity in his magazine. It was a matter of taste and practical good sense: obscenity was likely to put advertisers' noses out of joint.

Mailer's second installment brought Hayes up short. "I had a desire suddenly to forget the sea and dig the earth, a pure prong of desire believe me I felt not that often, there was canny hard-packed evil in the butt, that I knew," Mailer had written.

Hayes and Mailer had talked about the magazine's linguistic limits before, and Mailer tried to convince Hayes that he was giving *Esquire* a chance to lay low language barriers that had gotten in magazines' way for years. But there was a clause in the contract on *An American Dream* promising that the novel would be conventional enough to appear in a magazine.

Hayes handed the chapter over to Rust Hills, then together they took the problem to Gingrich. Not to worry, Gingrich said. Never mind that *Esquire* had published one installment and promised its readers seven more. *Esquire* could simply tell its readers that *Esquire* had changed its plans: there would be no second installment, or third, or fourth. Readers could buy the book in the bookstores.

Faced with that prospect, Mailer was not happy, but he did not see how he could change the chapter to satisfy Gingrich. He did not really want to change the chapter anyway. And he did not have time to change the chapter.

Hills was not ready to give up, even though this was his last week at *Esquire;* he had taken the job of fiction editor at the *Saturday Evening Post.* His years at *Esquire* had been good years for him. For a while he had reveled in seeking out and publishing a new generation of superb fiction writers—Saul Bellow, Bernard Malamud, John Cheever, and dozens of others. But after seven years, boredom was setting in, and, besides, nonfiction was crowding out fiction in *Esquire.* The *Saturday Evening Post* was doubling his salary and offering him a chance to publish as many stories in a week as he published in *Esquire* in a month.

Still, Hills cared what happened to Mailer's novel. Once you started publishing a serial, you ought to finish it. Stopping after the first installment would embarrass the magazine and embarrass Mailer. Hills had

always felt protective of Mailer: he thought that the magazine had sometimes treated him cavalierly, that Mailer had a right to be miffed by the
treatment. Surely a serious magazine ought to be able to publish serious
fiction that dealt with such subjects.

Hills's honor as a fiction editor was at stake: it was still his job to get
the fiction he had commissioned for *Esquire* into the magazine. He ran off
several photocopies and took the manuscript home with him for the weekend. Then he began a pruning job as delicate as any in the annals of
magazine editing: clipping a twig here, a branch there, until the episode
was clean enough to win Gingrich's approval. As Hayes said later, the
chapter as published in *Esquire* presented "a struggle between God, the
devil, Stephen Rojack, and Rust Hills, all of which had *something* to do
with a German maid. No one—author, editor or reader—could be quite
sure what."

Gingrich was surprised by reader reaction. With two installments out,
the letters coming in were more in favor of the book than against it.
Mailer had been doing "finger exercises" in his columns, Gingrich wrote
one reader; now he was sitting down to play something—although, he had
to add, the main character did seem to him "pretty sick."

The rest of the book, which ran January through August, 1964, was
comparatively smooth sailing for the editors, although Hayes once left a
chapter in a taxicab (he recovered it), and Bamberger plied Mailer with
legal queries. Mailer responded to them, Hayes noted, with "grace and
patience," more than lesser and less volatile authors often displayed.
Mailer did not give up on his efforts to widen the range of language at
Esquire. In installment seven, he put "shit" in, by his recollection, at least
twenty-five times—including some extras so he'd have room to negotiate.
Esquire immediately cut most of them out, but he negotiated to add back
a few more. Several witnesses claim to have heard Hayes's side of the
bargaining: "I'll trade two 'shits' for a 'fuck'." (Mailer said later that,
thinking back, he realized he had pushed *Esquire* pretty hard.)

Writing a novel on a monthly schedule wasn't easy. Mailer had to
meet deadlines regardless of what happened in his life—divorce, remar-
riage, a decision to stop smoking, a bruising debate with William F. Buckley. He was distracted from installment six by Cassius Clay's defeat of
Sonny Liston; he really wanted to skip the novel that month and just write
about the fight, but Hayes said no. When the installment came in, at the
last minute as usual, Hayes found it thin, shapeless, as if Mailer were

treading water until he could figure out which way to swim. Hayes talked the weaknesses over with him, hoping Mailer could figure out how to shore up the chapter. Mailer agreed the chapter had problems, but he couldn't fix them. "It would be like tearing down a motor and then trying to get it together again," he told Hayes. "All the parts are on the floor of the garage. There isn't enough time." In the last installment, Mailer took 25,000 words to tie up all the plot ends—twice as many as he usually wrote. To get them all in, the magazine printed the chapter in 6-point type.

An American Dream was a virtuoso improvisational performance written out of the mood of Norman Mailer and America in the months immediately before and after the Kennedy assassination: intense, giddy, as if Mailer were balancing on a high wire. Mailer wanted to be sure readers knew they were reading *in medias res.* After installment six he asked *Esquire* to remind readers that this was not simply a serialization of a book already written.

When the book came out later, reviews were mixed. Joan Didion thought Mailer, like Fitzgerald, had "some deep feeling for the mysteries of power," while to Conrad Knickerbocker in the *New York Times Book Review,* reading the novel was "like flying an airplane with the instruments cross-wired." The reviewer for *Harper's,* Paul Pickrel, found the experience of reading the book different from the experience of reading it a chapter a month, when it seemed "hardly more than a series of cheaply lurid episodes. . . ."

An American Dream did not have many fans at the magazine, although for once, advertisers did not complain (they seldom complained about text—just things they could see in a flash: images, cartoons). Arnold Gingrich hated it, although Hayes thought he was glad *Esquire* had published it. Bob Brown had to write summaries of the story thus far, which Mailer then edited, and Newman wrote a parody of Brown's summaries to pass around the office:

Summary of Norman's *An American (Wet) Dream*

Stephen Rojack is an ex-congressman, professor at NYU, author The Naked and The Dead, The Big Bite and other works. He comes back to New York and has a bad marriage with Deborah (Rojack), a pale skinned nympho who makes it all kinds of deviant ways. So far, so good, right? Well, this Rojack splits up with her, with fighting and yelling, and then, like some kind of a nut (he is a nut, I think) he almost jumps off a balcony at a party. This reminds him of killing Germans in the war. But he don't jump. Not him, that piker. He figures to himself, "If the full moon puts cancer cells in my body, then all mankind begins rotting away with some spiritual disease which I can help out." So then he goes to see his old lady, but such a terrible thing happens! (Did you read it in issues past? It was a crying shame, wasn't it?) He gets in a real squabble, you know what we mean, and crack! he chokes, and crack! he smashes and crack! he kills, the nut. So funny thing is, he feels like a terrific person afterward.

Now, imagine this. He walks into the maid's room and he sees this German maid, Ruta or Gruta, with all five fingers mashed into her privates, she's playing with it. Also, a dirty book she reads. So he leaps onto the maid and before you know it, Rojack is playing with it, and then he turns the girl over, and crack! he puts it in her ass, crack! in her cut, crack! in her ass again, and crack!! in her crack. So then the devil is happy because mankind's cancerous sense of evil is satisfied, sort of. Then back he goes, pleased as punch, and like a rat he tosses his wife out the window to make it look like she did a Brody.

And so on.

In August, the novel behind him, Mailer decided he wanted to cover the Republican Convention in San Francisco for *Esquire,* as he had covered the Democratic Convention four years before. The deadline was tight. He would have just about two weeks to write the article. That was hard enough—but as he was writing he also found himself negotiating with *Esquire*'s lawyers, who had, Hayes observed later, many objections. By this time, Mailer was accustomed to handling *Esquire*'s lawyers' objections, which he parried with guile. When *Esquire*'s lawyers told him he could not call Nelson Algren a son of a bitch in his column, Mailer suggested calling him a son of a bitch and then adding a line taking it back. Not good enough, said the lawyers. When the convention piece came around, though, he recycled the ploy and this time succeeded.

Mailer had written, "Goldwater was a demagogue—he permitted his supporters to sell a drink called Gold Water, twenty-five cents a can for orange concentrate and warm soda—it went down like piss—he was a demagogue. . . ."

Passing over the reference to Goldwater as a demagogue (he was, after all, a public figure), the lawyers fixed on Mailer's comparison of Gold Water to piss. That, the lawyers thought, came uneasily close to commercial libel. Hayes came to Mailer's defense. Why couldn't Mailer say it tasted like piss if that was what it tasted like to him?

The lawyers held firm: It was an unfair analogy.

Hayes knew that he ought to defend Mailer's right to say what he wanted, but the disputed passage seemed trivial, and besides, the policy at *Esquire* was to avoid inviting libel suits, not simply avoid losing them. Mailer wasn't happy about making a change, but an hour after their conversation he called in his solution: he had added four words—*"let no one say* it went down like piss." The amendment stood.

Other objections arose as, section by section, the piece came in. Mailer grew impatient. The last straw came at the end. Beyond deadline, he called *Esquire* with his title: "Cannibals and Christians. A History of the Republican Convention in 1964." To Hayes, the references were obscure. Who, in the piece, were cannibals? Who Christians? The lawyers thought they knew: Mailer did not like right-wingers—the cannibals must be right-wingers. The lawyers objected. But how, Hayes argued, could Mailer libel a whole group when in the past the lawyers had taught him that libel must be specific? They explained: Mailer had already pressed his luck several times in the piece, making remarks that a judge and jury might not consider fair comment. Litigants might claim that the title "Cannibals and Christians" demonstrated malicious intent.

Mailer gave in and changed the title to "In the Red Light." But he did not agree with the lawyers, and he thought the time had come to break off his relationship with *Esquire.* That relationship had always been ambivalent. Arnold Gingrich had disliked both "Superman Comes to the Supermart" and *An American Dream.* Mailer, on his part, thought Gingrich was an "old church warden"—the best thing he could say for him, even long after Gingrich's death, was that "he was always immaculately dressed." As for Hayes, Mailer found him "cold"; it seemed to Mailer that he and Hayes had trouble knowing what to say to each other. Hayes, in turn, found Mailer difficult. He felt there were times he had to reason with Mailer "like a child." He found the experience demeaning, for Mailer, for himself, and for *Esquire.* Yet he believed losing Mailer was a serious loss for *Esquire.* He would write later:

"His imagination and courage; his tenacity with a difficult problem; his commitment to his ideas (however fashion-oriented they might prove to be); the ambivalent loyalty he later developed for the magazine—these were all unique aspects of this writer. And then there were times when the heart of all our efforts—his writing—transcended considerations of business or profession. When he wrote well he wrote very well."

Mailer had not, Hayes noted, made *Esquire* a commercial success. His years with *Esquire* had been a low period for the magazine, financially. Yet his contribution to the magazine had been "inestimable." He had brought boldness to the personality of the magazine. Hayes spoke of the loss with regret: *"Esquire* had held to its legal restrictions for responsible publishing—and lost one of its strongest voices."

There was another major loss to come. In August 1964, *Esquire* published a profile of James Baldwin that offended him deeply. Baldwin had become a visible figure in the civil rights movement—*Time* magazine had put him on its cover the year before as a symbol of the movement. With a Broadway play in the works—*Blues for Mister Charlie*—Baldwin had turned into a full-fledged celebrity, the kind of figure *Esquire* liked to put under the microscope. Hayes gave the job to a writer named Marvin Elkoff, who had submitted a short story to *Esquire*, "Playing Off Keefe" (June 1964), a brash, freewheeling assault on political correctness.

Elkoff considered himself a radical, free of liberal guilt about blacks, and he approached Baldwin in an unfettered frame of mind. He laid out a sequence of scenes featuring a needy, exhibitionist Baldwin, then posed the question: "How does a man of so unorthodox and disorderly a mode of life become so persuasive and pertinent a spokesman for the Negro protest movement . . . ?" Elkoff's answer: Baldwin was voicing feelings middle-class whites were not accustomed to hearing from middle-class blacks— using "his blackness as a battering ram assaulting the mind mercilessly with an idea of suffering, a quality of life and experience that he maintains no white man can fully appreciate." The piece reached a climax with an account of a dinner party in the home of an unnamed white writer, where six or seven white liberal couples gathered to meet Baldwin. The scene, supplied by a source Gay Talese had suggested, was a revealing set piece: Baldwin attacked one guest unrelentingly as a white liberal "albatross."

Neither white liberals nor Baldwin himself emerged from the article with much dignity, although Baldwin emerged as more of a flesh-and-blood character than in other, more respectful accounts. The article opened with the title "Everybody Knows His Name" and an unflattering photograph of Baldwin, his eyes popping at a host of hands extended toward him. The photographer, Bob Adelman, recalled that his instructions were simple: "Get him." There's no evidence that Hayes assigned the piece itself to "get" Baldwin, although, given the audacity of Elkoff's short story, Hayes could not have imagined Elkoff would handle Baldwin gently. Why was Hayes willing to cast such an unflattering light on one of *Esquire*'s own contributors?

In fact, by 1964 Baldwin had not published anything in *Esquire* for a couple of years, but he had made a very big splash in *The New Yorker* in November 1962 with an essay later published in the book *The Fire Next Time*. Hayes thought *The Fire Next Time* was a polemic, and Hayes did not like polemics. He did not like the whole direction Baldwin's work was taking. A few months after Elkoff's article ran, and likely under its influence, Hayes spoke of "a virulent strain in some of Baldwin's recent work, more related to the political philosophy of RAM [Revolutionary Action Movement] than to that of Martin Luther King." Hayes seldom showed his political colors, but Baldwin brought them out.

The very special enemy of the Negro, argues Baldwin, is the white liberal, one who *knows* better but does nothing. Out of this argument a strange phenomenon has ensued: a whole body of readers, most of them white liberals, pleading for Baldwin to show them ever more clearly how terrible they are. As a matter of fact, many of us believe the so-called white liberal constitutes the better part of Baldwin's audience. Baldwin's proposition here, I respectfully submit, is dead wrong. . . . The white liberal who does not attend the picket line or sit-down in front of the attorney general's office goes to the polls nevertheless, articulates his commitment by voicing his opinion as well as his vote, and asserts in a thousand ways within this densely populated nation his influence. Without him, there truly would be blood in the streets.

Baldwin had struck a nerve.

The *Esquire* article so distressed Baldwin in turn that—Hayes told Elkoff—he threatened to sue. Although eventually he apologized to Hayes for overreacting, he did not publish in *Esquire* again for several years.

Baldwin and Mailer had come into the magazine around the same time, and had talked to each other on *Esquire*'s pages, with Baldwin on Mailer in "The Black Boy Looks at the White Boy" (May 1961) and Mailer on Baldwin in "Ten Thousand Words a Minute" (February 1963)—his report of Floyd Patterson's fight with Sonny Liston—then again in the literary issue of July 1963. They had sparred like fighters, their relationship highly conflicted, crossed by their differences in race and sexual preference—Baldwin homosexual, Mailer noisily heterosexual— and streaked with professional jealousy.

Esquire had profited from their mutual presence. As a magazine identifying itself as a magazine for men, *Esquire* had a mission to define what men were and what they could be. Baldwin and Mailer both expanded the range of possibility. *Esquire* in turn had helped make Baldwin and Mailer what they were—public figures. Writers had not always been public figures in America, nor would they continue to be, but in these years, Baldwin and Mailer came to stand for something in public life. They were more than celebrities, although they were that. They were serious men, but flamboyant of mind and imagination, deeply engaged in the American experiment, passionate about democracy. For a few years, *Esquire* had given them a platform from which to speak to an audience far wider than the little magazines where Baldwin and Mailer had started as journalists. Now both were gone.

A few months later—apparently after Mailer had said his goodbye, which gives the story an ironic twist—Hayes lost another writer who had written more for *Esquire* than either Baldwin or Mailer, and had played a key role in opening *Esquire* up to more imaginative journalism, especially in celebrity pieces: Tom Morgan. Morgan never forgot his last lunch with Hayes.

"Harold," he said, "I've been getting $1,350 for a piece, a profile, and you know how long it takes me to do—it took me longer than anybody else. I really would like to have some more money for my profiles."

"What do you have in mind?"

"Well, I got $6,000 for a profile I wrote of Sukarno for *Life*. I get $4,000 from *Look*. I think it would be nice if I got $1,500 from *Esquire*, even though an *Esquire* piece takes me six times longer than it takes to do either one. I'm an *Esquire* writer, and everything else is to fund my *Esquire* habit."

"Tom," Hayes replied, drawling the words out and sucking on his pipe, "we all think you're wonderful—but you know the only person at *Esquire* who gets $1,500 is Norman Mailer."

"But Norman Mailer has written like five pieces for you. I've written forty for you and Clay and Ralph and everybody—"

"I know Tom, I know, but it wouldn't be right. Norman Mailer is going to win the Nobel Prize."

"Well, I'm not through yet. If I can get somebody to publish my novel—no, Harold, I really gotta have $1,500."

"Tom," he said, "I'll tell you what. I'll give you $1,450."

It didn't really matter to Morgan what anyone else was paying him. He wanted to write for *Esquire*. But he felt boxed into a corner.

"Harold," he said, "I gotta have $1,500 or I don't think I'm gonna be able to continue."

"Tom, let me tell you something."

And this was to be the end of Morgan's long relationship with *Esquire*. Hayes didn't mean it to end, Morgan thought. That was just how Hayes played his hand—right up to the border, the way he always played his hand.

"Tom," Hayes said, "I understand what you're saying, but I want you to know one thing. When I die and they're lowering me into my grave, just before they close my casket, my last words are going to be"—and he sang out the words—"fourteen fifty for Morgan, fifteen hundred for Mailer."

The way he sang out the words in that restaurant—Morgan never forgot it. Almost thirty years later he said, "I felt so humiliated. I don't know how to explain it. Maybe somebody else wouldn't have been. Maybe somebody else would have socked him. It just humiliated me.

"And I said, 'Okay, Harold. Let's talk about something else.' I never wrote for him again."

Despite the defections, *Esquire* had a talented workforce in 1964, drawn partly from the ranks of newspaper writers who did not care that *Esquire* couldn't match the rates of the big-circulation magazines like *Look*. It had been a fine year, with Tom Wicker on Lyndon Baines Johnson, Gloria Steinem on Jacqueline Kennedy, Rebecca West on the Profumo affair in England, Peter Bogdanovich on Humphrey Bogart, Gay Talese on Floyd Patterson, Tom Wolfe on Junior Johnson, and David Halberstam on John Paul Vann, a former military adviser in Vietnam, now critical of the conduct of the war. Bruce Davidson took photographs of the new Verrazano-Narrows Bridge—something he had wanted to do since he and Sam Antupit had driven under it on their way somewhere else; Gay Talese wrote the text. *Esquire* got hold of Lee Harvey Oswald's letters to his mother, who came up to *Esquire* so Bob Sherrill could interview her and Diane Arbus could take her picture. And Gore Vidal's article on Attorney General Robert Kennedy, published the year before, was still rippling across the political scene. On August 13, 1964, the *New York Times* reported a movement among Reform Democrats to block Kennedy's unannounced candidacy for the United States Senate. Copies of Vidal's *Esquire* article were circulating "in plain, brown manila envelopes with an unsigned covering letter."

That fall, the *Columbia Journalism Review* judged *Esquire* and found it good. "A policy of letting writers say what they wanted to say has set off *Esquire* from the frightened-rabbit school of magazine journalism." *Es-*

quire was "never conformist and rarely dull." In a memorandum dated October 27, Hayes told his staff that *Esquire* might not have the resources of the big magazines, but *Esquire*, operating in the tradition of guerrilla fighter Francis Marion the Swamp Fox, could "touch a nerve." He urged editors to be "daring, original, bold, controversial, authoritative and responsible. . . . If you understand our personality, and I think nearly all of you do by now, we can literally do a story about anything in the world." The question they should ask of a story: "Will it shake people up?"

FIVE

Editor Hayes

O N FEBRUARY 21, 1965, Malcolm X was shot down in the Audubon Ballroom in Harlem. As his body lay in state, Harold Hayes and James Hicks, editor of the Harlem newspaper *Amsterdam News,* visited the funeral home together. Hayes had come to talk with Hicks about "the media and race relations," the subject of a seminar Hayes had been asked to take part in, but under the shadow of the assassination, their conversation turned to the rumors circulating, the sort of information that rarely makes its way into the newspapers.

There had been reports first that Malcolm X had been shot by other Black Muslims, but now there were contradictory reports. Hicks told Hayes he had heard that an international group—its identity left vague— had a plan to kill off a series of leaders of the American civil rights movement. Hayes brought up an article *Esquire* had run in October linking the most militant civil rights leaders with the Red Chinese. Together Hicks, the moderate black editor, and Hayes, the liberal white one, pondered the signs of something Hayes thought of as "Black Internationalism." The evidence for an international liberation movement made them both nervous, mutually troubled by what Hayes described as "the rumbling underground."

Against the backdrop of their conversation, the next day Hayes read a story in *Challenge,* which described itself as "the revolutionary weekly." The story joined the deaths of Malcolm X, U.N. Secretary General Dag Hammarskjöld, and John F. Kennedy in what seemed to Hayes a paranoid web, suggesting that the ruling class had ordered Malcolm X's death, and Hammarskjöld and Kennedy had died as a result of internal power struggles in the ruling class. To Hayes, here was ominous evidence of a twilight world of "rumor and semi-fact." He was troubled, too, by calls from black militants, even before the death of Malcolm X, to take up arms in self-defense.

Esquire had given the civil rights movement steady support, in its own way, running sober portraits of Black Muslims by Eve Arnold and a biting, funny tour of the South by Jessica Mitford. "The Segs," those long crazed monologues in which five southern segregationists spoke for themselves, had so provoked the editor of the *Geneva County Reaper*, in Geneva, Alabama, that he ran a long editorial offering *Esquire* a Dubious Achievement Award for completing "another twelve months of propaganda publication":

Blithely they continue to slam "bigotry in the South" in every issue, usually by means of Hitler's "big-lie" technique, assuming that integration of the races and Federal control of every facet of society is virtually an accomplished fact and only a batch of Southern Slobs, in their pitiful ignorance, are holding out against the establishment of a universal utopia in which everyone is color-blind except Martin Luther King and *Esquire,* Inc.

But Hayes, a southern liberal on race, was also a moderate American: he believed in reason, electoral politics, the system. He had never been "hip," and now, as America moved into a period when the word "revolution" would fall casually from many lips, he was not a revolutionary. He was troubled by radical rhetoric, yet in remarks he wrote up for the seminar after his visit with Hicks, he called on the press "to open up the gray areas, to explore the reasons behind them, to allow the most radical opinions—from either side—into print so that the nation's readers may understand, and *then* attempt to cope. Otherwise, there come to be undergrounds, and undergrounds usually lead to open rebellion, violence, hatred—and worse."

Just a few years earlier the challenge had been to break up the ice of fifties culture. Now the culture was fragmenting on its own at a quickening pace. The challenge was to keep up with the changes—to reflect the fragments into which American history seemed to be shattering: the disintegrating civil rights movement and the troubling war in Vietnam, the subject of a caustic first-person piece *Esquire* ran in August 1965, "The Ambush," by Captain James Morris, illustrated with small black-and-white pictures of dead Vietcong. In fall 1964, the free-speech movement at the University of California at Berkeley had drawn national attention.

In spring 1965, President Johnson began bombing raids on North Vietnam and draft calls went up; campus anti-war groups organized teach-ins. On April 17, 25,000 anti-war protestors, responding to a call by Students for a Democratic Society, demonstrated in Washington.

For the college issue for 1965, George Lois planned a composite face representing the new campus heroes: Bob Dylan, Malcolm X, Fidel Castro, and John F. Kennedy. Inside, some of the articles were serious attempts to describe a real change in campus life, but notes of disdain also crept in. "What *do* you want?" Cal Kid asks an activist, in a comic strip produced by Robert Benton and David Newman. "Don't bug me with goals, Kid! goals corrupt! we want power and revolt and freedom and that stuff!"

And at this turn in the road, this challenging time, *Esquire* suddenly faltered. Advertising revenues, rising steadily since 1962, abruptly dropped in the first four months of 1965. The Publishers Information Bureau reported a decline of 13 percent in advertising pages, while the industry average for ad pages in monthlies was up 7 percent. In a draft for a memorandum to Gingrich, Hayes referred to questions that had arisen about *Esquire*'s editorial direction. The biggest question appeared to be whether *Esquire* would make more money if the editorial focus shifted to "service"—lifestyle and consumer advice articles presumed to appeal to advertisers. Hayes staked his claim for long-term success on following the editorial line the editors had laid down several years before: reaching a literate, affluent audience with a magazine covering a variety of subjects. What set *Esquire* apart from *Life* and *Look,* which also covered a variety of subjects, was *Esquire*'s attitude—its assumption that its readers were "smarter, brighter, more original and better off."

This was a smart commercial approach in the long run, Hayes argued, because it built up the reader's faith in the magazine's authority. Only in the areas of fashion and travel did *Esquire* deviate from its policy of not "bullshitting a knowledgeable reader." And in spite of its slavish efforts to please advertisers in those areas, *Esquire* was losing fashion pages. "Why? In my opinion it's because we've tried to please everyone but the reader."

No shift in editorial direction occurred. Plenty of service features showed up—guides to gift-buying, fashion, travel, motorcycles, cars—but in no greater abundance than before. Hayes still had plenty of room for articles with attitude, like a guide to football ("The Fifteen Dirtiest Plays"), or an audacious musical comedy, "The Making of the President,

1968!"—pairing black comedian Godfrey Cambridge as the Democratic candidate with white comedienne Phyllis Diller as the Republican candidate: they marry and run the country together.

Hayes apparently did not feel his leadership was in serious jeopardy: in late spring he and his wife Susan left their son and new daughter at home and traveled to Europe on a kind of second honeymoon. Harold had been to Europe once before, in 1958, but this trip was more ambitious. For three weeks they drove 3,000 miles on the continent—"drove like hell," Hayes wrote Gingrich, "and saw lots." They started in London, where the daffodils were wildly in bloom. The city was vibrant. For Susan, visiting London was like revisiting her youth, when she was David Merrick's girl. From Merrick, a theatrical producer, Susan had learned where to buy tailor-made shoes and shirts and suits. Now, trying to see to it that Harold looked more like the editor of *Esquire,* she took him around to a shoemaker off Bond Street. They lunched with Malcolm Muggeridge, *Esquire*'s book reviewer, then headed for the continent on a tourist's vacation.

When an *Esquire* reporter and photographer went to Europe in early 1965 in search of "the hipster," they had found instead "something new"—a floating community of meditative rebels, high on pot, hanging out together in bare rooms equipped with a few books and knapsacks. Susan and Harold were more conventional travelers. Bypassing Paris, they toured the castles of the Loire Valley, drove through Switzerland, Italy, Germany—stopping at Berchtesgaden, Hitler's mountain retreat—then back to France. It was not easy for Harold to put work aside: he found himself waking up every morning talking to himself about the magazine.

One night in early June, they were driving a Triumph through the countryside of southeast England, headed back from Dover to London and looking for a place to spend the night. It was late, and they had stopped at several inns. Each time, Harold would go in, come out again, and say it might look charming outside but it was awful inside. "Not there," he would say, and they would go on. Finally Susan told him they had to stay somewhere. Impatient, Harold turned the car around, and just as Susan reminded him to take the left side of the road, they crashed head-on into a car coming from the opposite direction.

They were lucky, Hayes wrote Gingrich. "If the point of collision had been 15 degrees farther to the center somebody would have had it." The other car was totaled, although the driver was not injured. Susan and Harold were taken to a hospital at nearby Canterbury. Susan had a concussion, but the next morning the doctor was ready to release them. "How are your children?" he asked Susan. "What children?" she asked. He kept her in the hospital for a week.

Back at *Esquire* the staff was solicitous. Byron Dobell sent Susan a cable the morning after the accident; Bob Sherrill called the next morning. Muggeridge drove over from Robertsbridge to pick Harold up and take him back to his country home for lunch with Christopher Booker, the first editor of *Private Eye,* a satire magazine. Hayes enjoyed the afternoon—he got Booker to report for *Esquire* on the lively British cultural scene and he settled into a long and warm relationship with Muggeridge, even naming him his daughter Carrie's godfather.

Newspaperman, novelist, critic, television celebrity, former spy, and former editor of *Punch,* Muggeridge had lived through World War I and served in the British Secret Service during the Second World War. He appeared often on the BBC as an interviewer. He described himself as "a knockabout journalist" but was in fact an elegant writer with decided views.

With Muggeridge on books and Dwight Macdonald on movies, *Esquire* had in-house two of the more formidable critics on both sides of the Atlantic. They were also both mature men, but there was never a hint that Hayes or anyone else at *Esquire* thought their age a drawback in a magazine trying to appeal to young men. Years later one of *Esquire*'s young readers, Hayes's cousin Hayes McNeill, in college at Wake Forest during the mid-sixties, spoke of the importance of Dorothy Parker, Dwight Macdonald, and Malcolm Muggeridge to readers of his generation: They had "shone klieg lights into the '60s and taught a bunch of us what a high art criticism ought to be," he wrote to Hayes.

Hayes had been Muggeridge's editor for several years before the trip to England, and they had met when Muggeridge had come through New York, but he had never seen the man in his natural surroundings.

"It's impossible to measure the range of his involvement and influence over here," Hayes wrote Gingrich on this trip to England. "We lunched with him before we left for the continent three weeks ago, and that night heard him over BBC. Today he has the lead review in *The Observer* and is on BBC TV tonight interviewing P. G. Wodehouse. Last Tuesday he did a special TV show on America. His name seems to turn up in the literary and political press here more often than Harold Wilson's. A formidable man and completely without pretense."

That afternoon at Muggeridge's home, their conversation turned to

F. Scott Fitzgerald, and Hayes found himself sneering at the Max Perkins concept of the nurturing editor, then found himself "in a most defensive position" when, later, back home, he wanted to compliment Muggeridge for a piece he had done on the Left in *The New Statesman.*

Hayes had been back in the States only a few months when he came across a story he wanted Muggeridge to take up. Hayes had gone to Washington to talk with writers for an ambitious project: ferreting out information on the Central Intelligence Agency. Spying had become an obsession of the popular culture, and *Esquire* had fed at the trough—offering readers a spate of articles on James Bond and other spies. The question *Esquire* was asking itself for its May 1966 issue: What did it all mean—this conjunction of sex and science and spying?

"Ever since Jack Kennedy died the people have been desperate for something to distract them," he wrote Muggeridge. "Our thesis, to be rendered in this special issue, is that the fix is now on spying, science and sex. All three are related (the Bond films are a good oversimplified example). That this happens to be the quality of the American imagination right now is discouraging but fascinating; and we are trying to show some of the realities upon which much of the fantasy is based."

In pursuit of reality in Washington, Hayes had run across a toy manufacturer who had worked for the CIA until two or three years before; he reminded Hayes of a Southern Baptist minister, and Hayes liked him for it. The man gave Hayes a critique he had done of the agency while he was still working there, but he also told Hayes a story about a woman named Sylvia Press. As Hayes told the story to Muggeridge, Press had been a longtime CIA employee who had been investigated and then fired. She had written a novel about her experiences, and, according to his informant, the agency had spent between $50,000 and $100,000 to suppress the novel, which had been published by Beacon Press.

In New York, Hayes called Beacon and "cagily asked if they knew anything about the book." He was told the copyright had been transferred to first one press, then another, both out of existence. Then he discovered that Sylvia Press was living in New York. He called her and invited her to come in to *Esquire.* When he told her what he had heard, it was new to her. She *had* had trouble getting the book published, and then her editor had left suddenly; she had noticed the book had somehow never gotten into bookstores. She had thought the editor's departure had had something to do with that, but she wasn't surprised by the story Hayes had heard. She wasn't sure she wanted the whole thing dug up again—she had suffered enough from her interrogation by the agency. Besides, she was still hoping to receive an agency pension when she reached retirement age; bringing the matter up again might jeopardize her chances.

Hayes did not want to run anything without her consent, but he suggested he send the book to Malcolm Muggeridge to review, just as he reviewed other books; Hayes would call the review "Book Review of a Very Limited Edition."

Press said she would think it over, and left Hayes with a copy of the book: *The Care of Devils.* He read it. She was not Norman Mailer, but she had told the story in a convincing way, and her story raised interesting questions: "what right does the employee of such an agency have to privacy, justice, etc.?" Hayes was convinced *Esquire* should do something, and Muggeridge should do it.

The next day Press returned to say she would risk an article in *Esquire* because she still hoped to bring public attention to the book. Hayes was still troubled: Would the CIA really go to such lengths to suppress a critical book? He talked to a publisher who said Beacon Press, a small house, might simply have faltered in its distribution—those things happened. He tracked down the editor who had handled the book, and he said if the CIA had been throwing money around, none had come his way. If it had, he would have taken it and published anyway, he told Hayes. But he did not dismiss the possibility of intervention at the distribution level. And he did add information as to why the agency had subjected Press to investigation—she was apparently a victim of mistaken identity, and was perhaps, too, a bone thrown to Senator Joseph McCarthy.

Passing the ball to Muggeridge, Hayes knew he was handing him a challenge: his approach to the story would have to be somewhat oblique.

"Obviously you can say it's about the CIA and their methods, though, since it is presented as fiction, any specific relating to real people possibly could stir up a suit. But I'm reluctant to have you worry very much about all that. If you'll leave it to me I'll see that any bloodletting is kept to a minimum."

Muggeridge took Hayes up on the assignment and handled it gracefully, but came down clearly on Press's side. *"The Care of Devils* will assuredly *not* please the pros. From their point of view it has the truly appalling disability of being true."

In *The Man Who Kept the Secrets* (1979), Thomas Powers reported what happened next. Muggeridge's piece prompted Bantam to put out a paperback edition of Press's book five months after Muggeridge's review appeared. That version, said Powers, "fell stillborn from the press as well." The following year, 1967, Press wrote Richard Helms, director of the CIA, to ask if she could receive a pension. Helms sent a representative from the Office of Security, Howard Osborn, to meet with her in New York. Over dinner she made her case for herself: that she had been dismissed without a hearing and had never seen a list of charges or confronted a witness. She was old enough to receive a pension now and thought her fifteen years of work entitled her to it. Powers reported Osborn's response:

"Dick doesn't think there's anything wrong with you," Osborn said.

"Then why am I having so much trouble?" asked Miss Press.

"The thing is, Sylvia," said Osborn, "if only you hadn't written *that book!*"

Over the next two years, she met him again a number of times—"perhaps a dozen," Powers said—but she never received a pension.

Hayes had returned from England to a modest uproar on several fronts. In the June issue, *Esquire* had run an article on the relationship between President Lyndon Johnson and Abe Fortas, nominated by President Johnson to the Supreme Court. The article, written by Charles B. Seib, assistant managing editor of the *Washington Star,* and Alan L. Otten, a Washington correspondent for the *Wall Street Journal,* was scarcely a hard-hitting investigative report. But a couple of Republican congressmen used it to speak against Fortas in the House. One Democratic congressman leaped to Fortas's defense, suggesting that articles in *Esquire* were not the best basis for evaluating a Supreme Court Justice's qualifications. Another agreed that attacks based on an article like that "are not in the best tradition of the House of Representatives." Meanwhile, in June, *Esquire*'s movie critic, Dwight Macdonald, invited by the White House to a Festival of the Arts, created his own drama by going around asking other guests to sign a statement supporting poet Robert Lowell's decision to protest the Vietnam War by boycotting the festival.

Back in New York, Tom Wolfe was under attack. "Tom Wolfe really stood 'em all on their ears by two installments of a really vicious attack on *The New Yorker* in the *New York* Sunday magazine section of the *Herald Tribune,*" Gingrich wrote Helen Lawrenson on April 23, 1965. Further-

Esquire

EDITORS AND WRITERS

Harold Hayes, with the head of art director Robert Benton under his left arm. *Dan Wynn photo*

Clay Felker, Hayes's competitor and editor about town. *Irving Schild photo*

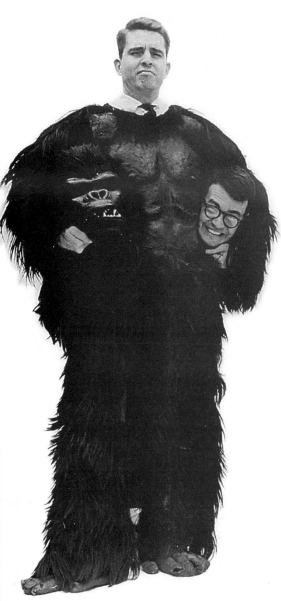

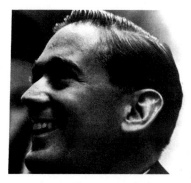

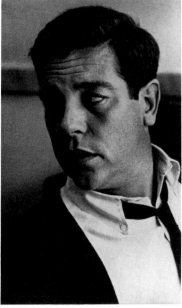

Rust Hills, fiction editor and organizer of literary symposia. *Irving Schild photo*

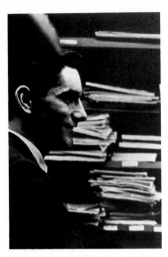

Harvard Lampoon alumnus
John Berendt. *Irving Schild photo*

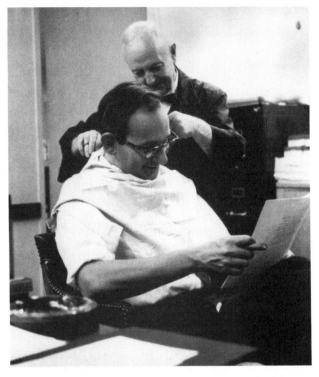

Byron Dobell, managing editor and steadying influence.

On the opposite page: David Newman, editor (*left*), and Robert Benton, art director, creators of "Dubious Achievements" and the movie ***Bonnie and Clyde***. *Burton Berinsky photo*

Editor Bob Sherrill, Hayes's friend from college. *Reine Turner photo*

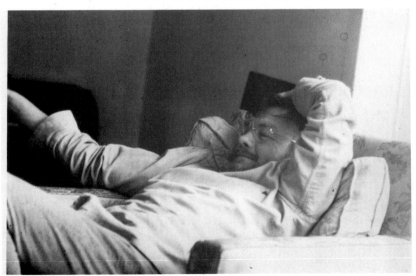

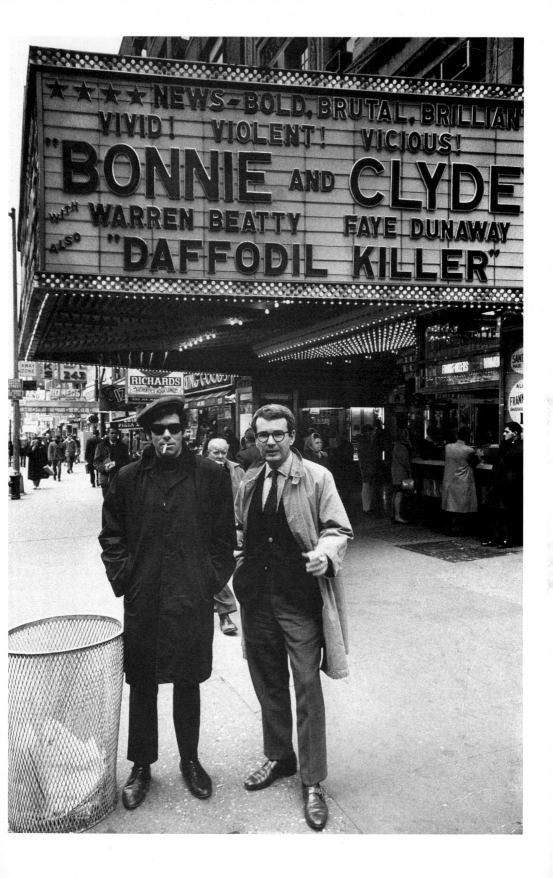

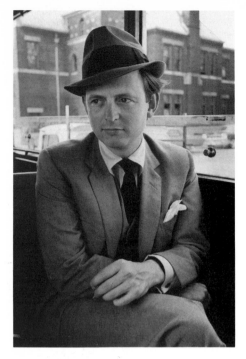 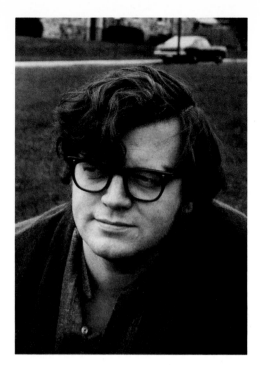

Above, left: **Tom Wolfe, chronicler of the cultural revolution.** *Photo © 1994 by Jill Krementz*
Above, right: **Garry Wills, who re-created the world of Jack Ruby and rode the bus to Martin Luther King, Jr.'s funeral.** *Photo © 1994 by Jill Krementz*

Gay Talese, *Esquire*'s most stylish man on men, among them (*shown here on right*) baseball hero Joe DiMaggio.
Ernie Sisto photo

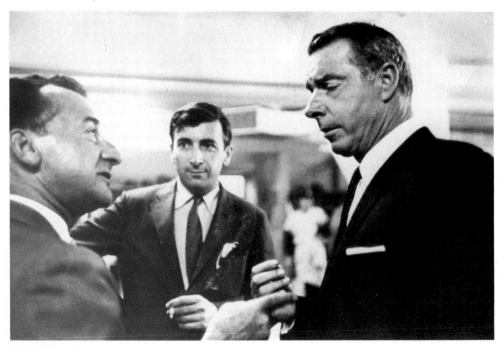

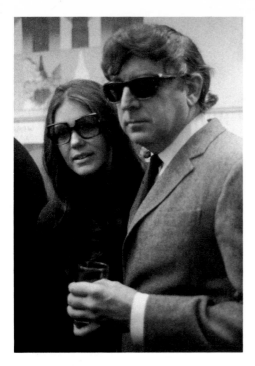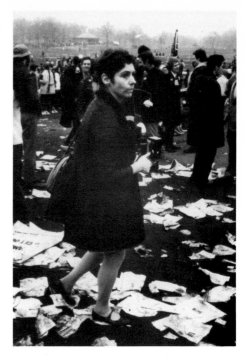

Above, left: Gloria Steinem, for a short time an *Esquire* writer, with Terry Southern, novelist, who also reported for *Esquire*. *Photo © 1994 by Jill Krementz*
Above, right: Diane Arbus, photographer, here at a peace march. *Photo © 1994 by Jill Krementz*

French playwright Jean Genet (*left*) and American beat novelist William Burroughs (*center*), who with Terry Southern represented *Esquire* at the 1968 Democratic Convention in Chicago. Allen Ginsberg (*right*) enjoyed their company but was not part of the team. *Photo © 1994 by Jill Krementz*

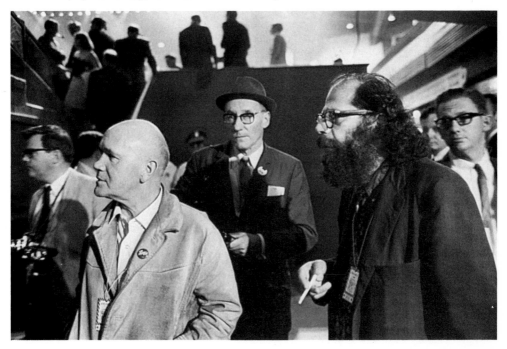

Michael Herr, whose reports on the Vietnam War became the book *Dispatches*.

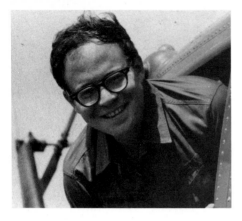

Gordon Lish, advocate for Raymond Carver and other unknown fiction writers.

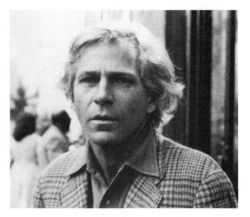

On the opposite page, above: Editorial staff 1968. Front row (*left to right, sitting*): Tom Hedley, Harold Hayes, Arnold Gingrich, Chip Tolbert. Second row (*left to right*): John Berendt, Richard Joseph, Bob Brown, Cathie McBride, Virginia Reilly, Sam Antupit, Alice Glaser, Don Erickson. Third row (*left to right*): Sheila Berger, George Frazier IV, Tom Ferrell, Jill Goldstein, Bob Sherrill. *Steinbicker / Houghton photo*
Below: Editorial staff 1973. Front row (*left to right*): Margaret Falk, Harold Hayes, Jill Goldstein. Second row (*left to right*): Virginia Reilly, Lee Eisenberg, Don Erickson, Rebecca Bartlett, Julie Schwartz. Third row (*left to right*): Ben Pesta, Richard Weigand, Tom Ferrell, Bill Ryan. *Dan Wynn photo*

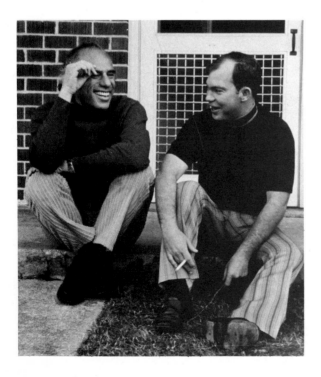

John Sack (*left*) with Lieutenant William Calley, Jr., convicted of killing civilians at Mylai, who sold his "confession" to *Esquire. Peter Ross Range photo*

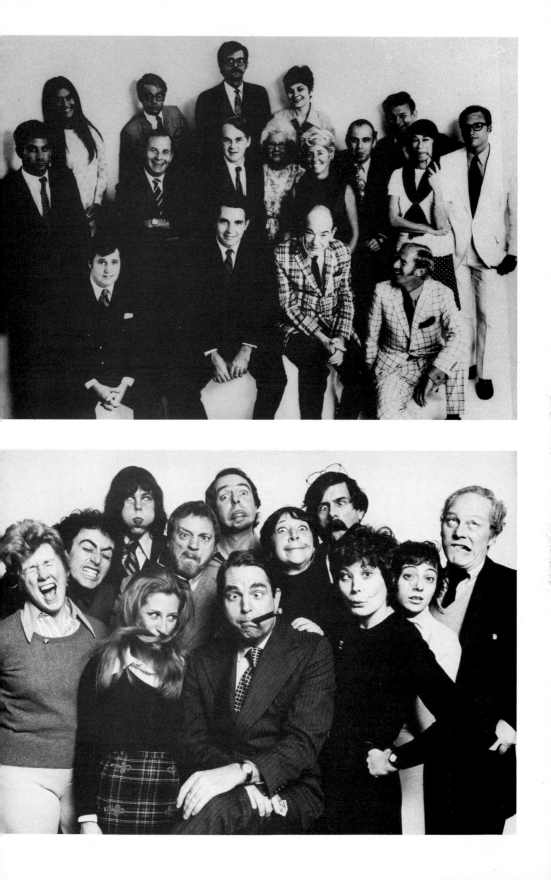

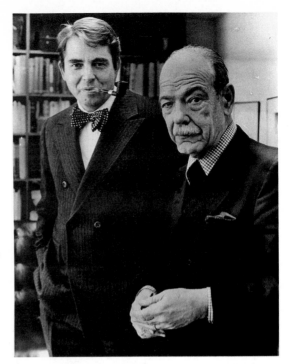

Harold Hayes (*left*) and *Esquire* publisher Arnold Gingrich, in the picture *Newsweek* ran when they parted.
NEWSWEEK—Tony Rollo photo

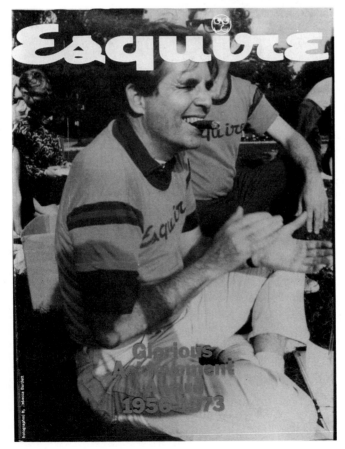

Hayes suited up in commemorative cover, not actually published.
Becky Bartlett photo

more, Wolfe had dragged *Esquire* into the fray. As proof that *The New Yorker* was not such hot stuff, Wolfe had claimed for *Esquire* a long list of writers that his critics said later *The New Yorker* could just as easily claim. He had said, further, *"The New Yorker* comes out once a week, it has overwhelming cultural prestige, it pays top prices to writers—and for 40 years it has maintained a strikingly low level of literary achievement. *Esquire* comes out only once a month, yet it has completely outclassed *The New Yorker* in literary contribution even during its cheesecake days." The fellows in *Esquire's* promotion department wanted to make use of these "almost embarrassingly flattering" remarks, Gingrich told Lawrenson, but Gingrich talked them out of it.

Wolfe's *New Yorker* pieces, written in retaliation for *The New Yorker's* own sniping at Wolfe and *New York* magazine, drew the serious wrath of literary New York. *New Yorker* writers were particularly peeved by the first installment (April 11, 1965), which dragged *The New Yorker's* reclusive editor, William Shawn, through a field of anecdotes that had little or no basis in fact. Shawn even sent a telegram to the newspaper's owner, John Hay Whitney, asking him to suppress the piece. *New Yorker* writers E. B. White and J. D. Salinger were among many who took Wolfe to task.

Fresh on the heels of *The New Yorker* fray, Wolfe published a collection of articles from *New York* and *Esquire,* its title taken from that *Esquire* piece on customized cars: *The Kandy-Kolored Tangerine-Flake Streamline Baby.* The book made a splash, earning more reviews than a newspaper feature writer had a right to expect. One of the reviewers was *Esquire's* own Dwight Macdonald.

Macdonald was practically a living history of American magazines. He had been a writer at *Fortune* magazine in the thirties, an editor at *The Partisan Review* in the late thirties and early forties, then editor of his own magazine, *Politics,* from 1944 to 1949. He had been on the staff of *The New Yorker* since 1951 and film critic at *Esquire* since 1960. He had published several collections: *Memoirs of a Revolutionist* (1956); *Masscult and Midcult* (1961); *Against the American Grain* (1962). He was a smart, pugnacious writer, whose political sympathies had veered, by his own account, from liberal to radical to Communist sympathizer to anti-Stalinist to conservative anarchist.

During Macdonald's years at *Esquire,* Arnold Gingrich wrote a correspondent in 1969, he had inspired more readers to write angry letters than

any other writer besides Norman Mailer, and *Esquire* valued him for it. In
an early review, Macdonald slashed his way through *Ben-Hur*—"bloody
bloody and bloody boring"—until he came finally to a point that most
riled great numbers of readers: that the film falsified the Bible, making the
Romans, not the Jews, responsible for the crucifixion. His explanation for
that transfiguration: "there are no ancient Romans around and there are
many Jews and $15,000,000 is $15,000,000."

The letters poured in to *Esquire*—so many that Gingrich prepared a
form letter in response. Later, when a piece from Leslie Fiedler contained
a statement Gingrich thought might be comparably troublesome, Gingrich told Hayes to dilute it by cutting three words; he would just as soon
avoid the flood of letters the *Ben-Hur* article had brought in. But to
Macdonald, he professed delight. "Dwight, I love your column, and one
of the things I like most about it is that it makes the cash customers sit
down at their desks, pen in hand, and holler and yell."

There was no question about it: Macdonald loved a fight. "Blast and
let blast, that's my motto," he once told Hayes after an irritable exchange
of letters between them. Now, in the *New York Review of Books,* which in
two years had edged out *Commentary* and *The Partisan Review* to
become the nation's leading intellectual journal, he took on Tom Wolfe.
The Kandy-Kolored Tangerine-Flake Streamline Baby was "a nice little
book," Macdonald said in a review on August 26, 1965. But all the praise
heaped on it worried him, especially the idea that this was a new kind of
journalism: "parajournalism," he called it, reminiscent of parody, or para-
noia—"a bastard form, having it both ways, exploiting the factual authority of journalism and the atmospheric license of fiction."

The form had started out at *Esquire* and was now thriving at the *New
York Herald Tribune,* where Dick Schaap and Jimmy Breslin were practitioners, but Tom Wolfe, with his "practically symbiotic" relationship with
Clay Felker, was "king of the cats." Macdonald was not wholly unkind to
Wolfe—he could be fun, Macdonald allowed, if you skipped enough—but
he doubted that Wolfe would be read much in the future: his subjects
were ephemeral, his style too eccentric. There was something manufactured about Wolfe's pieces, Macdonald thought: Marianne Moore had
said poets put real toads in imaginary gardens, but "Wolfe has reversed the
process; his decor is real but his toads are synthetic."

Macdonald followed his review up, in a later article, with a stern refutation, pseudo-fact by pseudo-fact, of Wolfe's articles on *The New Yorker*. What would later be called New Journalism was off to a guilty start: it was new, but was it journalism?

Hayes watched as one of his star writers savaged another. He did not admire Shawn's attempt to block publication. Nor did he admire the writers' assault when he failed: "—all the great elephants stampeded into print with trumpeting denunciations. . . ." He thought he detected ritual overtones: the burial of the myth of the great editor.

In an unpublished manuscript Hayes pronounced his own judgment:

"Certainly the loyalty Shawn has inspired among his staff is to be envied by any magazine editor at any time. Part of this loyalty must surely derive from the fact that the man has sacrificed much of his time, and his life, to the work of his writers. Certainly *The New Yorker* is a great institution. It is always well written, thoroughly researched, reliable, authoritative—and urbane. But Wolfe's central point was that, for the most part, it is irrelevant; and even if Shawn hadn't sent that telegram (hardly the act of a Great Editor), I would be inclined to agree with him. To be a great editor one must, at the very least, edit a relevant magazine."

The controversy was still rippling when Truman Capote, who had published *Breakfast at Tiffany's* in *Esquire,* brought out his "nonfiction novel," *In Cold Blood,* first as a serial in *The New Yorker,* then in book form. Malcolm Muggeridge reviewed it in his books column and Dwight Macdonald reviewed it in his movie column in the same issue, "perversely," Hayes wrote Muggeridge, "on the tenuous grounds that it will eventually be made into a movie." Then in June 1966 *Esquire* ran two features: one on Capote—"In Cold Comfort"—and one on the "nonfiction novel"—"In Cold Fact." They began on facing pages, flanking a parody portrait of an aging Capote in his sultry-boy-on-a-couch pose, itself a parody. Each, in its way, took apart Capote's claim to be a rigorous truth-teller.

Over three days with Capote, a sportswriter named Barbara Long unearthed no deep secrets, but several small telling ones. Her Capote, who had claimed almost total recall of what people told him (92 percent, 95 percent, or 90 percent, depending on whom he was talking to), could not remember his own lawyer's name. The man who made such strong claims to truth-telling in *In Cold Blood* told little fibs ("Oh Truman," said his neighbor Piedy Gimbel, "how *could* you tell her that?"). In the companion piece, Philip K. Tompkins argued that Capote played fast and loose with the evidence that Perry Smith really was a cold-blooded killer who never repented.

The same month the Capote pieces appeared in *Esquire, The Atlantic Monthly* ran an essay by *Esquire* writer Dan Wakefield disputing Capote's claim to have done something original. Wakefield pointed to other writers who had been practicing journalism as art since the fifties: Murray Kempton, James Baldwin, Harvey Swados, Gore Vidal, George P. Elliott, Norman Mailer—especially Norman Mailer, in his long *Esquire* pieces— but also Brock Brower, Gay Talese, Thomas B. Morgan, and—"later," he noted carefully—Tom Wolfe. All of them appeared "most often in the pages of *Esquire.*" There were others as well, writing elsewhere—Meg Greenfield in *The Reporter,* Willie Morris at *Harper's.* Still, Wakefield gave the credit to *Esquire* "for leading the way to many of the newer, freer, more imaginative forms of nonfiction." Why was *Esquire* the magazine leading the way? Because *Esquire* had an editorial attitude: "Anything goes as long as it is interesting and true."

To Tom Wolfe, what some journalists were doing was more specific than Wakefield let on; eventually Wolfe would launch an entire theory of the New Journalism. He started thinking the theory out after Macdonald's attack on him in the *New York Review of Books,* and finally wrote out some of his thoughts for the April 1969 issue of *Dateline,* a publication of the Overseas Press Club. (His girlfriend, *Esquire* art associate Sheila Berger, was designing the issue.) A couple of years later, he expanded the theory for an introduction to a collection of *The New Journalism,* laying out a range of realist techniques that defined the genre— scene-setting, dialogue, details of status life, manipulation of point of view. He would suggest that New Journalism owed its status, maybe even its very existence, to the novelists' failure to respond to the rich, rambunctious sixties culture, leaving the field to journalists.

Hayes ran the theory in *Esquire* but he never bought it—thought it was pretentious, Wolfe imagined. In an introduction Hayes wrote for a collection of *Esquire* pieces from the sixties, he called the whole idea of "New Journalism" (or "the nonfiction novel" or "history as literature and literature as history") a "symptom" of the writer's "unstrung condition" in the sixties, when the mass media could make writers celebrities, even millionaires. In other words, these claims to new forms were publicity ploys. When even the *Wall Street Journal* and *Newsweek* started referring to the New Journalism in the early seventies, Hayes spoke his piece in the "Editor's Notes" he sometimes wrote for the front of the magazine. No one could seem to agree on what New Journalism was, he said, only that it was new and that Gay Talese, Norman Mailer, and Tom Wolfe were its leading practitioners. "Yet except for their admiration for one another, Talese and Wolfe have very little in common. The work of neither man is related to that of Norman Mailer, each of the three having arrived at his station by following different routes."

Talese had more in common with *New Yorker* writers Lillian Ross and Joseph Mitchell than he did with either of his two contemporaries, and Tom Wolfe was literary kin to J. D. Salinger's Holden Caulfield. Mailer "owes more to past influences than present." Taking a line similar to Wakefield's, Hayes argued that if these three writers constituted a school, then it was a "school of coincidence" and not new at all. Consider Edmund Wilson, James Agee, George Orwell—all used the techniques of fiction as reporters. *The American Mercury, Vanity Fair,* the pre-sixties *Harper's, The New Yorker*—all were full of the kind of journalism now being designated "New."

The truth, Hayes concluded, was that all of these writers were engaged in a venerable form of journalism that could travel under the term "literary journalism," and that was what Old New Journalists like Dwight Macdonald called their work. There was no need to call literary journalism New Journalism just because Old Journalists had never seen it. Old Journalists tried to convey information in a style familiar to their readers. Literary journalists engaged in "conceptual writing," which was something else, but not new. What was new was not the journalism but the writer, exercising his singular originality: "a Mailer, a Talese, a Wolfe."

"Anything goes as long as it is interesting and true," Wakefield had said. If *Esquire* had a program for unleashing all this originality, then the program was having no program, Bob Sherrill believed. Hayes was a lot like Harold Ross, the founder of *The New Yorker,* Sherrill thought—"except smarter and never as boorish. I don't mean he didn't have a deep streak of SOB in him, I mean he wasn't day-after-day a lout. . . . Like Ross, he found these strange, tetchy, bodacious people (I'm not comparing them with Thurber, Woollcott, White, etc.) who fed him ideas, and so on. He made them his own and put them into the magazine. If it was right, he just got out of the way and let it happen, or shepherded it along."

If editorial ideas began falling in line, Hayes would nudge them out of line. Take him a story idea, Sherrill recalled, and he would hold his hand up and slowly turn it: rotate the idea just the right number of degrees to make it unique and therefore *Esquire*'s. He improvised. A young editor who came along later, Lee Eisenberg, would always remember Hayes showing him how to write copy for a spread on the Black Panthers. It was Eisenberg's first feature for *Esquire,* and he approached the subject with mixed feelings. The Panthers' rhetoric bothered him, but, on the other hand, he wasn't a fan of the establishment that the Panthers were terrorizing. He tried headline after headline—maybe fifty in all, all predictable, pedestrian—until, finally, Hayes took over.

Hayes thought for a moment, his lips moving silently as he parsed out the headline in his mind. Then he took a piece of yellow paper and blocked out this question in large letters: "IS IT TOO LATE FOR YOU TO BE PALS WITH A BLACK PANTHER?" Then below that, in smaller letters, he wrote: "Maybe not if you are able to know one when you see one. Test yourself. Take a sharp pencil and cross out those who are not Panthers. Then turn the page for some bad news."

But we don't have a picture, Eisenberg protested.

Hayes reassured him: They would—and none of the people in the picture would be Black Panthers.

Hayes worked with a loose script and made up his lines as he went along. There was nothing careless about the process. He was relentless in his demands for perfection, but his creative mode was improvisational rather than programmatic.

"We weren't locked into any structure," Bob Brown recalled. "Mostly any magazine then and now, if you came up with some great idea, the editor would say, 'That's an interesting idea, but it's not the sort of thing we do.' At *Esquire,* there *was* no sort of thing we do." When Brown read that young Candice Bergen wanted to be a photographer, he wrote her and told her to stop by when she came to New York. By the time she did, she had been hired to star in the movie *The Group.* She had never wanted to be an actress, she told him; she wanted to be a photographer and writer. If she kept a journal of what happened on the set, Brown said, *Esquire* would publish it, and *Esquire* did, under the title "What I Did Last Summer."

Hayes liked surprise: that was one reason he liked to send fiction writers on reporting assignments—who knew what they would come back with? When Brown asked that nice, quiet fiction writer Gina Berriault, out in California, if she would like to try a reporting piece, she came up with a surreal display of topless waitresses, including one, Carol Doda, who had pumped up her breasts with silicone injections. Surprise could come from pairing writers with unlikely subjects. William F. Buckley, Jr., told Dan Wakefield that Hayes had asked him to write an introduction to a special issue on sports, and when Buckley said he didn't know anything about sports, Hayes replied, "That's why we want you." A writer never knows his best idea, Hayes would say. Find an idea that a writer would never write; that's exactly the piece that writer ought to write.

Hayes would give his editors pep talks on originality, urging them, for instance, in a June 24, 1965, memo "not to write to any pre-conceived idea of a form" when they contributed items to a new section that would be called "Adversaria." They should ignore similar sections in *The New Yorker* and *The New Statesman* and write their items as if they were writing comments on the buck sheets they used to comment on manuscripts. Each of them had his own unique tone and point of view. "It is not at all important to sound alike." He suggested they approach their items as he had been taught by military intelligence to interrogate prisoners of war:

"They pick up a dumb-assed buck private from the other side, who would be perfectly willing to tell everything but is in so lowly a position he knows nothing to give away. But the theory is that he knows much more than he is aware that he knows, and the trick to withdrawing helpful information from him is to review what he takes for granted is *not* information or knowledge. With patient handling, he is capable of sealing the defeat of all nations."

That was Hayes's approach to the whole magazine—the great secret, Sam Antupit thought, of his success at *Esquire:* he took what was known and, "with patient handling," teased out of it something unknown. Although sometimes he gave writers no special advice, leaving them to follow their own instincts, at other times he wrote assignment letters like the one he sent Richard Rovere on Joe McCarthy—carefully positioning the subject for the writer. If the writer turned in a piece that did not rise to Hayes's expectations, Hayes was capable of tinkering with the idea at length, hoping to get the writer to see what was wrong. When *Esquire's* records columnist, Martin Mayer, turned in an article on Leonard Bernstein that Hayes wasn't happy with, Hayes talked with him first, and then wrote him a four-page letter, insisting, "on the grounds of our long friendship," that Mayer pay attention to him.

The piece wasn't bad, he explained—he had asked Dobell to read it,

too, and Dobell had confirmed his own reaction: "Not a very penetrating
job, but one we won't be embarrassed to publish. Right. Which is exactly
what I *didn't* want. . . ." When they had first talked about this idea,
Mayer had been dazzling—Hayes had thought he would have difficulty
finding space for Mayer to say all he wanted to say. Now Hayes was
disappointed. He launched into a detailed critique, beginning with
Mayer's overhasty introduction of Bernstein's biography before the reader
had reason to care about it. Then he moved on to his second major objection:

> . . . I don't understand the nature of his talent. Stern says it is so great it frightens
> him. Reiner says he was the most talented of his students (but not as a conductor).
> You say he won't be remembered as a composer, and there's plenty wrong with
> his conducting. He's fine with contemporary 20th century music; he has a fine
> sense of complex rhythms; and there's that hocus pocus word, rayonnement, or
> projection. Like stage presence? Is that all there is to his talent? What could there
> possibly be to this that would frighten a man like Stern? (And why, oh why, didn't
> you give me some inner assurance that you poured lots of that high-level, three-
> hour chat with Stern into the piece? Maybe you did, but I don't get that feeling.)

He went on in that vein, until finally he said: "I guess an inherent flaw
for me is that you yourself don't really seem to have resolved Bernstein in
your own mind."

He wrote the letter on a Saturday, and he was still worrying over it that
evening when he ran into two conductors at a party. He talked with them
("off the record of course") about Bernstein's talent; then he passed on to
Mayer the substance of the conversation.

"Martin, damn it," Hayes said. "Go back to work on this piece. I can
give you ten days, maybe a little more. Approach it, please, as though
you'll never have another chance to profile Bernstein. If you need to do
more research, do so. I have closed the color illustration. I will take what
you give me, but I don't feel assured that you have as yet given me your
best."

Hayes could give a writer extraordinary backing—writing letters, making calls, clearing the way, as if the *Esquire* office were a support unit for
soldiers in battle. Writers would call him and report on what they were
turning up and he would say, "Fine, fine, wonderful." If they needed it, he
would run interference. He would love what they were getting and urge
them on. He gave them the feeling that writing for him was a personal act.

But when the manuscript came in, Hayes turned into what he believed
the editor must be: "representative for the harshest, most demanding

reader the writer would address." Sometimes he would dismiss a manuscript abruptly: "This stinks," he would say, and return it to the assigning
editor. (But please, he asked his editors once, don't pass on those exact
words to the writer.) *Esquire* killed 50 percent of articles assigned, Byron
Dobell recalled—a high rate. The policy was not to spend a lot of time
rewriting and editing to get a marginal manuscript into publishable shape.
Gingrich had always said that the editor edits best who edits least. Even if
a good writer was not writing well, it was presumptuous of the editor to
take pen in hand: better to talk the problems out with the writer until the
writer understood them and could fix them himself. If Hayes wanted a
piece—if he believed the writer was good and the piece could be good, or
(as happened often enough) if he had saved space for it in an issue—then
he would step into the ring and wrestle with the author.

Tom Wolfe described Hayes as editor-at-work in a letter he wrote to
Hayes on August 27, 1976, after Hayes had sent him a manuscript for a
book he had written on East Africa, *The Last Place on Earth.* Checking
off the many things he liked about the book—"wonderful things"—Wolfe
said:

And THEN I say to myself . . . "You know, what this book needs at this point,
before it is committed to the printer's hands, is a good going over by a skillful
editor who can clear out some of the tangles and the Lazy Writer spots, an editor
like that guy who used to star at *Esquire,* that guy who really knew how to cut the
fat off a manuscript and display the writer's choice cuts (right in the face of the
writer's own mindless attachment to certain pet but repetitive and irrelevant
passages)—that guy HAYES."

Harold, goddamn it, you've got to put that manuscript down on your desk,
turn around, walk to the other side of the room, speak softly to the wall or the
woodwork, saying: "I, Hayes, artist and philosopher, am now residing on top of
the desk across the room in the transmogrified state of *manuscript.* When I turn
around, I, through astral projection, will have become Hayes the Now-Legendary
Editor, and I am going to approach Hayes the Artist and Philosopher, who is on
that desk, with the same fierce visage that used to move 'em and shake 'em when
I walked down the aisles at *Esquire."* (For it is true, there are those who quaked,
because they knew Play Period was now over! This IS real life!)

Almost three decades later, Norman Mailer could recall the experience of confronting Hayes's editorial eye. He told Dan Wakefield, "He
was like a doctor poking his finger in a part of your body, like poking very
unhealthy tissue, and he did it so it hurt, the place where he poked really
hurt."

Hayes was no respecter of friendship—if anything, as in the case of

Mayer on Bernstein, friendship with the writer made him more critical, more determined to get the writer's best out of him. Hayes had "a long and powerful relationship" with Peter Bogdanovich, according to Robert Benton, who worked with Bogdanovich later when both had become movie directors. In 1965, Bogdanovich had left the Museum of Modern Art for Hollywood, but before he left, he would come by for Friday-night drinks at Hayes's office, and Hayes had looked on him as *Esquire*'s expert on film. Later on, as *Esquire*'s Hollywood representative (he could get into screenings free that way), he wrote several pieces for *Esquire*, but one piece Hayes killed—a profile of Sonny and Cher. Bogdanovich was angry about the editorial response, and wrote Hayes a long letter defending the piece as the story of two people who had gotten what they wanted— fame—and found it empty. Bogdanovich revised the piece in an effort to get it through, and Hayes said it was better, but he still rejected it. Hayes never let friendship sway his editorial judgment, Gingrich once wrote Helen Lawrenson; he had a "whim of iron."

Many of the writers Hayes worked with admired him and understood his gifts as an editor, especially as years passed and they never encountered any other editor as good. Few, in fact, could count themselves his personal friends. Hayes kept his distance. His longtime friend Bob Sherrill thought circumstances had a lot to do with that: he simply did not have much time to devote to friendship. But in Hayes's comments on the writer-editor relationship, Hayes kept friendship firmly apart. Once, later on, he angered William Humphrey by leaving him out of an ad featuring *Esquire* authors—a disloyal act, Humphrey thought, that required an end to both his relationship with *Esquire* and his friendship with Hayes.

Hayes protested:

As an editor, my responsibility to you or any other writer is to respect your problems and authority as a writer, nothing more. I have no obligation to choose you or anyone else for any list on the basis of our friendship (*especially* on the basis of our friendship). It is not a question of my loyalty to you as a friend, or as an editor. My loyalty as an editor is reserved for the protection of your interests in publishing you—against advertisers, or management, or newsstand promoters or, as is sometimes the case, against those who disagree with my judgement about publishing you at all. My loyalty to you as a friend rests solely upon my interest in you as an individual I have come to respect and enjoy.

Clearly stung, Hayes defended his selection of writers for the ad, then said, "It never occurred to me that our friendship rested on my willingness to put you forward under any and all circumstances that might arise in my role as editor of this magazine. That's not loyalty, it's sycophancy."

On more than one occasion, Hayes rejected the Max Perkins model of the editor as pal—the model Gingrich had followed. An editor needed to keep writers off-balance—to be seen as unpredictable, he said once, and thus without limitations. As an editor, he was playing a role: straight man to the writer, countering the writer's vanity with indifference, the writer's loss of faith with confidence, shifting his own position to counter the shifting moods of the writer. How could editor and writer be friends? Only a few writers crossed the line over to friendship with Hayes: Peter Bogdanovich, Martin Mayer, and, closer than any, Gay Talese, whose life would have been substantially different without him.

Talese had quit the *New York Times* in the spring of 1965, and was now writing for *Esquire* for $15,000 a year—less than he had been making at the *Times,* but enough, and better pay than *Esquire* was offering to anyone else for assigned pieces. His first piece under contract was a profile of the *Times'* obituary writer, Alden Whitman, a kindly piece, in which, over Whitman's objection, Talese revealed that Whitman's teeth were all false; he had lost his own teeth in an attack in an alley back in 1936. Whitman had not been as cooperative as he might have been: he would not let Talese see obituaries he had written for people not yet dead. Talese's second subject as contract writer turned out to be exponentially more difficult.

Hayes had set up the job for Talese, or thought he had. It was a delicate matter. *Esquire* had approached Frank Sinatra's representatives several times over recent years, asking if Sinatra would cooperate on a story. Always the answer had come back: only if Sinatra could approve the manuscript. And always *Esquire,* unwilling to accept that condition, would turn away. Now, in late 1965, Hayes thought he had broken through the impasse. He had talked several times with Sinatra's agent, Jim Mahoney, and he thought Mahoney liked the idea of a major piece, in Hayes's terms, a "definitive profile." To produce it, Hayes explained to Mahoney, Talese would need access to Sinatra because Talese preferred observing to interviewing. Hayes promised in writing that this would not be "a 'hatchet' job." *Esquire* would accept any areas of Sinatra's life that Sinatra wanted to designate off-limits. But Hayes would still not let Sinatra read the piece before publishing.

Hayes thought the prospects were sufficiently promising to send Talese to Los Angeles. Talese arrived on a Wednesday evening, November 3, 1965, checked into the hotel, and settled down with a steak, a bottle of wine, and a packet of background material. For two weeks, he played cat and mouse with Sinatra. He kept Hayes informed of what was going on, portraying himself as frozen out of a town where Frank Sinatra seemed to wield awesome power, even controlling the menus in Italian restaurants. When further interventions by Hayes did not unlock the door, Hayes finally had had enough. On November 16, he dictated an angry letter to Sinatra's agent, Mahoney:

I am most distressed by the manner in which you have operated in processing our request for an interview with Frank Sinatra, and I really don't think I ought to let your actions go by unrecorded and without complaint.

You will recall that *Esquire* has, over the past few years, expressed an interest in doing a story on Mr. Sinatra. Upon requesting cooperation from Mr. Sinatra's representatives, however, we have always been informed that Mr. Sinatra would not cooperate without assurance from the magazine that he would have a chance to approve the manuscript. On each of these occasions, then, we have withdrawn our request.

Recently, however, I was led by you to believe you would welcome an assignment by *Esquire* to Gay Talese to prepare a major story. In each of our several conversations, we discussed the question of manuscript approval, and I repeated our policy on this matter. Finally, two weeks ago, when the possibility of assigning Talese was imminent, we attempted to resolve this problem. You said you had a responsibility to your client; I said I had a responsibility to my magazine. You said you understood my position, and I said I understood yours. Fine, up to this point. But then, you said, or words to the effect:

"What could I tell Frank?"

And I said:

"Why don't you tell him exactly what I am proposing—that we are not out to do a hatchet job on him, and that we will abide religiously by any reservations or restrictions you may care to place on the writer and magazine—that is, any area you indicate as 'off the record' will not be touched upon."

You said that seemed reasonable to you, and then I asked—twice, I believe, because our movements from this point forward involved a considerable outlay of expense money—if you were sure this was a sound approach from your end. You said yes, and on the strength of that decision, I sent Talese to California.

This morning, thirteen days and some $1500 later, I have just received confirmation from Talese that our request for time with Mr. Sinatra has been denied. And that, further, Talese is not to be allowed on the set of the film Mr. Sinatra is preparing (even though he's finished shooting). And that, by implication, he is not to expect cooperation in preparing a story from any person close to, or sympathetic with, Mr. Sinatra.

As I told you earlier, it was our intention—and still is—to prepare a favorable story on Mr. Sinatra. We will now proceed on this story without your cooperation, and presumably without Mr. Sinatra's, since I can only assume from what you have told Talese over the last few days that, somehow, this *contretemps* is all our making, and that you are damned sore that we've put you in such a position with your boss, and by extension, he's sore too.

Let me assure you that I'm not sore, but I do feel I've gained some insight into the way the ball bounces at Jim Mahoney Associates.

There probably ought to be a squadron of seeing-eye dogs assigned to those of us back here in the East, groping our way through the great Western darkness. In lieu of such, however, I think the most humane gesture I could make would be this modest notification to some of my colleagues of the general vicinity of at least some of the things that go bump in the night.

He cc'ed the letter to the editors of *McCall's, Saturday Evening Post, Holiday,* and *Redbook,* and to Gay Talese and Frank Sinatra.

Sinatra eventually did let Talese into his dressing room—he even let Talese watch him take off his toupee—but that was three weeks into the story, and expenses were mounting. Talese offered to share the costs.

"It's a real gamble for you, I realize," he wrote Hayes, "and yet I have a feeling that things will work out. I may not get the piece we'd hoped for—the Real Frank Sinatra . . . but perhaps, by not getting it—and by getting rejected constantly and by seeing his flunkies protecting his flanks—we will be getting close to the truth about the man . . ."

He turned that intuition into the theme of his story, "Frank Sinatra Has a Cold"—Sinatra's effect on the lives that revolved around him. The charm of the piece derived from the perfect match: two crooners, Gay Talese on Frank Sinatra, who had given America "music to make love by, and doubtless much love was made by it all over America at night in cars, while the batteries burned down, in cottages by the lake, on beaches during balmy summer evenings, in secluded parks and exclusive penthouses and furnished rooms; in cabin cruisers and cabs and cabanas—in all places where Sinatra's songs could be heard were these words that warmed women, wooed and won them, snipped the final thread of inhibition and gratified the male egos of ungrateful lovers; two generations of men had been the beneficiaries of such ballads, for which they were eternally in his debt, for which they may eternally hate him."

It was one of the best of a parade of *Esquire* pieces that paid homage to the great stars whose lights were dimming—the music and movie and sports heroes of the thirties and forties. It was as good as it was partly because Talese wrote it, and partly because Hayes gave him what he needed to write it. In 1987, in his introduction to *Best American Essays,* Talese looked back at the time and research and money he had spent on that Sinatra piece—close to $5,000 of *Esquire's* money and three months on research and writing—and noticed how things had changed in the magazine world. Editors had become less willing to underwrite such detailed reporting, and writers had become more reluctant to undertake it. Writers satisfied themselves, instead, with transcribing their tape-recorded interviews and passing their collected quotations off as profiles, which were acceptable to editors because they were cheap. What editor in these later times was willing to compensate a thoughtful writer to spend six weeks just writing a piece, after the research, as Talese had spent writing "Sinatra"?

Without the kind of financial support Hayes had provided, a magazine writer could not afford to do the kind of reporting Talese's pieces required: "lingering and careful listening and describing scenes that offer insight into the individual's character and personality"—the method that became identified with "New Journalism," although it contained, as Talese noted, a component of the Old Journalism: "tireless legwork and fidelity to factual accuracy."

After Sinatra, Talese pursued Joe DiMaggio, the great baseball player who had been his own boyhood hero, and who had also been married, for a time, to Marilyn Monroe. DiMaggio was not, at first, any more cooperative. This time Talese put some of his troubles into the piece, introducing himself into the story as a man DiMaggio "did not wish to see." DiMaggio's attempts to evade him became part of the plot, DiMaggio's ambivalence toward the limelight a theme of the story. *Esquire* gave the piece a title so inspired that two editors, Bob Brown and Byron Dobell, would later lay claim to it:

"Joe," Said Marilyn Monroe, Just Back from Korea, "You Never Heard Such Cheering."
"Yes, I Have," Joe DiMaggio Answered.

At Hayes's suggestion, Talese turned next to Clifton Daniel, the managing editor of the *New York Times*—it was a case, Talese supposed, of one editor from North Carolina eyeing another editor from North Carolina. Bob Brown came up with the title: "The Kingdoms, the Powers, and the Glories of the *New York Times*" (November 1966), and set Talese on a track of biblical titles. In the end, Talese did three *Esquire* pieces on *New York Times* men, and they became the start of a book on the *Times, The Kingdom and the Power,* a rich, detailed narrative of life at the nation's leading newspaper. It was a history like no other, moving inside minds and through the cobwebby thicket of daily life with the assurance Talese had earned at *Esquire* and the assurance, too, of a writer who really knew what he was talking about—this time not because he had gone in as an observer and lingered on the margins, but because he had been part of the action. He would say later, "I was right there sitting in the center of the story, on Forty-third Street. I was right there, I wasn't working for the Washington bureau or coming back every two years. I was there, and I saw the change."

The Kingdom and the Power, published in 1969, put Talese over the top as a best-selling author. After his next book, *Honor Thy Father* (1971), an account of life inside a Mafia family, Doubleday gave him a contract for his next two books that carried a $1.2-million advance. *Esquire* would have the opportunity to publish excerpts from *Honor Thy Father* and did, but Talese was no longer on call for assignments. He and Hayes remained friends and Hayes remained, in a sense, his editor, providing a detailed critique of *Honor Thy Father,* as he would later provide one for Tom Wolfe's *The Right Stuff* and *Bonfire of the Vanities.* Hayes would write about Talese's rise to prominence as a writer with apparent pride in the role *Esquire* had played. Although Talese would have become a respected journalist in New York City if he had stayed at the *Times,* he would not have been able to push his talents to their limits, Hayes said; he would not have become one of the best and best-paid journalists in the nation.

"Writers need editors," Hayes wrote—and magazines provide writers with the environment in which a symbiotic relationship can develop between writers and editors. Not only can editors give writers evaluation after the fact; they can, if they are imaginative, provide better subjects than the writers can come up with themselves—most of the ideas for Talese's articles had come from editors at *Esquire.* The magazine editor "holds the writer's hand as he works on voice, structure, syntax and the more complex techniques of prose which he will need to advance in his profession."

Hayes made a less definable contribution to Talese's work as well: he provided an editorial attitude that suited Talese. Hayes brought to New York a wide-open view of the North's racial hypocrisy and of New Yorkers' vanity and pretense, Talese believed. "He was an Anglo-Saxon Protestant, but he was from the South. Therefore, he was the majority's minority." He brought that outsider's stance to *Esquire*, Talese thought—small-town, in a way, not sardonic or cynical—and it became the stance of those who worked with him.

"He was the only editor that played a role in my life, and I never had anyone like that before or since," Talese would say. But he also said, "I had a very tricky relationship with him. A lot of love was there, and a lot of mistrust was there. I never trusted him. Because he was tricky. He looked like a wolf. He had that tricky eye, he was selling you something. He was coming to town with a wagon full of snake oil, and he was going to do the huckstering, and you were going to be the buyer, he hoped, and I'd buy a little bit, but I didn't want to buy the whole carton, the whole wagon load of his shit, I didn't want to buy that.

"I liked him. And I loved him in a way. And I liked working for him, I loved working for him."

Part Two

What? Has it really been just six years, or are we all
going crazy? It seems like it's been the Sixties *forever*. . . .
We have had enough! Enough! . . . Let six years be a
decade. Let the next four be a vacation.

ROBERT BENTON AND DAVID NEWMAN, *Esquire,* AUGUST 1966

SIX

History All Around

*I*N THE FALL OF 1965, John Sack, former CBS bureau chief at Madrid, was sitting around CBS in New York without very much to do but read magazines. He would sign up for whatever office magazine he wanted to read, and when he got finished reading the magazine, he would cross off his name and a mail boy would deliver it to the next name on the list. The routine varied for only one magazine: *Esquire,* which had to be passed around in an interoffice envelope—otherwise the mail boys would divert it.

One day toward the end of October, Sack was reading *Time* magazine, and he came to an article that described soldiers getting off a troop ship in Vietnam as "lean, laconic, and looking for a fight." He didn't believe it. He had been a soldier in Korea. A night or two after he read the *Time* article, Sack woke up in his apartment on East 63rd Street at four o'clock in the morning, and he knew what he was going to do. He would do the same thing he had done in his book on the Korean War, *From Here to Shimbashi*—he would follow a company through infantry training into their first combat in Vietnam. Now that he thought of it, it seemed obvious—the only way to report a war, the way Mailer did it in *The Naked and the Dead,* the way Joseph Heller did it in *Catch-22:* show soldiers in a context readers can identify with, then follow them into the strange world of war.

He would do it as a documentary for CBS News—then he had second thoughts. As soon as he proposed the idea he would be told, "Great idea, you're the associate producer." He could guess how the producer in charge would do the piece, and he wanted none of it. Better he should take a leave of absence from CBS, and write the story as an article for *Esquire*.

On October 25, he wrote to Harold Hayes, as chattily—although they had met only once—as if they were buddies.

"All right, it happened, after four happy years as a writer, producer, and special correspondent there is something I want to just plain write.

"It's this. I just can't bring myself to believe in the soldiers said to be doing duty for us in Vietnam." He mentioned *Time,* he mentioned the afternoon paper, he even mentioned *Esquire,* which had somewhere called the soldiers "cool." "Where in this outfit is Beetle Bailey? Willie and Joe? Dammit, I know they're there . . . where is Private Hargrove?

"Look, this is the Army, I've got to assume that a couple of things are still snafu, that the cooks are getting eggshells in the scrambled eggs, that the back-of-the-barracks conversation is about making it with girls, that a sergeant's most awful anxiety is over the sheen of his combat boots, that one or two privates haven't learned dress-right-dress from right-about march, that a certain number of them haven't the foggiest of where Vietnam is or why they're going there. . . ."

Why wasn't anyone saying anything about the "sad sacks, boneheads, goldbricks, loudmouths, paranoiacs, catatonics, incompetents, semi-conscientious objectors, malingerers, cry-babies, yahoos, vulgarians, big time operators, butterfingers, sadists, and surly bastards"?

Would Hayes give him an assignment to follow a company into Vietnam?

Hayes answered right away:

> Dear John,
> Jesus Christ, how much would all this cost?

A thousand dollars? suggested Sack, going for what he thought he could get.

By early January 1966 he was out at Fort Dix, New Jersey, on assignment for *Esquire.* By the second day, he was glad he had not done the story for CBS News. No one on the base was talking about Vietnam. Everyone was more concerned with the captain's inspection on Saturday, or getting off on the weekend. Vietnam never came up, except now and then when a sergeant would say, "You'd better shape up because you're going to Vietnam." And everybody would just groan.

If he were working on the story under a CBS producer, after one day with the company the producer would come back shaking his head and saying, "No one's saying anything about Vietnam, they're not talking about Vietnam."

And Sack would say, "Yes, that's the whole story."

The producer might give it another day, and on the second day when nobody was saying anything about Vietnam he would break into a sweat. His face would turn red, and he would say, "We've gotta get in there with a correspondent." And he'd have Charlie Kuralt go up to the soldiers and say, "Well, in one month you're going to Vietnam. What do you think about that?"

Sack was glad he was writing the story for *Esquire.* Like the television producer he was, he passed his days at camp collecting scenes: M Company firing its first real ammunition in a mock attack—guns stalling, guns going off, soldiers running in front of other soldiers with loaded and unpredictable guns. He went around scribbling notes and thinking he'd walked into a goldmine. He'd clutch his notebooks and say, "It's gold, it's gold."

The story was falling into place just as he imagined it—a gallery of real, true enlisted men was taking shape in front of his eyes. There was Demirgian, who wanted more than anything else to get out of the army—he even hired a former policeman to break his jaw. Then someone said, just in time, that a broken jaw wouldn't get him out of the army. He'd have to break his foot. "Can you break my foot?" There was Mason, a Harlem street-fighter who figured he had the skills to come out of Vietnam alive. There was Smith, a God-fearing farmboy who wanted to be a minister and joined the army to test his ability to follow the Lord's will and *not to kill.*

Sack's plan was to go with the company on its first operation, and that would be the end of the article. He flew with the men to Saigon and rode with the company up country. For the first operation helicopters were going to take M Company into a Michelin rubber plantation. M expected the plantation to be wired just for them—staked with poisoned bamboo, mined with explosives. When the time came to board a helicopter, Sack changed his mind. Under ordinary circumstances he was a fit, cheerful, confident man. But the prospect seemed a lot more dangerous than anything he'd been through in Korea. He went out to the airstrip to see the guys off and ran into Dan Rather, who had worked with him at CBS. "Don't worry about it, you'll be okay," Rather told him. Sack climbed into a helicopter.

The operation began on Monday; it was Friday before, as Sack wrote later, "M's battalion killed somebody, at last." A soldier tossed a grenade into what looked like a bunker, and the grenade exploded inside. A dozen or so women and children came running out, screaming, but no one seemed hurt.

. . . A Negro specialist-four, his black rifle in his hands, warily extended his head in, peering through the darkness one or two seconds before he cried, *"Oh my god!"*
"What's the matter," said a second specialist. . . .
"They hit a little girl," and in his muscular black arms the first specialist carried out a seven-year-old, long black hair and little earrings, staring eyes—*eyes*, her eyes are what froze themselves onto M's memory, it seemed there was no white to those eyes, nothing but black ellipses like black goldfish. The child's nose was bleeding—there was a hole in the back of her skull.

She died moments later.
Back at the brigade, Sack apologized to an officer, a lieutenant colonel. "You know," explained Sack, "I'm really sorry, the plan was to get with this company, hang out with it, go on this first operation, and the book would end there. But the first operation was a big mess. That's the story, and I'm stuck with it. I know it isn't typical."
The officer thought a second or two, then said, "It's typical."
Sack couldn't believe it. He couldn't believe that with this vast army in Vietnam—with thousands of flights landing and taking off every day from the airport at Tan Son Nhut—the result would be the death of seven-year-old girls. He just couldn't believe it.
As he wrote the article out by hand back in Saigon, at the Hotel Continental, he still supported the war. He thought it was a bad war, but he thought the United States had to fight it. He had grown up during World War II, and served in Korea, and he had never heard anybody suggest that America might fight a war that it shouldn't fight. He wrote in an ironic mode, the beginning light as a literate sitcom, the middle mock heroic as Company M embarked on the ancient ship of war, the ending a black comedy:

The captains told their lieutenants, don't burn those houses if there's no VC in them—the lieutenants told their sergeants, if you burn those houses there better be VC in them—the sergeants told their men, better go burn those houses because there's VC in them, and Morton kept striking his C-ration matches.

He sent the first half of the article to Candida Donadio, his agent, to see if she thought he could turn the article into a book, and then he ran across an article that Michael Herr had written on Fort Dix for *Holiday* magazine. Reading Herr's piece Sack realized he had left out something important—description. He had been so used to writing television documentaries that he had forgotten there would be no camera to show his readers the scenes. He had produced a narrative bare to the bone. He started going back through the manuscript putting in sentences to describe the people and places. He still hadn't heard from Donadio by the time he had finished the whole article, so he sent it all in to her and to Hayes. He heard back from her first. She had read the first half, she said, and she didn't think there was a book in it.

So he had failed. What he had tried to do hadn't worked. He wasn't really despondent about it. He still had a job making more money than a book would earn. He just thought: I've tried, I've failed. It was a good try. The next day a cable came from Harold Hayes. *Esquire* liked the article. It would run in the next possible issue.

Now Hayes wanted pictures of Company M.

Sack borrowed a camera from a photographer who worked for Associated Press and joined the company for a helicopter assault. So deep was he into this story by now that the night before they went out he found himself thinking, tears in his eyes, that the most wonderful thing he could do would be die with these men the next morning. He did jump out of the helicopter first when it landed so he could get pictures of the guys coming out, but there was nobody around to shoot at him. He took hundreds of pictures and sent them in; *Esquire* didn't use any of them.

On June 21, another cable came from Hayes: "Stringent invasion of privacy legal problems must be corrected at source." Hayes asked Sack to call him. When he did, Hayes told him the plan: *Esquire*'s lawyer wanted Sack to get releases from the ten major characters in the story. Then if any of the others took *Esquire* to court, the lawyer would use the ten releases to demonstrate the faith the more important figures had in Sack and undercut the credibility of complaints.

By this time, M Company had moved into War Zone C, on the Cambodian border—a really dangerous area. Not all of the men Sack had written about were in Zone C, but two important ones were. The only way to get there was by helicopter. To reserve the press helicopter, Sack had to come up with four other journalists who wanted to go where he wanted to go. The first was easy. He had a French girlfriend, a baroness, and she had shown up in Saigon one day, equipped herself with press credentials and a tailor-made tiger suit, and set about covering the war. She would make one of the five. He learned that a big cache of rice was about to be burned in War Zone C—obviously good television. He went to Dan Rather.

"They're going to burn the biggest cache of rice they've ever found. We *hope* it's VC rice."

Rather thought about it and said he would come along. With a sound-man and a cameraman that made five. Sack reserved the press helicopter for early in the morning.

The five of them showed up and told the pilot they wanted to go to War Zone C.

No way, said he.

But it was his job to take them where they wanted to go, Sack argued.

The pilot reflected. Look, he said, it's too hot, it's too dangerous. I'll get you in, I'll just touch the ground and you jump out and I'll fly out immediately. You're going to have to find your own way out.

They flew in, right up on the Cambodian border, and as they landed, machine-gun fire sent a .50-caliber bullet through one of the blades. The helicopter touched down, they all jumped out, the helicopter lifted off.

As Rather and his crew and the Baroness went on down the road where the rice was supposed to be, the two men Sack came to see showed up. They signed the releases, and when a brigadier general landed in a small bubble helicopter to check out the scene, Sack hitched a ride back to Saigon with him. The Baroness, Rather, and his crew would have to find their own way home.

Sack was back in Saigon by lunchtime. Around five in the afternoon, he sat down at the Hotel Continental to have a beer with a friend, a radio correspondent. Sack told him about leaving the Baroness and Rather behind, and his friend said, "Aren't you worried about these people?"

Not at all, Sack assured him. He predicted that within the next hour the Baroness would come walking up in her tailor-made tiger suit saying, "How could you do this to me? How could you leave me there? How could you abandon me with all of the people shooting the machines at me? This is a terrible thing—you call yourself a friend."

"I'd be worried," said his friend.

"No," said Sack, "I promise you."

About half an hour later the Baroness walked across the square in her tiger suit, stomped up to Sack, and said, "How could you do this? I have dinner tonight with the French ambassador, it's a dress party, I have to get my hair done, it is six o'clock, I do not have time to put on my dress and my makeup. How could you do this?"

In spite of what he had already seen in Vietnam, Sack could still laugh. He still had not fully understood what it all meant. He understood there were no iron-jawed heroes—he did not yet understand the horror, the wrongness of the war. When he talked with Hayes about a cover for his story, Sack suggested getting a color photograph of helicopters landing and soldiers jumping out, and over the face of each soldier, painting or gluing the face of Beetle Bailey.

"No," Hayes said, "you don't understand your article at all."

The cover George Lois would create for "M" would be large white words on a black background:

"OH MY GOD—WE HIT A LITTLE GIRL."

Then, across the bottom, in smaller type:

THE TRUE STORY OF M COMPANY.
FROM FORT DIX TO VIETNAM.

Esquire's Vietnam articles in the preceding months had treated the war with skeptical humor: "An Armchair Guide to Guerrilla Warfare" or, as a cover for a campus issue, Jerry Lewis putting on lipstick ("How our red blooded campus heroes are beating the draft"). In austere black and white, the "M" cover was like a formal announcement of a change of heart.

After Sack got back to New York, *Esquire* gave a party for him in the offices, and Candida Donadio came. She had read the second half of the article by then and could see there really was a book here. She sold it to the New American Library and Sack spent the rest of the summer writing the book on Fire Island, then finishing up back at his apartment on East 63rd Street. "M" appeared in the October issue, 1966; Sack's father died on October 7, three days before the book manuscript was due—he was making final changes at the funeral. Later, basking in the Indian summer, sitting with friends at the cafe at the Central Park Zoo, he began to feel like a deserter. The *New York Times Book Review* even wrote a little item about him in a roundup of publishing news: Company M was still in Vietnam but John Sack was in New York. Sack told Hayes he wanted to go back and write about M's last battle.

By the time he got to Vietnam late that fall, the men were so close to

ending their tour of duty that they were being kept out of the fighting, but
Sack interviewed Demirgian and others who were around and visited the
scenes of the stories they described. Then he reconstructed a night when
Demirgian slept through an attack on his own nearby camp. Demirgian,
who had once wanted out so badly he had asked another soldier to break
his foot, had become obsessed with the idea of—finally—killing a Communist, but he had slept on as a squad of Communists went by on the
trail. He woke up to learn he had missed the whole battle, his last chance.
As he walked past the Communist dead, one moved an arm.

A living breathing communist, a boy of about eighteen, a Vietnamese in black,
Demirgian brought down his foot on his face and *crunch,* Demirgian felt his little
nose go like a macaroon, he said to the communist, "Bastard—well, was it worth
it," kicking him in his eyeballs. "Stupid bastard—what did it get you," kicking
him on his Adam's apple. "Goddamn bastard. . . ."

Finally, the boy was dead.

"Well," Demirgian said to another soldier, "I finally killed me a gook," and
Demirgian smiled satisfiedly, Demirgian's soul was at peace, Demirgian, a little
later, had started back to the country in whose interests he had been posted to
Asia, to his green gabled home in Newton, to the sign in the living room *welcome
home* in red, white, and blue! Safe and sound, Demirgian came marching home
again! Let's give him a hearty welcome then! Hurrah! Hurrah!

In "M," the American men were still innocents, stumbling into a
black comedy. "When Demirgian Comes Marching Home Again. (Hurray? Hurrah?)" was an infinitely more bitter story. The comic-strip out-
lines of "M" had disappeared. Sack was no longer describing soldiers who
inflicted death by chance, but soldiers who had learned to hate. The story
builds to the revelation of "Demirgian's Secret":

Demirgian hates the Vietnamese people—well, so does every soldier, but Demirgian hates and hates! The goddam bastards! Goddam people! Come to help their
miserable country and what? Anyone get a word of thanks? Dead or alive—
crippled, I could be blind, a basket case and they wouldn't care, not if they'd had
my damn piastres first! Money is all they'd care, the crooked bastards! . . . A really
and truly detestable race of people. Demirgian's year of duty among the Vietnamese had taught him to loathe them, the earth and Demirgian would be better
rid of them, Vietnamese go to your damnable ancestors, die! Demirgian wants to
kill communists because they're the only native people the Army's regulations
allow him to kill.

By the time John Sack's "M" appeared in *Esquire* in October 1966, American troops in Vietnam outnumbered South Vietnamese and opposition to the war was rising sharply. Other magazines not conceived as political had stepped into the fray. The *New York Review of Books* was raising questions about the war in a barrage of articles, bringing out I. F. Stone, America's leading iconoclast, to lead the charge. On the West Coast, *Ramparts*, once a small lay Catholic literary magazine, featured Special Forces Master Sergeant Donald W. Duncan on its February 1966 cover, bedecked with Bronze Star and other medals, announcing "I quit! The whole thing was a lie!"

Faith in the credibility of the American government, already put severely to test by the war, was being tried on another front. Speculation over the assassination of President John F. Kennedy had turned into a national parlor game, played for serious stakes. The Warren Commission Report, which Dwight Macdonald reviewed at length in the March 1965 *Esquire*, had simply set more wheels turning. *Esquire* collected a whole set of assassination theories for the December 1966 issue and was working on a second set.

Of the three principals in the Dallas drama, only Jack Ruby survived, his killing of Oswald still a major mystery. It was an act that, no matter how Ruby explained it, remained unaccountable. Why had this very ordinary apolitical man, the owner of a Dallas nightclub, gunned Oswald down in full view of police and millions of witnesses watching on television? Hayes wanted Ruby's story, and he put the proposition to Garry Wills in a single sentence: "Make a human being out of Jack Ruby . . ."

Garry Wills was never sure why Hayes thought he was the man to send to Dallas at the end of 1966 to write about Jack Ruby: maybe because Hayes liked the way Wills did scenes in the profile of William F. Buckley that Buckley himself sent over to Hayes. Wills had been writing reviews for Buckley's *National Review;* his review of James Baldwin's *The Fire Next Time* had been "very possibly our finest hour," Buckley said.

A classics professor at Johns Hopkins University in Baltimore, Wills was an unlikely writer for *Esquire*—and certainly an unlikely writer for a piece on Jack Ruby, the man convicted of shooting Lee Harvey Oswald. But Hayes spotted in the Buckley piece a reporter's eye at work. Wills had not actually had much experience as a reporter, but he would be working with a great investigative reporter, Ovid Demaris, who knew Dallas, the underworld, and Las Vegas, and had been standing near Ruby at the mo-

ment Ruby shot Oswald. Demaris had taped interviews then with people
Ruby knew but had not done anything with the tapes until three years
later when Wills showed up in Dallas. For a week before Wills got there,
Demaris looked up his sources and taped new interviews.

When Wills got to Dallas, Demaris gave him the bad news: they could
not get to Jack Ruby, who was dying in Parkland Hospital. But there was
this good news, too: "I've got these wonderful tapes of all these other
people. Sit down and listen." So Wills sat down and listened to the voices
of people who had known Jack Ruby—among them the strippers who
worked in his club, the Carousel. Then he called Hayes and filled him in
on the situation: no interview with Ruby, but all these other interviews.
Hayes liked the sound of it; they should proceed with the story.

They did, operating from radically different premises. Demaris believed a conspiracy lay behind the assassination. Wills, on the other hand,
had read everything the Warren Commission Report said about Jack
Ruby, and he did not believe the conspiracy theories. It didn't matter.
Together they retraced the steps of Ruby's daily life, talking to the people
who knew him well; and many seemed to know him well—he was a socia-
ble man, immersed in a world that for all its meanness was intensely social.
They spent days in lawyers' offices and nights in nightclubs. The Wills-
Demaris partnership was, Demaris would say, a marriage "like the kind
that used to be made in heaven." He enjoyed watching Wills enjoy himself, as when a drummer named Bill Willis was telling them stories in a
stripper's dressing room while Wills sat "yogi-style inside a tiny doorless
closet in a tiny room, a sleazy red dress brushing against his head every
time he rocked in laughter."

Who could have predicted the ease with which Wills settled into Jack
Ruby's world? Not only was the writing not hard, but Wills found himself
having fun. All those Dickensian characters—they leaped right out at
him. Years later he would still remember one of Ruby's lawyers, out with
Demaris and Wills at a nightclub, blowing his nose on paper napkins, then
on the doilies that came with the drinks, and finally, in desperation, on the
little paper packets the sugar came in, "the detritus of this extraordinary
sequence" (as Wills wrote later) "all the while gooily silting up, both sides
of his chair, upon the floor."

Wills wrote about Ruby's nightclub life in a babble of voices. Unlike
Talese, who preferred not to do interviews and disguised those he did do,
Wills put the interview process at center stage. He made no attempt to

characterize himself and Demaris, although the two of them did occasionally appear as "we," but they were indubitably there, asking the questions that punctuated the quotes: "Was Jack a good fighter?" "Did you get along with him?" "What about the view that he fought in sudden fits, not knowing what he did?" Not only were they asking the questions, they were judging the answers. You knew from the start that the voice telling this story, the voice behind that unidentified "we," came from another world, betraying itself in the rich, precise language, the sudden thrust of a different moral point of view:

The pasteboard star on Jada's dressing room shrivels at its corners. A sequiny gold horse in bas-relief is punctured at two points and shows its papery insides. There is more (and more efficient) punching than in the club's old days, but less fighting. It is still, as in Ruby's lifetime, a policeman's world, but no longer a girl's world. Ruby's club was electric with the violence of exploited women.

In spite of his years as an academic, Wills, a fan of G. K. Chesterton's Father Brown stories, had no trouble at all producing a vivid vocabulary—a singer mouths "syllables as unshaped as the drum thuds." Sometimes Wills dropped into Wolfean prose—"girls with Tower-of-Pisa hairdos, raspberry-popsicle pants, dragonfly eyelashes." But mostly his style seemed uniquely his own, a tumble of scene and talk, his versatile voice segueing easily into the voices of all these people he had gathered to bear witness to Ruby's life.

Jack Ruby emerged from this din of testimony as a man who plunged without thinking into whatever drama he found at hand; who took matters into his own hands without thinking twice; who liked to say, "You have to take the play away"; who wanted class and had none; who liked being the king of his world but wished he could be an emperor. "He always thought his next deal would be the one to make him a big man."

At the end of the piece, Wills slipped into straight dramatic narrative to tell the story of Jack Ruby's day, Sunday, November 24, 1963, the day he shot Oswald. Now, suddenly, Wills wrote as Gay Talese would have written—the writer obscured, no signs of the sources or interviews, tapes or notepads; just a story, the kind fiction writers create: "As usual, he cannot sleep after the call. Others, this morning, want to linger underwater in their sleep world, but Ruby is anxious to break the surface. He feels History all around him. . . ."

Coming after the many pages of reported interviews, that final section carried great credibility: imagined though it was, it was based on detailed research, which Wills had just laid out for the reader. It appeared to be a creative solution to the problem some readers—especially old-style journalists—saw in New Journalism: without any evidence of the reporting, how do we know all this is true? Later, Wills said he structured the piece the way he did simply because it seemed more suspenseful.

William Humphrey, the fiction writer who would later break with *Esquire,* wrote Hayes that he had started reading the article and had not been able to put it down. Theodore Peterson, magazine historian, singled out the Ruby piece, along with Sack's "M," when he spoke on contemporary magazine journalism the next spring. "If you think that no one could possibly interest you in Jack Ruby after all of the millions of words that have been written about him, read the pieces about him by Garry Wills and Ovid Demaris. . . ."

The cover for the May 1967 issue, when the story appeared, showed a young boy who looked like Dennis the Menace—archetypically American—sitting mouth agape, hamburger in hand, Coca-Cola bottle clutched between his knees, on a braided rug—in color—watching a black-and-white television screen filled with that famous scene: Jack Ruby shooting Lee Harvey Oswald. The boy's open mouth mirrored the victim's. As Gingrich explained in his publisher's column, the cover was a comment "on the new age of violence that our kids are growing up in."

Two months later, the July cover asked—skimming the question over the top of actress Ursula Andress's head, bearing a Band-Aid—"Why are we suddenly obsessed with violence?" David Newman has recalled the theory behind the issue—that "sitting and watching Jack Ruby on your television set come through that door and pump that bullet changed everything, changed television, it changed the climate of expectation, it changed the kind of things that we imagined could go on." Or as he and Benton explained it in a memorandum at the time, "The event which crystallized [violence] into a total preoccupation of our times was the shooting by Ruby of Oswald, watched on T.V. by millions of viewers as it happened."

Benton and Newman were still doing special projects for *Esquire,* and they laid out a set of story ideas for the entire issue. Not all of them materialized, and some of those that didn't would have been good to have: a major piece by Norman Mailer, who "called the shots on this American love affair with violence years ago," or Stokely Carmichael on Malcolm X, or Diane Arbus photographing men on death row. One proposal that did make its way into the issue was a Tom Wolfe essay on porno-violence; another was a big spread on "VIOLENCE AS AN ART FORM," including *Bonnie and Clyde,* its release imminent, "written by you know who, which, take it from us, is about violence and is violent. . . ."

Around the time the issue on violence was in the works, Bob Sherrill made his own existential contribution to *Esquire's* understanding of violence. One afternoon, a woman writer staged a demonstration in the hall at *Esquire;* although the *Wall Street Journal* later reported the incident as the work of hippies claiming the magazine was square, the woman actually had a personal bone to pick with Hayes. After it was all over, Sherrill went out drinking with her at the Four Seasons, and drank seriously indeed. On his way home, he got in a fight with some street workers and nearly had his ear taken off. The police took him to the hospital for stitches, then to the police station, where he called Gay Talese because he figured Talese knew how to deal with New York—Sherrill had never quite gotten the hang of it. Talese showed up with his cousin, Nick Pileggi, a police reporter who wrote for *Esquire,* and Byron Dobell. After a night in jail, Sherrill was released. ("Looks to me like you've had enough punishment," the judge said.)

Arnold Gingrich was ready to fire him, but Hayes talked Gingrich out of it, arranging for Sherrill to see a psychiatrist instead. He did for a while, but couldn't see that it did much good. "It was one of those impossible things. Whatever my sanity is—I was not nutty, that's what I am: I'm exaggerated."

When the violence issue came out, *Time* featured its cover in a July 14, 1967, report on *Esquire,* which *Time* found "bold and occasionally brilliant, and sometimes superficial or old hat or appallingly tasteless." Whatever *Esquire* was, it was doing well: circulation had risen monthly for twenty-eight months and, pushed upward by cut-rate subscriptions, had topped a million. One-fourth of the readership was female. Advertising had risen spectacularly, by 25 percent in 1966—the year in which the Sunday *Times* in London featured *Esquire* on its cover as one of "the world's great magazines"—and *Esquire* had reported advertising revenue of $10.5 million, way behind *Playboy's* more than $17 million, but ahead of *Holiday's* $10 million. In fiscal 1967, Esquire, Inc., posted profits of $3,450,000, a big shift from a company loss of $431,175 in 1962.

The magazine was reaping less tangible rewards, too. In March 1967,

Arnold Gingrich received a special George Polk Memorial Award. For creating a magazine that gave freedom to editors and writers, Gingrich was named "a shatterer of contemporary myths," a designation that, in these acrimonious times, itself produced dissent. *Esquire* had just carried a myth-shattering article by Ben H. Bagdikian, "The American Newspaper Is Neither Record, Mirror, Journal, Ledger, Bulletin, Telegram, Examiner, Register, Chronicle, Gazette, Observer, Monitor, Transcript nor Herald of the Day's Events," a critique strong enough to provoke a newspaper company in one southern town to buy up all the copies of the issue before anyone else could get to them. Customers had had to add their names to long waiting lists while the dealers ordered more. When Gingrich received his Polk Award, the chief speaker at the luncheon, Dwight E. Sargent, curator of the Nieman Foundation, launched into a fifteen-minute criticism of the article for what he called its "gross exaggeration" and "myths."

But if *Esquire* was on the forefront in some areas, it had difficulty keeping up with the developing anti-war movement, even though some *Esquire* staff members sympathized. On April 15, 1967, Bob Sherrill had joined peace marchers walking from the Sheep Meadow in Central Park, just a block from his apartment, to the United Nations. He wrote to his old college friend Bynum Shaw, now teaching at Wake Forest, that he'd never seen so many people—more, he thought, than the estimates of 125,000—and they came in all kinds, "from plain old slobs like me to hippies decorated like Easter Islanders. . . .

"I wore my Legion cap and troo eggs at dat buncha commie punks. Halla bastahds. Ho, ho. What weeda done to dat Reverant Martin Luther Pink if heeda said anything like dat when we was in World War I, I mean, World War II. Yeah."

He was being funny, but the truth was that Sherrill, Hayes, and Dobell belonged to the World War II generation, and even younger editors at the magazine had gone through college before the great sweep of political energy had touched most campuses. As conflict intensified over war and race, and the college generation supplied the ranks of militants, *Esquire* maintained the outsider's stance it had staked out for itself. "We had the catbird seat," Bob Brown recalled. "We didn't have to participate, we didn't have to be hippies. . . . 'Power to the people'—'power to the people' is a phrase maybe we can use as a joke somewhere."

Hayes himself was impatient with the student movement that had collected strength around a number of issues—free speech, social justice, relevant education, the war in Vietnam; he was antagonistic even, betraying, Sam Antupit thought, a genteel southerner's contempt for people who did not know their place. Nor was Hayes much interested in the drug-based counterculture. John Berendt led off his idea list for June 13, 1967, with an impatient proposal for a special section on "The Pot Generation": "Harold, whether or not we approve of it or like it, marijuana has become an important current issue and it is ripe for us to deal with."

Berendt laid out a run of ideas, then passed on a prediction from the health director at Michigan State University that marijuana would become legal within five years. "And if this happens, you can bet there will be a dramatic shift in the patterns of American leisure time. (Do you notice the casual pot-smoking scene in *Blow Up*? Have you read the June 17th issue of *The New Republic* [an argument for decriminalizing marijuana]?) What are we waiting for?"

It was difficult to see what they were holding back, Hayes replied, considering the September issue coming up, the campus issue Berendt had put together after a spring tour of universities. The issue included "Confessions of a Campus Pot Dealer," psychedelic art by the artists who did posters for Filmore East, Gina Berriault's profile of activist Stanford leader David Harris, and "Room-mates": four full-page portraits of couples who lived together, unwed, on college campuses. Gingrich balked at showing one of the women bare-breasted; the whole idea, Hayes explained to Berendt, who was not happy about the decision, was to show "reasonably presentable young folks" living in this unconventional way. *Esquire* did not need to add in bare breasts to have an effect—such domestic arrangements were so unexpected that television interviewer David Susskind called *Esquire* up and insisted the spread must be a spoof (when he found out it wasn't, he invited the couples to appear on his show). For the cover of the issue, George Lois posed a helmeted student with the declaration, "If you think the war in Vietnam is hell, you ought to see what's happening on campus, baby."

By the summer of 1967, even moderate liberals of Hayes's generation were turning out to oppose the war; Arthur Schlesinger, Jr., the Harvard intellectual who had written gentlemanly essays for *Esquire*, took to the road, addressing anti-war meetings across the country. Meanwhile, police actions in urban black ghettos provoked looting and burning so fierce and prolonged that the National Guard was sent into Detroit and Newark.

Millions of dollars' worth of property was destroyed and sixty-six people died in those two cities, the majority of them at the hands of the forces of law.

Esquire had considered sending a war correspondent to cover the riots but settled instead for William Worthy's report on Negro resistance to the draft: How could American Negroes fight in Vietnam if they saw the war as a colonial war? Worthy, a correspondent for the *Baltimore Afro-American,* had published articles in magazines as far apart as the *Saturday Evening Post* and *Ramparts,* which was firmly on the left. Like Hayes, he had been a Nieman Fellow. He had also successfully challenged the State Department's ban on travel in designated Communist countries, a challenge that had the support of journalists like Edward R. Murrow who thought Americans had a right to know what was going on everywhere, even in Communist countries.

Worthy had written for *Esquire* before—he was the author of that October 1964 piece on links between black militants and Third World revolutionaries, the one Hayes talked over with James Hicks in Harlem in the wake of Malcolm X's death. In this newest article, on draft resisters, he took a stance that was nonjudgmental, if anything sympathetic. He also produced a Black Power establishment chart, made up of lists in the mode of earlier power charts: "Negro Dropouts" (Ralph Bunche, Sammy Davis, Jr., Joe Louis . . .), "Whiter Than White" (Bayard Rustin . . .), "They Hire Negroes" (U.S. Armed Forces, C.I.A.).

"If there are 'villains' in the chart," Worthy explained in the accompanying text, "they would have to be the church, the educational system, and most of the white press. . . . Thanks to these three institutions, most white Americans didn't truly realize until the Sixties that the country had a serious racial problem. They still don't know that we have a colonial problem."

At midnight on October 17, 1967, sitting in bed, William Worthy read "in complete dismay" this advertisement in the *Boston Globe* for his article in *Esquire:*

GROWING DANGERS IN
THE BLACK POWER
MOVEMENT

Is the American Negro being tricked into subversion by Communist-backed reactionaries? Has the Black Power movement developed into a "Red Power" movement? Why are Ho Chi Minh and Fidel Castro serving as inspirational "heroes" to certain key Negro militants? Now, in *ESQUIRE* Magazine, Negro author William Worthy reveals shocking inside facts about a definite Black Power link with North Vietnam. Here are explosive, behind-the-scenes details that probe deep inside the reactionary movement. Learn how the Black Power underground force has become a world wide organization. Read, in *ESQUIRE*, why Joe Louis, Ralph Bunche, Bobby Short and Sammy Davis Jr. are now known as "Negro dropouts." Discover the crucial significance in the latest draft resistance. Find out about the international non-white pact—the hottest new powder-keg of all. Learn why the most powerful, best organized and best financial [*sic*] Black Power groups are still unknown. For complete, provocative details on the Black Power Establishment, plus a two-page chart of who's really who in the Negro powerhouse, don't miss the November *ESQUIRE*. Now on sale.

The ad had rotated the political frame of his piece 180 degrees. Worthy would learn, to his horror, that *Esquire*'s publicity department—a wing of the company, not of the magazine—had run it in twenty-three newspapers. He had spent months on these pieces, and *Esquire*'s research department had subjected them to its usual close scrutiny. He had been prepared to defend what he had said. But he could not defend this advertising. Repercussions came tumbling down upon him. He learned, as he said later in *Esquire*, "the fate of truth, news and information in a revolutionary era." It was like wartime: nobody wanted to hear it. As he reported all this a few months later in an *Esquire* column, "Aftermath," some of his strongest critics did not even read his article: they did not question whether the advertisement represented it fairly. In fact, he pointed out, his only exposé involved the CIA's support of the Black Power movement, featured in one corner of the power chart.

Worthy believed the editors had not seen the advertisement, and Hayes did not, in fact, routinely see all ads. Several years later he would protest vigorously an *Esquire* ad that went into the *New York Times* without his seeing it first. Yet Hayes himself, however supportive he had been of integration, was not necessarily out of sympathy with the sentiments of the ad. He was put off by the Black Power movement and militant rhetoric. "For all his toughness and his bravado and the shouting and the screaming and the stomping, he was not a violent person," Sam Antupit recalled, and he would not countenance or glorify the rising violence, rhetorical and real. He had been disturbed by the implications of Worthy's first piece on what Hayes called "Colored Internationalism," which seemed to him "racism of another color." Yet, critical as he might be of the movement Worthy was describing, it is difficult to believe Hayes would have countenanced the publicity department's outright betrayal of one of his writers.

These were tricky times for a magazine that defined itself as apolitical but provocative. When *Esquire* columnist Dwight Macdonald switched from movies to politics at the start of 1967, Fritz Bamberger, watching over company interests, questioned the move. Running a political column represented a "radical change" in *Esquire*'s policy, he told Byron Dobell. Did management know about it? Might not Macdonald's monopoly be taken as proof that *Esquire* had become a "leftist" magazine? Bamberger's instincts were right, not simply because what Macdonald would say in his column did swing *Esquire* leftward but also because Macdonald was such a visible member of the anti-war left, speaking, writing public letters, showing up at demonstrations.

Dobell had assured Bamberger that Gingrich was writing a "Publisher's Page" that would "set the column in the context of an apolitical magazine consciously choosing to do a political column." Gingrich did the job nicely. In his "Publisher's Page" for January 1967, he framed Macdonald as a kind of reviewer of politics, pointing out that Macdonald was always disappointed in movies and would likely be just as disappointed in politics.

Esquire, of course, has no politics of its own, which is why its only possible choice for a political essayist would have to be "a conservative anarchist." . . .

This magazine's only ism is, and has always been, againstism. So, when a nonpolitical magazine looks for a political columnist, it naturally figures that it couldn't settle for less than a man who, in the long run, can be depended upon to be against everybody.

It was not strictly true that *Esquire* had "no politics," although Gingrich himself, Hayes once said, was "apolitical to the point of indifference." In the November issue, the same issue in which Worthy's piece appeared, Gingrich found it useful to describe *Esquire* as a "liberal magazine." But its liberalism was loosely libertarian: a support for civil liberties, which translated at the magazine into a willingness to run widely variant points of view. "Any point of view was welcome as long as the writer was sufficiently skillful to carry it off," Hayes wrote in his introduction to *Smiling Through the Apocalypse,* "but we tended to avoid committing ourselves to doctrinaire programs. . . . None of the programs available would permit us consistently to keep our lines open to the reader, so we stayed loose."

Hayes himself usually preferred an evenhanded approach in features, but regular columnists had more of a license to say what they wanted to say. Dwight Macdonald once thanked Hayes in a letter for the freedom Hayes and Gingrich had given him—"showing interest and editorial respect (no interference, hands off, a passive but essential virtue editors don't always have) for my stuff. . . ."

Macdonald and fellow columnist George Frazier, who wrote on style, both tested editorial tolerance in their columns for that November 1967 issue, the first chance *Esquire* had to respond to the terrible riots of the summer, the worst of a series of summer riots in black ghettos. Frazier, one of *Esquire*'s best prose stylists, poured out his anger over the "bloodshed and strife," which he thought had done more damage to Negro identity than all the degradation of preceding years. "Now in so many minds that were once sympathetic to his plight, the Negro seems an inciter to riot, a savage obsessed by dread dreams of the desolation and destruction of all white people—a figure of unimaginable evil, a being hardly human." In the midst of all this, white readers might forget Negroes had "immense style"—in music and dance and sport and words. Like a man taking small treasures carefully out of his pocket, Frazier offered stylish moments and figures, one by one, until he came quietly at the end to an evening with Duke Ellington.

"I looked up at the sky and said, 'I hope it's a good day tomorrow. I want to wake up early.' "

"Any day I wake up," said Ellington, "is a good day."

Macdonald gave no comparable quarter. He laid waste right and left, taking aim at President Lyndon Johnson ("No. 1 White House Bungler and Most Disastrous President") and American Jews who had supported Israel's war and now turned their backs on the war's Palestinian refugees. Then his attention settled on the black radical group SNCC, which had done the right thing in supporting the refugees and attacking Israel, but had nevertheless gotten the facts wrong ("they're not strong on library work"). As for all their talk of revolution, he'd hate to be around if "the boys" were going to be running the show.

The deterioration of Snick has been appallingly rapid even for these speedy times: racial hatred, a neurotic delight in violence, corny melodrama, ignorant fantaticism—how did all that dedication and idealism sour so rankly in two or three years? To think I gave them $25 once! This honky wants a refund, blackey.

Herb Mayes, president of the McCall's company, thought Frazier's "stunning piece" ought to be compulsory reading—it "would have a more salutary effect on white racists than all the psalm-singing members of the Urban League put together." But compared to the Kerner Commission's later response to the riots—a powerful indictment of racism in America— *Esquire*'s November issue containing those two columns and Worthy's set of pieces did not rise to the moral challenge of the moment. As black communities counted their dead in Detroit and Newark, *Esquire* titled Worthy's feature "THE AMERICAN NEGRO IS DEAD . . . and risen as a black man of the world, soul brother to non-whites everywhere. Don't look now, honky, but some of his best friends are Vietcong."

Police were arming themselves for war. When Garry Wills came up from Baltimore that summer, Hayes had showed him brochures on armored cars, and they had talked about the reports that police were buying tanks and heavy armaments. Wills had quit teaching and gone on contract for *Esquire;* in return for a monthly retainer, Hayes would expect three or four pieces a year. For his first assignment, how would he like to go to some city, any city, now that the riots were over, and get the riot plans of the police? The idea grew, and Hayes started sending Wills more material on exotic weapons. Wills went to arms gatherings where they were selling this military-style equipment and got police contacts in various cities. "Do you want me to follow up on these?" he asked Hayes, and Hayes said, "Sure."

Wills did Baltimore, where he lived, and Detroit, and Hayes said, "Well, why don't you do Los Angeles, I'm sure they're really prepared." So, in the fall of 1967, the story grew, born at first out of a suspicion that police were overreacting—was this Hungary, where the military crushed the people with tanks?—but the meaning of it all deepening over time. Norman Mailer had come to *Esquire* for a luncheon and had said something that impressed Hayes:

"I have advocated more violence in American life, and now I have to live with that. But when men shoot at the firemen who are trying to put out the fire in their own homes, isn't that a civilization's way of committing suicide?"

To document what *Esquire* would call "The Second Civil War," Wills went out traveling for about two months, starting that September 1967. He paid visits to nine cities, telling police he was looking at urban unrest: Would there be trouble? Could they contain it? He was not an aggressive questioner—not like Ovid Demaris; he would hang around, wait, sit, listen, stay overnight if he could, and people would tell him all sorts of things. In the guise of a curious innocent, he asked simple questions of officers, riot control experts, and militants—black and white, left and right.

What would have happened if the fighting had crossed over into white neighborhoods?

"The police would have to be neutral, fighting both sides. . . ."

To a private guard who had shot a Negro: Was this the only man he had shot?

"Hell, no, I emptied my Luger over and over."

The police filled Wills in on their plans for riot control: how they would deploy their men, in what numbers and what vehicles; how they obtained intelligence. Sometimes they showed him, in confidence, intelligence reports. He examined the merchandise available in what was now a big business: armored vehicles designed for Vietnam were being marketed for riot control. Wills tried out the Stoner gun, designed to shoot through walls, flew over Watts in a bubble helicopter, sniffed samples of gas outside the home of the inventor of Mace, let a man marketing a flame thrower shoot the flame at his wet shoes, and described it all—absurd as some of it seemed to be—in a kind of deadpan. But always he returned to the theme of the title: absurd as it might seem, this was war.

When Wills set out on this assignment, he had thought the idea was to do some tsk-tsking about the disparity between the kids on the streets and the cops in their tanks. By the end of his journey, Wills had gone further than he could have imagined: He had lost his sense of America as a familiar home. He had found, instead, "an alien, armed place, not at all the one I had thought I was living in. . . ." This America contained two nations, one holding the other in thrall; but the subordinate nation was rising up in revolt. The only question was: How far would it go?

Wills had worked now with Harold Hayes on three major stories— Jack Ruby, Svetlana Stalin, and this latest—and had come to know his ways. There was something of a kid in Hayes—a kid wide-eyed and wondering at all the strange things going on. He would lean back and make a dramatic gesture out the window and say, "Oh, it's a strange world that goes by here every day." When Wills would check in by phone to tell him what he was turning up, Hayes would say (his inflection "pleasantly in-credulous"), *"Really?"* And Wills would want to go out and bring in more so as to make him amazed. Despite the enthusiasm, the encouragement, even the flattery, despite the big gestures, the jaunty little walk, his shoes tapping on the floor, Hayes was soft-spoken. He gave minimal direction, although he thought Wills was slow getting started in those early pieces, and he would cut the leads down. He would say, sometimes, "I like this, give me more—"

They were comfortable together. Wills's family was from the South, and Wills had an interest in the South. He thought that made a bond, but he never knew, really, what attracted Hayes to his work. He recalled Hayes saying, "You're a reporter, you're a reporter." Wills would suggest doing a profile of someone—say, opera singer Beverly Sills—a quick way, he thought, of meeting the obligations of his contract, and Hayes would say, "No, no, no, no, no, what you're good at is going out and describing a whole scene of action." And so these assignments for *Esquire* became very time consuming, and very long. Wills turned the Ruby pieces and "The Second Civil War" into books, and later did the research for a third book, *Nixon Agonistes,* with the idea of publishing sections in *Esquire,* which he did.

Hayes was demanding: he expected so much reporting for an article that the *Esquire* fees—decent as they were, Wills thought, by the stan-dards of the time—did not really compensate the writer. So *Esquire* writ-ers were happy to turn their *Esquire* work into books, and publishers would read *Esquire* to find nascent books—"one of the indirect ways Harold shaped the perception of his times," said Wills.

Hayes's great gift, he thought, was the "gift, amid chaos, for imagin-ing the chaos." It was a gift monthly magazine editors had to have, work-ing under their long lead times, assigning articles six months or more before the articles ever appeared. Magazine editors had to stand back from the fast flow of events in the sixties and imagine what a writer could say that would be fresh after all the media attention that had already gone into the event. Maybe, Wills thought later, that lead time had more to do than anything else with the development of what was called "New Jour-nalism." The challenge of living in two levels of time—the present in which he was reporting and the future when the piece would appear—produced an intense state of mind. Wills looked at all he saw with double vision: seeing whatever he was seeing at the time and seeing it, too, through the filter of all the other accounts that would come to readers' attention before his.

Hayes had found ways to deal with the long lead time, Wills observed. He nudged his writers to the edge of the current: "His instinct was centrifugal—get to the sidelines and watch." It had been Hayes's idea to approach the controversy over riot control by finding the inventor of Mace. Hayes liked *characters*—would ante up more expense money to add good ones to the story. He liked hearing about them when Wills called—would sometimes find them more interesting than Wills himself did, and Wills would wonder, What was he missing? Hayes encouraged him to move around in time: to explore past events in a story that would ripple into the future. Hayes himself lived, Wills observed, in multiple layers of time, embodied in the plans of future issues that lined his walls. The very speed at which one layer gave way to the next seemed to stimulate him.

In late 1967, public life was moving at a high rate of speed. There was a move afoot among Democrats to dump Johnson in the 1968 election. Draft deferments for students who had spent four years in college ended in the summer, eliminating graduate school as a safe haven, and the antiwar movement gained thousands of supporters. On October 21, approximately 100,000 anti-war demonstrators marched on the Pentagon.

Garry Wills went on the march on the Pentagon, and Hayes gave his secretary, Connie Wood, the day off to go down, too. She wound up marching with the Yippies—she hadn't meant to, didn't even know who they were, really. At one point she heard people saying, "Don't look, don't look left." She looked left, and saw the American flag going down and the Vietcong flag going up. It was dusk, the time when the American flag would have been lowered anyway, so nobody thought anything of its coming down. But when the Vietcong flag went up she heard a roar from the cops and saw them walking elbow to elbow with their truncheons, walking all around the entire building—saw them coming at her and the rest swinging their truncheons and blowing pepper gas. "My God," she recalled, "we had to run like hell."

Macdonald and Mailer had spoken at a rally the night before with the poet Robert Lowell, and over dinner all three had decided they would get arrested together, but only Mailer succeeded. Mailer wrote about the march for *Harper's* magazine, which devoted an entire issue to the account that became the book *Armies of the Night.* Macdonald wrote in *Esquire* about what Mailer wrote in *Harper's.* Mailer's piece was "a journalistic masterpiece by any standards and, by contemporary ones, a literary triumph," Macdonald said. Unlike Truman Capote, who had made the mistake of removing himself from the narrative of *In Cold Blood,* Mailer had carried "journalism into literature in the way that Agee had done in *Let Us Now Praise Famous Men:* by planting himself squarely in the foreground and relating the whole composition to his own sensibility." Revealing a mind "more complex and interesting" than he had demonstrated before, Mailer had rivaled Henry James in his rhetorical control, his "density of style," "his baroque comic touch."

Comedy did play through Mailer's account, as it did through Garry Wills's "Second Civil War" and John Sack's "M"—all responding to the American apocalypse with parody, mock epic, black humor; bringing to events of the later sixties the sensibility of the earlier sixties, when satire helped thaw a postwar world. But a new writer for *Esquire* was about to drop the comic mask and face front-on America's heart of darkness.

SEVEN

Hell-bent

B ACK IN MAY 1967, Michael Herr had come to Hayes with a request: he wanted to go to Vietnam and cover the war for *Esquire*. He spoke in grand terms of "the best kind of journalism . . . dramatic value of the war . . . a chance to make it seem more real." A few days later, on June 1, 1967, he wrote Hayes a letter outlining six specific ideas in detail—the press in Vietnam; the Green Berets; a profile of General William Westmoreland, or maybe of Major General Edward Lansdale, Graham Greene's quiet American . . . all in the weary spirit of a war that had dragged on too long.

What he wanted, he told Hayes, was to be *Esquire*'s correspondent in Vietnam, roaming the country for several months. He would send Hayes a kind of journal, which Hayes could run as a regular column—"extended vignettes, set pieces, geographical sketches, personality portraits (it would be full of people), even battle reportage." He would not send Hayes news. There had been news enough out of the war, and it had missed the mark. The news had made "conventional propaganda look innocent." Where were the honest voices of soldiers in Vietnam? The men sounded "programmed, one more symptom of a packaged war." The news had deadened reality, concealed truth, made the war "look canned and hopelessly remote."

With the exception of John Sack's "M" and academic political analysis, no "higher journalism" had come out of this war. Could Herr do better? "For good reason, you've been skeptical about what I could do for *Esquire*," Herr acknowledged. They had known each other for six years, ever since Herr had asked Hayes for a job; they had met every now and then at cocktail parties at the *Esquire* office or over lunch. But, aside from his early work on a college issue, Herr had never had an assignment from Hayes. His friend John Berendt, who had taught Hayes to call Herr by his boyhood name, "Mickey," had suggested a couple of pieces for him, but nothing ever came of the suggestions. Now Herr rolled out his credits— his articles for *Holiday,* including the long feature on Fort Dix that had sent John Sack back to revise "M." He wanted very badly for Hayes to like this idea.

It was a big idea, he knew it, and he knew, too, he would run a professional risk—more a professional risk, he thought, than a physical risk. If he failed, it would be a big failure. Yet he felt confident, even arrogant, he admitted: he wanted to take the risk and take it for *Esquire.* He was not after money; he wanted editorial respect and the right audience. ". . . *Esquire* and any writing that I do in Vietnam are all tied together in my head, and it would take some terrible desperation to separate them for me. This is one of those weird, magic equations that writers make up for themselves, an illogical arrangement of symbols that has been known to generate first-rate work." Somehow, in spite of the friendly relations between them, he and Hayes had failed to connect. "I think, finally, that this might be our time."

There was one question he could not answer: Should *Esquire* devote that much space to Vietnam? He was not the one to say—but he could say this about the war:

"As an overwhelming, unavoidable fact of our time, it goes deeper than anything my generation has known, even deeper, I'm afraid, than Kennedy's murder. No matter when it ends or how it ends, it will leave a mark on this country like the trail of slime that a sand slug leaves, a lasting taint."

Considering the proposal, Hayes knew Herr was not asking for much from *Esquire.* Herr had an assignment from *Holiday* that would pay his way across the Pacific, and his agent, Candida Donadio, had gotten Knopf to convert a contract for a book of short stories ("Found Objects") into a contract for a book on Vietnam. Hayes knew Herr was going to Vietnam to write a book—the book was, really, always the main thing. But accreditation from *Esquire* would get him into Vietnam as a journalist (he had been once before, briefly, tagging along with Marine officers he had met in Manila); he would be able to travel around with the military. In a note to Gingrich later, Hayes said, "I got him a visa and advanced him $500, then forgot about him."

Herr did not arrive in Vietnam until late in 1967, after a delay of several months. He told Hayes that *Holiday* had kept him waiting for nearly two months for money he needed before he left the United States, but, years later, he speculated that he was probably delayed by a failure of nerve. He spent three or four weeks with friends in San Francisco, where he bought a gun to take with him; it took him four months to get from New York to Vietnam, a delay that left him sitting "bolt upright in the middle of the night, all sweats and bad nerves," he confided to Hayes. He arrived in Saigon, finally, around December 1.

In a letter from Saigon on January 7, 1968, he wrote that everything was going "fantastically well," but it didn't seem to be, really. He and Hayes had talked about doing a power chart of the American establishment in Saigon, like the other power charts *Esquire* had done, and Herr had brought with him a list of names he had gotten from another writer, but the list was outdated. Herr and Hayes had imagined Herr would find "irregularities in the use of power," and Herr hadn't. "The power of Americans in Saigon is boring, it is shabby," he wrote. Still, he was producing a chart and a map of American Saigon, along with a cover piece on Saigon. He had been on four operations, two not really dangerous, one spooky, one terrifying. He would be sending a column.

The truth was, the war Herr was seeing now was different from the war he thought he had seen before, different from the one the press and the government had been saying was being fought. This war was no quagmire, half-lit by the light at the end of the tunnel. This war was terrifying: the military situation was "desperate," Herr wrote to Hayes. And the worst was yet to come, he said: despite the epic scale of war, the superb fighting men, no part of Vietnam was secure. Yet no one there would talk about it. Herr himself was keeping silent, except with a few journalists like Bernie Weinraub or John Apple. He had to keep his pessimism to himself if he wanted cooperation from the military. But he expected spring to bring the worst: "the bloodiest time of all."

For several months the North Vietnamese had been building up forces around the American base at Khesanh, a plateau in the Highlands, and the United States had responded by sending in reinforcements, drawn from posts elsewhere in South Vietnam. That was just what the North Vietnamese command had hoped the United States would do. On the last day of January 1968, less than a month after Herr's bleak prediction, the Vietcong and North Vietnamese launched the Tet offensive—an attack

on Saigon and other cities, towns, and villages, a broad sweep across the
central Highlands and the Mekong Delta.

Herr was with the Special Forces at Cantho, in the thick of fighting.
He knew, now, that the power chart and column material he had sent in
the last week in January—enough for two columns, he had thought—were
all wrong: Tet had changed everything—made what he had sent "seem
like it had been written from a different war." During that five days of
fighting in Cantho, he had no time to sleep, no time even to take off his
boots, but he managed to make a call to Saigon to have a cable sent to
Hayes, telling him not to publish the material he had sent. Back in Saigon,
he found much of the city occupied by Vietcong. Mail was not going out,
and he wondered if the copy he had sent in, or the cable, had even reached
Hayes. After a couple of days in Saigon, he left for the city of Hué.

It had been storming for days. On February 5, Herr rode toward Hué
under a dark sky. All along the road the men in the trucks had seen shell-
shattered houses, hundreds of refugees, many of them wounded. That
night, camped outside the city, Herr wrote to Hayes, asking him again not
to run the pieces he had sent. Too much had changed.

There is no similarity between the Saigon I left this morning and the Saigon I
wrote about in January. . . .

The last ten days have been incredible. Even the most experienced correspondents here have been shattered by the offensive and, even more, by the insane
American reaction to it. . . . I have passed through so many decimated towns and
cities that they get all mixed up in my mind. Here in Hué . . . the destruction has
been incredible, air strikes knocking out whole blocks of the one really lovely city
in Vietnam, destroying the university, the walls around the Citadel and, probably
tomorrow, the Citadel itself. Yesterday morning, in Cholon, I was riding on the
left side of an armored jeep when a mortar round exploded ten yards away. I had
my field pack slung over my shoulder and a four-inch piece of shrapnel burned
into it, and another fragment hit the driver, blinding him in the left eye. [The
Vietcong] fight at least as well in the cities as they do in the jungles, and I think
they could, eventually, take Saigon. Right now, with about 1500 men, they have
crippled the city, and no American with any power will admit it, will even give the
Vietcong the respect they've earned by this offensive. Where we have not been
smug, we have been hysterical, and we will pay for all of it.

The next morning Herr and the others with him crossed the canal on a
plank and strolled toward the Perfume River. South Vietnamese officers
drove by in jeeps on looting raids. There was something almost comic
about the scene. One ARVN soldier wore his booty, an oversized hat and

overcoat that trailed in the mud. Then Herr saw the first of the hundreds of civilian dead he would see in the weeks to come: "a little girl who had been hit while riding her bicycle and an old man who lay arched over his straw hat." Soon there were more: in a park, "four fat green dead lay sprawled around a tall ornate cage, inside of which sat a small, shivering monkey." The worst dead of all the ones he would see—not just in Hué but all over Vietnam—was the Vietnamese man killed near a canal in the southern part of the city.

The very top of his head had been shaved off by a piece of debris, so that only the back of his scalp remained connected to the skull. It was like a lidded container whose contents had poured out into the road to be washed away by the rains. Perhaps something had driven over it, or perhaps it had just collapsed during the ten days or more that it had lain there, but I couldn't get the image of it out of my mind.

Herr was now part of the long, grueling battle for Hué, which the North Vietnamese had occupied and the Americans and South Vietnamese were trying to retake. It was cold, dark, and—he wrote later— "that damp gloom was the background for all the footage that we took out of the Citadel. What little sunlight there was caught the heavy motes of dust that blew up from the wreckage of the east wall, held it until everything you saw was filtered through it." A block away from the American compound where he was staying, civilians lay dead on sidewalks and in the park by the river, their bodies rotting in the rain.

After Hué he went to Khesanh, the embattled base on a plateau in the Highlands, then to Danang and back to Saigon, now a "desolate city whose long avenues held nothing but refuse, windblown papers, small, distinct piles of human excrement and the dead flowers and spent firecracker casings of the Lunar New Year." He had run out of money. In a borrowed room at the Hotel Continental, he slept for forty-eight hours. He got up feeling completely empty, traumatized beyond belief. Smoking pot, in an extreme psychological state, he began to write.

There is a map of Vietnam on the wall of my apartment in Saigon, and some nights, coming back late to the city, I'll lie out on my bed and look at it, too tired to do anything more than just get my boots off. The map is a marvel, especially absorbing because it is not real. For one thing, it is very old. It was left here years ago by a previous tenant, probably a Frenchman since the map was made in Paris. The paper has buckled, and much of the color has gone out of it, laying a kind of veil over the countries it depicts. Vietnam is divided into its older territories of

Tonkin, Annam and Cochin China, and to the west, past Laos and Cambodge, sits Siam, a kingdom. That's old, I told the General. That's a really old map.

The General is drawn to it too, and whenever he stops by for a drink he'll regard it silently, undoubtedly noting inaccuracies which the maps available to him have corrected. The waters that wash around my Indochine are a placid, Disney blue, unlike the intense metallic blues of the General's maps. But all of that aside, we both agree to the obsolescence of my map, to the final unreality of it. We know that for years now, there has been no country here but the war.

Within a couple of days, he had finished his report for *Esquire* on the battle of Hué, the Tet offensive, the Vietnam War—"the only war we've got," as he had himself say, at the end, to the General.

When the article came in to *Esquire,* Hayes passed it on to Gingrich with a note:

"A John Sack-type sleeper. . . . This came in Friday, obviously dated—but despite that, an extraordinarily perceptive and thoughtful battle report. I think it holds up for whatever issue we might tack it in. 'Impressions of the only war we've got' or something like that. Meanwhile, Herr is hardpressed for dough over there. I'd appreciate your reaction to it at your earliest convenience."

Then in a parenthetical postscript, he added, "Obviously not a column. Better as a straight piece." Gingrich circled "straight piece" and wrote "good." The article ran into one problem when the legal department expressed concern about the unnamed general. In a letter dated May 18 from Hong Kong, where he was taking a break with the help of funds sent by Hayes, Herr explained about the General: "He's fiction—I hoped that would be obvious—made up out of a dozen odd types I've run into around Vietnam." Bob Brown gave the piece its title, drawn from the words on a Marine's helmet—"Hell Sucks"—and the piece was scheduled for the August 1968 issue.

The "Backstage" comments on Herr were oddly cautious, as if *Esquire* were not quite willing to claim him fully—certainly not as its Vietnam correspondent: *"Hell Sucks* (page 66) was sent to *Esquire* from Vietnam by Syracuse University graduate, erstwhile movie reviewer for *The New Leader,* and magazine writer Mike Herr, and it was written partly in an effort to convince *Esquire* that we should publish a regular column from Vietnam."

Hayes himself did not talk much about the war—not to John Sack or to Michael Herr or even to his secretary, Connie Wood. Tom Wolfe, who had little sympathy himself for the anti-war movement, was never aware that Hayes had any politics at all. For Hayes, Wolfe thought, "Journalism was paramount. . . . First came the journalism, the excitement, the story."

The evidence bears him out. In late 1967, Hayes wrote a letter to President Johnson's former national security adviser, McGeorge Bundy, in which he managed to convey his intense interest in what Bundy said at an off-the-record talk at *Esquire* without offering his opinions of what Bundy said, then went on to the point he cared about most: Would Bundy write an article in Johnson's favor, setting forth his achievements and potential achievements as president? Such an article in *Esquire* would be surprising to readers, Hayes admitted, given *Esquire*'s record—Johnson had been an easy mark of *Esquire* mockery, particularly in illustrations. On the other hand, Hayes observed, "we are sometimes assumed to be deliberately inconsistent." At no point in the letter, respectful though it was, did Hayes suggest any political sympathy with either Johnson or his opponents on the war question.

True, back in January 1960, Hayes had actually offered his services to the Democratic National Committee to help defeat Richard Nixon; he did not favor any particular Democratic candidate, he said then, "I'm just against Mr. Nixon and I'm a Democrat." But nothing apparently came of the offer, and it was uncharacteristic of Hayes, who did not share political thoughts even with his wife. When people would ask Susan Hayes what Harold thought about developing events, she would not know what to say.

To Bill McIlwain, Hayes's good friend from college, Hayes was simply not a very political man. While McIlwain was editing at Long Island *Newsday*, they talked often, but they didn't spend much time talking about politics. Once Hayes told him about getting a critical letter from a military officer in which the officer made some political remarks. Hayes remembered from the Marine Corps that an officer was not supposed to make public political remarks. He wrote a letter to the defense secretary reporting the incident, and then didn't mail the letter; he just sent a carbon to the officer. "I just let that son of a bitch worry about that for a while," Hayes told McIlwain. Maybe Hayes himself had found Marine policy useful at *Esquire.* In some positions, it was sensible for a man to keep whatever political views he had to himself.

John Berendt, who opposed the war, chose his words carefully when he put Vietnam on his idea lists. On June 13, 1967, he had proposed a "very simple, straightforward unimpassioned piece on just what compa-

nies are profiting from Vietnam." And on January 26, 1968, on the eve of
the Tet offensive, when a news item on body bags being unloaded at
Khesanh prompted another idea, again his wording was cautious:

A copy editor at the *New York Times* told me a long time ago that the newspaper's Vietnam correspondents were avoiding one subject that the paper did not
think fit to print. It was any copy about the Graves Registration Teams. It's
horrible to think about, and I got a queasy feeling in my stomach when I came
across it last week. But I think we should be the ones to do it. Without editorializing of course; completely objective. I'm sure we can count on [Charles] Mohr not
only for a good job of reporting but for a neutral tone.

"Unimpassioned," "completely objective," "neutral tone"—careful
words for a volatile time. Then while Herr was still in Vietnam, Berendt
was leafing through his mail one spring day and came across the *Vietnam
GI,* an anti-war newspaper published in Chicago—one of the many little
publications he regularly skimmed for story ideas. There, on the front
page, was a picture of four young GIs posed, crouched, cradling their guns.
Two of them held two severed heads upright by the hair. In the foreground were two headless bodies. Berendt stared at the photograph, and
the thought formed: *This is one way to end the war.*

He set about getting as much information as he could about the photograph. He tracked down the army photographer who had developed the
film, and the photographer told him the squadron the men belonged to.
He told Berendt a platoon sergeant had asked him to develop the roll, but
when the photographer's commander saw the film, he ordered it destroyed. Instead, the photographer had brought the negatives back to the
United States.

Berendt wrote to the army's chief of information at the Pentagon.
Enclosing the photograph, he informed Major General Wendell J. Coats
of the magazine's intention to publish the photograph.

In doing so, it is not our intention to attack the role of the United States in
the Vietnamese War, but to show what war in general can do to the men who are
forced to fight it. We are aware that strict rules prohibit such mutilation of
prisoners; nevertheless, this sort of thing happens on both sides. And, in order to
be perfectly fair, we would have to print alongside this photograph another showing Vietcong atrocities being perpetrated on American G.I.s.

Admitting his request was unusual, Berendt asked for a selection of
Vietcong atrocity photos to choose from.

Berendt soon had his reply. General Coats expressed the hope that *Esquire* had "irrefutable evidence" that these apparent atrocities and the GIs' apparent responsibility for them were all that they seemed. If they were, then the guilty parties were subject to trial. Therefore, *Esquire* had a strong moral and legal obligation to give the army all information it had on the circumstances under which the photograph was taken and the individuals involved.

General Coats pointed out that the photograph, alone, did not prove the GIs' guilt. The victims might have been South Vietnamese soldiers or civilians who had been mutilated by the enemy. The army would be investigating the incident, he said. Meanwhile, unless *Esquire* could fully substantiate the meaning of the photograph, he suggested *Esquire* "reconsider the propriety of its publication."

Esquire prepared the photograph for publication and Berendt wrote the copy to go with it—a one-page draft in which Berendt wrestled with the blanks in the story. Byron Dobell had left *Esquire* to edit a newspaper book-review supplement, so Berendt gave his draft to Don Erickson, the new managing editor, who forwarded it, with the photograph, to *Esquire's* lawyer. At the top of his letter to the lawyer, a handwritten note said, "*Rush* HH wants for Nov."—the issue that would coincide with the next election, when the Democrats' conduct of the war would be up for renewal.

The lawyer identified two problems.

One, the magazine did not own rights to the photograph and could not buy them from the photographer who had the prints, since he maintained he did not take the pictures. The sergeant who gave him the film to develop was now denying any knowledge of the incident. If the army wanted to punish *Esquire* for running the pictures, the army could locate the person who took them and promise him immunity if he took action against *Esquire* for publishing his work without permission. The lawyer thought this chain of events was unlikely.

Second, the army quite possibly would discover the identities of the men in the photograph and hold a hearing or court-martial. If the men were found guilty of a war crime, *Esquire* would not need to worry. But if instead they were found not guilty, they could sue *Esquire*.

Summing up the lawyer's comments to Hayes, Erickson concluded: "Is the feature valuable enough editorially to justify the risk involved? Would you take up with Mr. Blinder?"

It was customary, during this period, for management—Gingrich, Blinder, and Smart—to see manuscripts that might prove controversial. The year before, on June 19, 1967, John Smart had complained to Gingrich when he did not receive a copy of James Deaken's article "The Dark Side of L.B.J." until it had already been typeset and put into page form. Smart was not comfortable showing so much disrespect to the president, and he thought there were seven or eight points at which the article should have been cut. He had been distressed enough to talk the matter over with Blinder, and they had both talked to Hayes. Bamberger had told Smart he had raised questions about many of the points that troubled Smart, but apparently his questioning had not had much effect. Smart told Gingrich he hoped future controversial articles would be sent around while there was still time to intervene.

Thus it was that the photograph of the GIs had to be submitted to Blinder. The photograph did not run, but not, as Berendt recalled, for legal reasons; it was a question, really, of taste—a feeling that the picture was too gory for *Esquire*. Years later, Blinder recalled that *Esquire*'s coverage of the war, unopinionated though it was, troubled advertisers, but the agencies told their clients "they should advertise in this magazine even if they didn't like it, because the young people were going to be such an important part of their market in the future." Blinder did not remember the picture of severed heads at all.

When *Esquire*'s newest editor, Tom Hedley, a towering Canadian, set out to test the water on campuses that spring of 1968, he found revolution brewing. On a trip to the West Coast, he attended meetings with the Students for a Democratic Society at San Francisco State and met members of the Black Panthers; he foresaw something approaching guerrilla warfare. Hayes and Erickson had a hard time believing it.

Then on April 4, the Reverend Martin Luther King was shot and killed in Memphis, where he had gone to support striking garbage workers. As soon as Garry Wills heard the news of King's death, he called *Esquire*. It was night, and nobody answered, but he caught a plane to Memphis anyway, arriving just hours after the shooting. He stopped at a hotel and the police station. At the motel where King was killed, "dawn was just disturbing the sky; flashbulbs around and under the balcony still blinked repeatedly against the room number—306—like summer lightning." Wills paid a call to the funeral home, heard a description of all the mortician had to do to restore King's face. The men working on King's body listened to his recorded voice on the radio as they worked.

Wills finally reached an editor at *Esquire,* and, without hesitation, the editor said yes, Wills should write about King's death for the magazine. At eight that evening, he was at the funeral home, watching hundreds of mourners file past the body, not a single white person from Memphis among them.

Wills had learned from Hayes to move to the margins of a story—out to the edges. As the rest of the press flew to Atlanta for King's funeral, Wills stayed behind and attended the meeting of mourning the day after King's death. He heard the most eloquent speech he had ever heard—the Reverend James Bevel speaking to the garbage workers whose cause had drawn King to Memphis—telling them (as they answered back in re-peated call and response):

"Martin Luther King is not our *leader!*"..."*Our* leader ... is the *man*—who led *Moses* out of *Israel.*"..."*Our* leader is the man who went with Daniel into the lions' den." ... "Our leader is the man who walked out of the grave on Easter morning." ..."Our leader never sleeps nor slumbers. He cannot be put in jail. He has never lost a war yet. *Our* leader is *still on the case.*"

Wills stayed on four days until the night before the funeral was to take place, when he joined the garbage collectors on their long bus ride from Memphis to Atlanta. To get to the church where the buses were to pick them up, he took a cab with a driver who kept a pistol next to him on his seat. "Nigger territory, eh?" the cabdriver said when Wills told him the address. "Well, get in," and the driver slapped down all four locks. Riots had ripped through America's cities after King's death; on the way to the church, Wills's taxi passed an armored personnel carrier. Inside the church, a hundred people waited. Some had waited for hours, afraid to try coming after curfew. They waited patiently, with "a quiet sense of pur-pose, dimly focused but, finally, undiscourageable." They were, Wills thought, "the world's least likely revolutionaries."

On the bus, where folding chairs had been placed in the aisles to accommodate all the passengers, one man, a tall man who had joked softly with the other riders, began musing over Dr. King, and the people around him murmured responses, "mingled but regular, like sleepy respirations, as if the bus's sides were breathing regularly in and out."

These were not luxury buses, and the ride took ten hours. By the time they all reached Atlanta, the funeral service at Ebenezer Church had already started. Nobody had time to change into the good clothes they had brought, and they could not get into the church. They had simply to stand in the crowd and watch, as celebrities passed by. But they did not regret coming, none of them did: they owed it to Dr. King. T. O. Jones, the president of the sanitation local, said he knew when King came to Memphis, he would be in danger. "He was in Memphis for only one reason—the Public Works Department's work stoppage. This is something I lay down with, something I wake up with. I know it will never wear away."

Later, Todd Gitlin, a leader in the Students for a Democratic Society, would write of King's death, "When he was murdered, it seemed that nonviolence went to the grave with him, and the movement was 'free at last' from restraint." In late April, a Columbia University plan to build a gymnasium in Harlem's Morningside Park set off days of demonstrations, fed by anger over racial and social injustice and the Vietnam War. Students occupied buildings, Dwight Macdonald climbed over windowsills to show his support, and the university called in the New York City police to make the students leave. The *Columbia Daily Spectator* reported nearly 700 arrests and 100 injured students and faculty members. In mid-May student riots shook Paris, France, raising specters of an international youth revolt.

On June 5, Robert Kennedy, campaigning for the presidency in California, was assassinated. *Esquire*'s July issue was already on its way to the stands, featuring an acerbic Murray Kempton piece on Robert Kennedy. The best *Esquire* could do was pull off the stickers attached to newsstand copies to call attention to main features. Some readers who did not know about *Esquire*'s long lead time expressed surprise that *Esquire* did not explain itself in the next issue, perhaps apologize, but, as Gingrich did explain in September, it had been already too late even to make changes in the August issue, which contained Garry Wills's article on Martin Luther King. "What can you do when the coverage of one assassination comes out *after* the next one?" Hayes asked Wills.

In the last week of August, Democratic delegates gathered in Chicago. The nomination of Hubert Humphrey, Johnson's stand-in, seemed assured. The surviving peace candidate, Eugene McCarthy, had lost heart.

The National Mobilization Committee to End the War in Vietnam, which had led the march on the Pentagon, had put out a call for anti-war protestors to come to Chicago, and so had the Yippies, an anti-war group with an almost *Esquire*-ish sense of humor. Many anti-war activists stayed away, but enough came to put Mayor Richard Daley and the Chicago police on guard. Daley refused protestors' requests for permission to camp in the city parks or march on the city streets. The FBI warned the city that the protestors might dump hallucinogenic drugs into the city's water supply. Peace movement leaders who were not going to Chicago warned that protestors who went might be killed. Harold Hayes had originally planned to go to Chicago with *Esquire*'s reporting team, but in the end, he thought better of it and sent John Berendt in his place.

Hayes had started out with the idea of sending novelist Terry Southern to cover the Democratic Convention, but as he and Southern talked about the assignment, they had come up with a better plan: assigning the Black Humorists of the Western World to go to Chicago for *Esquire*. So it was that Berendt accompanied Southern, Jean Genet, the French novelist and playwright who had also been a homosexual prostitute, thief, and convict; and William Burroughs, the American Beat writer and drug enthusiast who had tried to shoot a gin glass off his wife's head and killed her instead. (French playwright Eugene Ionesco had agreed to be part of the team, then thought better of it and withdrew.) Genet's editor at Grove Press, Richard Seaver, went along too, accompanied by his French wife, Jeanette, who interpreted for Genet.

Gathered in the downstairs bar of Chicago's Sheraton Hotel for their first evening together, *Esquire*'s correspondents seemed puzzled by their own presence, but they set themselves to work seriously—trekking out to the airport the next day to meet Senator Eugene McCarthy and finding Norman Mailer there, too, covering the convention for *Harper's*. Berendt had the job of observing their progress and letting Hayes know how things were going. His first report was cautious: There was some drinking and some smoking of grass, and he couldn't tell if the team had any idea of what was going on.

When John Sack called about something else, Hayes figured he had better put him on the story, too—just in case. Sack, the war correspondent, would follow the police around. On Sunday night, walking among anti-war demonstrators at Lincoln Park, Sack ran into Genet, Burroughs, and Southern, all talking to each other. Well, he thought, they're great writers—they can just walk through the park and get wonderful material, and I'm second-rate and I can't write without sitting with people hours on end, listening and talking to them. He went his own way. Norman Mailer, on his way out of the park (he had decided he could not afford getting arrested because he had to write this piece for *Harper's*), spotted the *Esquire* correspondents, too, and thought they "had the determined miserable look of infantrymen trudging to the front." Actually, Genet liked the Yippies. When he passed a group camped in a backyard he handed out dollars, and the young people gathered around him with hugs and kisses.

Around lunchtime Monday, Berendt called in to report to Hayes and left a long message: Genet was the toast of the town, the Yippies loved him and he was intrigued by them. He had already started writing his piece; Berendt thought it would be a classic. Burroughs was pleasant but afraid he might collapse and was not yet into the swing of things. Berendt had had to hire another car: they were adding celebrities—Allen Ginsberg had shown up that morning. A plainclothesman in a blue shirt was following them. And finally, Berendt reassured Hayes, "DON'T WORRY."

That afternoon, Ginsberg and Genet both made statements at a Yippie press conference in Lincoln Park. Ginsberg offered to march to the Amphitheatre on Wednesday if the Yippies would take off their clothes in front of the Hilton Hotel. Genet, with Ginsberg translating, admitted he was groggy from taking "a lot of Nembutals" the night before, and spoke fondly to the crowd:

> You children are living the life I used to lead, you know, and you are beautiful. Someday the buildings of Chicago will be covered with flowers and trees: then they too will be beautiful. But be careful now to guard your rights. You have a right to sleep in the park, to wear long hair and imaginative clothing. Certainly you are more pleasant to look at than the cops with their blue helmets, plexiglass masks, and revolvers. Your very presence here is a fitting antidote to the silly convention going on downtown.

Burroughs had been taping background noise on his tape recorder wherever he went. Applying a method he used to create manuscripts, he would break the recording up and reassemble it: he would record ten minutes or so, then back up to the start and record something else over what he had recorded, then skip over a few minutes of the original recording, then record over it for a while and so on, making, as he said, "a complete hash of it all." Then, he had explained over lunch, "you walk around with the damn thing under your jacket, playing it at low volume. It flips people out."

That night at the convention, Burroughs fiddled with his tape recorder while Ginsberg lit two sticks of incense. Ginsberg gave one to Genet and held the other himself, softly chanting a mantra. They were sitting in that part of the balcony reserved for the periodical press, and around them their fellow gentlemen and ladies of the press stared and took their pictures. After half an hour they stood up to go. Ginsberg raised both arms and, in a loud voice, boomed, "Hare Krishna!"

Shortly after eleven, they watched the scene at Lincoln Park. Several thousand young people stirred in the darkness while policemen in riot gear guarded the park's southwest corner. Hundreds more people were pouring into the park. Burroughs went off to the Oxford Club Bar on Clark Street. The others crossed onto the grass of the park, unlit in the cloudy night. They heard that police were massing by Lake Shore Drive.

Ginsberg, Genet, Southern, Berendt, and Seaver linked arms and walked through the crowd in that direction. Genet's presence rippled through the crowd.

"Hey, wow, Jean Genet's here."

"I didn't think he really existed. Oh, beautiful."

Ginsberg began to chant "Owwmmm" and others joined in. The sound filled the whole park. Even the protestors at the barricades gave up shouting "Hell, no, we won't go" and joined the chant.

Every now and then a move from the police would set off a wave of panic. There would be shouts of "Walk, walk, don't run, don't run!" The panic would die down.

Ginsberg sat down a hundred feet away from the barricade. He became the center of a couple hundred young people chanting, "Owwwmmmm."

At 12:30 a roar down the whole line of the barricades set off a stampede. Everyone was running, screaming through the dark, terrified. Berendt and Seaver took hold of Genet's arms and began to run. Tear gas grenades were exploding, and they ran through the pale smoke with the police running after them, swinging their billy clubs. The crowd fled into Clark Street, and the police came after them, swinging clubs. Bottles and rocks flew through the air, smashing car windows. Policemen fell upon a boy who had thrown a handful of stones, swinging down on him until their nightsticks were covered with blood. When a newsman took a picture, they grabbed his camera and destroyed it.

Seaver, Berendt, and Genet took refuge in a vestibule, with four other people. Four policemen descended upon them.

"Communists! You fucking commies! Get the hell out of here."

"Press!" someone shouted.

"Press my ass!" a policeman shouted and brought his club down on the man, who fell into the street. The policeman pursued him, pausing to slam the club across the back of a girl.

Back in the vestibule, a policeman shouted, "God damn you. You don't live here; get the fuck out before I let you have it!"

Terrified, Berendt held Genet, pressed against the wall. When the policeman, face contorted, raised his club above them, Berendt shouted, "Stop, he's an old man. Don't!"

He and the others groped toward an inner door and the policemen's attention passed to other victims.

Inside the building, people on floors above were calling for them to come up to safety. On the second floor a young Negro woman invited them into her apartment.

"My God, it's horrible," she said.

They escaped from the building out a back stairway onto Wells Street. At first they thought they were safe. Then they saw police running toward them. When they turned, police were coming from the other direction. They slid through a doorway into a front yard surrounded by a high wall. Safe now, beyond the wall they could hear shouts, running feet, the crash of glass. They waited for the noise to subside, then left.

As Berendt wrote later,

It had been a bad night for Chicago and a squeaker for the progress of Western literature. At the very moment Jean Genet had stood up against the wall, menaced by a club-wielding, half-crazed policeman, Terry Southern had ducked into an entranceway two doors down under a shower of broken glass; Allen Ginsberg had paused briefly in the middle of Clark Street for a last ditch "Owwmmm" before fleeing into the Lincoln Hotel where he was staying, and William Burroughs, having left the Oxford Club Bar, was flushed out of the back of a parked truck on Clark Street where he'd been invited by some of his young hippie-head fans for a smoke.

The next morning Genet, dressed in his kimono, went to the Seavers' hotel room to say he was furious at what had happened. He wanted to issue a public statement denouncing what the police had done. By mid-afternoon, Genet, Burroughs, Southern, and Ginsberg had all written statements condemning the police as "vicious guard dogs" (Burroughs), "mad dogs" (Genet), "swine" (Southern). Ginsberg's phrasing was more gentle: he condemned Chicago officials as "authors of loudmouth bad poetry."

Burroughs and Genet read their statements at an un-birthday party for Lyndon Johnson at the Coliseum that night. The emcee read Ginsberg's (he had almost lost his voice) and Southern's (he had begged off). They had meant to go to the convention after that, but Genet had a better idea: "Le parque," he said.

They arrived at Lincoln Park a little after curfew. Fewer people were there on this night, since many had gone to Grant Park to demonstrate before the Hilton Hotel, the headquarters of the candidates. Tonight, several hundred clergymen had gathered around a wooden cross. The crowd was singing "Kumbaya."

Jean Genet had found much that he saw beautiful—not the convention itself ("it babbles on"), but the policemen ("He is so handsome I could fall into his arms") and the hippies, and now the "very beautiful poetry" of the religious service. He fell into a sweet meditative state:

And what of the trees in the park? At night they bear strange fruit, clusters of young people suspended in their branches. . . . The clergymen invite us to be seated: they are singing hymns in front of an enormous wooden cross. . . . The cross, borne by several clergymen, moves away into the night, and this imitation of the Passion is very mov—

His thoughts broke off abruptly: the police were attacking, hurling tear gas canisters.

Arms linked, the *Esquire* contingent, including Ginsberg, moved through the smoke, surreal in the lights from police motorcycles, back to the crowded hotel lobby, filled with people coughing from the tear gas and bleary-eyed. A medic poured water over Genet's eyes to wash out the gas: first the Americans had tried to burn him, he reflected, now they were trying to drown him. The correspondents retired to Ginsberg's room and watched the convention on television.

On Wednesday, there were plans to defy the city's refusal of a march permit and march from Grant Park to the Amphitheatre. At the rally to start the march, Ginsberg spoke, then Burroughs and Genet. Norman Mailer stood in the crowd listening. He had already told peace movement leader David Dellinger that he would not march because he did not want to risk being arrested. And since he wasn't going to march he didn't want to speak, either. But when the time came for the rally, he felt drawn there. As he heard Ginsberg and Burroughs and Genet address the crowd, he approached Dellinger and asked to speak.

Ever since that first time Mailer had watched Burroughs and Genet and Southern going into the park as he was leaving on that earlier night, a fear had been growing inside him (he would confess in his *Harper's* account): a fear that he was losing his edge, that he was wrong not to join in, that he was compromised by the life he lived, which was in its way a good life after all: he wanted to go on writing, he wanted America to go on being a place where he could go on writing. Finally, he could not resist speaking. He explained to the crowd why he would not go with them on this march—he had to write.

For their part, Genet, Burroughs, Ginsberg, even Southern, were all going to march with the five or six thousand other marchers. Burroughs was impressed by the war gear of the demonstrators: crash helmets, shoulder pads. He took his place in the second row of the nonviolent march, feeling out of place: nonviolence was not his program. When the marchers reached the police line, for one awful moment he thought the police were going to let them march the whole five miles—and he already had blisters. Relieved to be stopped, he strolled through the park (as he wrote later) "recording and playing back, a beauteous evening calm and clear vapor trails over the lake youths washing tear gas out of their eyes in the fountain."

Later, in the Amphitheatre, where the *Esquire* team retired to watch the vote for the presidential candidate, Burroughs played back his Grant Park recordings. Ginsberg chanted "Owmms" and a security guard eventually ejected him, probably because his "Hare Krishna" had disrupted the benediction. Genet was deeply depressed: "These are rubber people; this is a rubber convention." He had an urge (he wrote) "to go outside and touch a tree, graze in the grass, screw a goat, in short do what I'm used to doing."

Southern had gotten separated from the others back at the park, and wound up in the bar of the Hilton Hotel, where demonstrators had gathered after police blocked the march. With what he called later "a certain undeniable decadence," he and writers William Styron and John Marquand, Jr., watched through the plate-glass windows as police pummeled the kids outside.

> . . . at the height of the slaughter five or six kids were pushed through a plate-glass window on one side of the bar. The cops rushed in after them.
> "Get the hell outta here!" a cop was yelling, which they were trying to do as fast as possible. But something was wrong with one of them, a thin blond boy about seventeen.
> "I can't walk," he said.
> "You'll walk outta here, you little son of a bitch!" said the cop and clubbed him across the side of the head with his stick. Two of the others seized him by the shirt and started dragging him across the floor of the bar through the lobby.

For nearly twenty minutes, police attacked with a brutality relayed to the nation by television cameras—finally close enough to a power source to plug in and broadcast live. While police attacked, the crowd chanted: "The whole world is watching, the whole world is watching."

The next day, Genet asked the Seavers to go for a drive with him out in the country. He was tired of the stink bombs, the tear gas, the litter, the weariness in the faces: he wanted to see trees and flowers. They went the wrong way and spent hours wandering through one of the most poisoned industrial landscapes in America—the broad polluted flats between Chicago and Gary, Indiana.

Meanwhile, the photographer Carl Fischer had been out scouting a location for the cover. When he had an art assistant lie down on the street like a fallen demonstrator while he climbed a post, the Chicago police—who had been following him and his assistants around—put them all in a paddy wagon and took them down to the station. He decided he had better take the *Esquire* team back to New York to shoot the cover.

The plan had not actually been to put the convention on the cover. The plan, according to Tom Hedley, had been to feature instead a package of pieces on Robert Kennedy's funeral. Carl Fischer, who usually took the photos for the George Lois covers, had been intrigued by the idea of showing the crucifixion in contemporary dress, as painters did during the Renaissance, and he had shot a photo that he had shown to Hayes. Hayes hadn't seen a way to use it, but when *Esquire* put together the package on the sanctification of Robert Kennedy, the idea was revived, and Fischer produced a cover showing Jesus Christ nailed to the cross, surrounded by television cameras, with a coverline that went something like this: "What if Jesus Christ got the coverage that Bobby Kennedy did? The canonization of a mediocre man." The cover had cost a lot to produce, but in the end Arnold Gingrich couldn't live with it, Hedley recalled. George Lois wasn't in on the decision—hadn't had anything to do with the idea, he said later; it sounded heavy-handed to him. Thinking back, Carl Fischer couldn't recall hearing objections from Gingrich; he just thought the convention had turned out to be such a dramatic event that Hayes wanted *Esquire*'s convention team on the cover.

On the plane going back to New York, John Sack was sitting next to Terry Southern. Sack thought Southern was a really good writer, but, boy, was Southern's attitude different from his: so contemptuous of the police. Sack had thought what the police were doing was disgusting and evil, but he liked them as individuals. He had what he thought was the true radical view: not that the police were pigs and needed to be straightened out but that the police were good Americans, doing their best by the American way, "and if those people can go out and break open heads in Chicago and do what they did in Chicago, then that's an indictment, not of the Chicago police, but of the whole American system."

In New York, Carl Fischer shot the picture under elevated tracks in Upper Manhattan. Then the writers settled down to write on a deadline tighter than any of them were used to. It was scary, Sack thought: here it was Friday, Labor Day weekend, he hadn't written a thing and he was already on the cover. He worked in the *Esquire* offices through Saturday, Sunday, and Monday, with a little time off to go to a party over the weekend at David Halberstam's. Tuesday the *Esquire* staff came back and he spent Tuesday, Wednesday, and Thursday rewriting.

Meanwhile, Genet's hatred and fear of America rose to a fever pitch. Unable to get a visa, he had entered the country without one, coming through Canada—a fact he alluded to in his piece. Now that he saw how American law officials could behave, he feared his fate if they caught him out. He fell into a paranoid tantrum. As Seaver was reporting to Berendt on the phone, Genet began tearing up his manuscript (which Seaver had already translated). The Seavers wrestled some of the pages away from him and pieced enough together to satisfy *Esquire*'s lawyers that the translation was accurate. A few days later Hayes called Sack and asked him if he knew anyone who spoke French who could take Genet to the Canadian border. Sack did know someone, but by the time he got hold of her Hayes had already found someone else. (Later, the FBI showed up at the *Esquire* offices to ask about *Esquire*'s involvement in Genet's illegal entry.)

Meanwhile, the articles themselves presented problems. As soon as Hayes saw them, he knew he was going to have to run interference. Southern's and Sack's contributions were comparatively mild—Hayes had warned Southern in advance to stay away from four-letter words, and Sack only dropped in a few "fucks." But Genet described the first day as "The day of the thighs":

"The thighs are very beautiful beneath the blue cloth, thick and muscular. It all must be hard. This policeman is also a boxer, a wrestler. His legs are long, and perhaps, as you approach his member, you would find a furry nest of long, tight, curly hair."

Later, he described a policeman "holding his billy club in his hand the way, exactly the way, I hold a black American's member."

He also said the world and America would be better off if America were "demolished," "reduced to powder."

Burroughs concluded his report with a speech by a purple-assed mandrill, candidate for president: a savage satire.

"Why when I was fourteen years old" [the mandrill said] "our old yard Nigrah Rover Jones got runned over by a laundry truck and I cried my decent American heart out. And I have a deep conviction that the overwhelming majority of Nigrahs in this country is good Darkies like Rover Jones. However we know that there is in this country today another kind of Nigrah and as long as there is a gas pump handy we all know the answer to that." (Thunderous applause) "And I would like to say this to followers of the Jewish religion. Always remember we like nice Jews with Jew jokes. As for Nigger-loving communistic agitating Sheenies well just watch yourself Jew boy or we'll cut the rest of it off." (That's telling em Homer)

Working on a tight deadline—the issue went to press more than a month after the usual date—Hayes sent all of the pieces to Fritz Bamberger, who screened them for taste and libel problems, and to Abe Blinder, president of the company. Along with the pieces, Hayes attached a memorandum to Blinder in which he made the strongest case he could make for minimal cuts in the articles. He began by acknowledging the material was "rough going" and would tax Blinder's sense of propriety.

But these were important writers, he argued, and they had approached their assignment seriously. He argued that Sack's use of "fuck," Genet's homosexual references, and Burroughs's fantasy of a purple baboon as president were all integral to their satiric point of view.

He staked *Esquire's* very identity on publication of these pieces with minimal tampering. If major deletions were made, he said, "we weaken the reputation of this magazine as a publication that practices what it preaches, and at a time serious issues call for the utmost strength and tolerance in permitting writers the opportunity and freedom to express themselves."

Blinder read the pieces and talked them over with Hayes. Hayes was willing to make some cuts. But they disagreed on one: Genet's line about holding the black American's member. Blinder didn't see it as necessary. Hayes tried to convince him it was "integral to Genet's perversion and perversity."

Hayes won out, and the articles ran, member and all; Genet's contribution was coyly titled "The Members of the Assembly." Hayes did agree to an editor's note distancing the magazine from the writers' views by identifying them as belonging to the writers. "They were given no instructions; it was their reaction to Chicago that was wanted and it is that which is printed below."

Maybe because the writing was too rushed, maybe because this time Hayes missed in his effort to match writers with unlikely subjects, maybe because each piece was too short, the results were disappointing, at least to Hayes, who thought that by 1968 events were moving so fast that the three-month lag time made the pieces hopelessly dated. Yet Genet, Burroughs, and Southern, working their way seriously through the week, had been part of events in a way Norman Mailer had not. Men much older than most of the demonstrators—men whose personal worlds had been vastly different from the worlds most of the demonstrators inhabited—they drifted through the dark, violent nights like specters in a film by Federico Fellini. Who were they and why were they there? History would not say. They appeared in the detailed *Walker Report to the National Commission on the Causes and Prevention of Violence,* but their presence went unexplained: they were just there, as if events had simply drawn them there—a French playwright and a Beat fiction writer living in London and an American satirist. In its own way, *Esquire* had made a contribution to the national drama that played itself out that last week in August of 1968.

In a television film he made later called *The Late Great '68,* Hayes heard, that year, "the sound of a world ending." In speeches he made at colleges in the late sixties, he would go down a list of the year's "disruptions to our public life": January 31, Tet offensive; March 1, dollar crisis; March 12, New Hampshire primary; March 14, Bobby Kennedy decides to run; April 1, LBJ withdraws; April 4, Martin Luther King assassinated; April 5–11, city riots resulting from death of King; April 18, riots at Columbia; May 16, riots in Paris; June 5, Bobby Kennedy shot; August 28, Chicago riots. It seemed to him that American history had taken a sharp turn in 1968—the culture altered in a definitive way. Unlike some of the others in the *Esquire* circle—David Newman was out demonstrating with his Afro and gas mask—Hayes looked on at the demonstrations, riots, and revolutionary rhetoric with growing distaste.

"There are manifestoes directed to the overthrow of any establishment that might come to mind—sexual, psychological, social, economic or political," he said in a speech to the Authors Guild on February 20, 1968. "Reason has been displaced by emotion. In the name of declaration and commitment, the orderly systematic progression of evidence toward the building of coherent ideas is being abandoned. Perhaps we are indeed on the eve of some revolution, if not of the law then certainly of the spirit."

Hayes had always had a wire service reporter's belief that truth was best arrived at through an objective approach; he had never favored polemics, unless they were expressions of personality, like Gore Vidal's attack on Bobby Kennedy. Now as writers were increasingly making assertions, he found himself increasingly wanting to see writers' evidence for their assertions. He rejected a piece on Vietnam by Jean Genet as "propaganda," and when Garry Wills began turning in pieces that sounded to Hayes like arguments, Hayes would say, "Why doesn't he go back and do a 'Second Civil War'?" When Dan Wakefield sent Hayes a piece on attempts to suppress the film *Titticut Follies,* Hayes rejected it, calling Wakefield's "seething state of indignation" not typical of *Esquire.* "Calm, reasoned, unruffled—letting the evidence accumulate so that the reader may not escape the author's intended (but unstated) conclusion—*that's* our ticket!" In the past, Hayes had held up Francis Marion the Swamp Fox as a hero; when actual revolution appeared on the horizon, he circled the wagons.

Hayes had always wanted every issue of *Esquire* to provoke a response. Now Americans had been exposed to too much provocation: they had turned numb. The *Esquire* attitude—irreverent, iconoclastic—was faltering in the face of a society that seemed to him "hell-bent on destroying itself." As 1968 neared its end, Hayes looked back over the year's issues and found himself disappointed. True, there had been good moments. In April, George Lois had put Muhammad Ali on the cover as Saint Sebastian, pierced with arrows, symbolizing the fighter's martyrdom for refusing to fight in Vietnam. Novelist Kurt Vonnegut, Jr., had appeared in June with an article memorably titled "Yes, We Have No Nirvanas." The July cover had featured an interview with an angry James Baldwin. For August, *Esquire*'s rock critic Robert Christgau had reported on radical efforts to organize a union in the U.S. military, and the issue had been briefly banned at Fort Hood, Texas. In September the Magazine Publishers Association gave Arnold Gingrich the Henry Johnson Fisher Award for individual achievement in magazine publishing.

But the next month Hayes reported to the editorial staff that newsstand sales were down—"roughly 20,000 an issue," and he was disappointed in *Esquire*'s editorial performance.

One reason we were doing better in '67 is that we seemed more sure about our materials and our approach to them. For another, the year was less turbulent than '68. For another, our efforts at establishing a satirical voice were somehow more effective than they now seem to be. And for still another, there seemed enthusiasm and exuberance coming out of our pages.

Every now and then Hayes gave the staff tongue-lashings in memos, castigating them for coming in late, being too lackadaisical. This was one of his fiercest laments. Editors were relying too much on "second-rate, professional free-lancers, whose level of work is without style, wit or perception; hacks mostly, who can be found in most other magazines." How many editors were asking fiction writers, who did have style, to write journalism? Only Sherrill seemed to be even out looking for new writers. And they weren't making their writers revise when they needed to. And they weren't giving Hayes ideas he asked for. "When you do go for big stuff, you tend to try only for politics or race—increasingly boring subjects these days."

Hayes rolled on to a dramatic conclusion:

. . . I suppose the reason behind this jeremiad is that I am frightened by our collective failure of response to the possibilities of this magazine—the lack of enthusiasm but also, of course, lack of imagination, resourcefulness and a special kind of effort as well. If most of the stuff that comes along bores me, and it does, I can only assume it must surely bore you—and a good proportion of our audience. Paradoxically, however, there are people who still think this is a hot shot magazine, and who would love to work here, and who presumably are bubbling over with enthusiasm for what we seem to be trying to do. Maybe they don't see all the periodicals.

I do, and I'm scared. In the past two years we've seen the emergence of *Ramparts,* the underground press, a new *Esquire*-approach at *Harper's, New York,* a much stronger *Village Voice* and still another re-organization at the *Post.* Some of these are deliberately competing editorially with us; others don't even bother, they see us as irrelevant and outmoded.

For several years *Esquire* had faced editorial competition in New York from Clay Felker's *New York* and the *Village Voice. Harper's* under its new editor, Willie Morris, was a national challenger, and Willie Morris himself was the hottest magazine editor in town. Just before Morris became editor, he had written a book expressly with the idea of establishing his reputation: *North Toward Home,* the story of Willie Morris's coming of age, was not just readable; it was eloquent. Here was a good writer and thoughtful man—like Hayes, a southerner, and like Hayes an editor with high ambitions.

Morris went after the best writers he could find, raising *Harper's* fees by a quantum leap to sign on David Halberstam, the *New York Times'* Pulitzer Prize–winning reporter, for $16,000 a year. As one of the first reporters to see through the veil of obfuscation on Vietnam, Halberstam brought to *Harper's* high credibility on the most pressing issue of the day. Morris put other talented writers on the payroll as well: Larry L. King, a Texan; Marshall Frady, another southerner; and John Corry, another refugee from the *New York Times.* As one of his editors he hired Midge Decter, wife of Norman Podhoretz, who as editor-in-chief of *Commentary* was one of the central figures of New York intellectual life. Morris brought in other bright lights when he could—Larry McMurtry, Norman Mailer. Working out of a very different magazine tradition—*Harper's* had a solid identity as a serious intellectual-literary magazine—Morris had a certain advantage over Hayes: he could focus on the political-cultural revolution without the distraction of coming up with the range of material, textual and visual, that Hayes had to come up with every month. Morris could even be forgiven if he imagined his job was not just to make money for the magazine's owners but to put out a magazine that made a serious contribution to the culture; Hayes had fewer illusions on that score.

Meanwhile, in San Francisco, a feisty editorial team had transformed *Ramparts,* once a small lay Catholic literary magazine, into a vehicle of no-holds-barred muckraking, spiced with political art and strong photographs. Operating in the red on donated funds, uninhibited by commercial constraints and by any pretense of political neutrality, Warren Hinckle and Robert Scheer unapologetically took on the American establishment. Beginning in July 1965 with an exposé of the "Vietnam Lobby"— academics, Catholic Church leaders, and anti-Communist intellectuals who had supported American involvement in Vietnam—*Ramparts* had fired off volley after volley, blasting away at the CIA ties of such apparently innocuous institutions as Michigan State University and the National Student Association. Hinckle took out full-page *New York Times* ads to announce *Ramparts'* findings, and the *Times* itself was quick to pick up on *Ramparts'* exposés in the news columns. Since *Ramparts* was virtually devoid of advertising, and, like *Harper's,* had a circulation a fraction of *Esquire'*s, it was never a commercial threat to *Esquire,* but, like *Harper's, Ramparts* offered a serious editorial challenge. In fact, *Ramparts* had only a few more months to live; it would go into bankruptcy in February 1969, but in late 1968 Hayes only saw what was before him— another iconoclastic magazine with a great flair for showmanship.

Another upstart went unmentioned by Hayes, probably because in 1968 it had not yet found its footing, but it would prove to be the mightiest and most enduring competitor of all: *Rolling Stone,* which had appeared the year before in San Francisco on the edge of the *Ramparts* circle. Under its founder Jan Wenner, *Rolling Stone* had been pretty much a rock fan's magazine during its first year, until Wenner hired John Burks as managing editor and *Rolling Stone* took on journalistic weight it hadn't had. Burks had learned his trade at *Newsweek* and the *Oakland Tribune,* but he had also been an *Esquire* reader. Years later he would remember reading a Tom Wolfe piece in *Esquire* while he was sitting at his *Tribune* desk, and idly typing a passage from the story onto the sheet of paper stuck in his typewriter, just to see how Wolfe did what he did— how he built those sentences. More than any other magazine, *Rolling Stone* picked up the beat of *Esquire'*s literary journalism, becoming, its historian Robert Draper said later, the home of New Journalism in the seventies that *Esquire* had been in the sixties.

Starting out when it did, *Rolling Stone* caught the youth culture wave at the optimal point; it packed political and cultural reporting around the core of rock 'n' roll. *Esquire* made token gestures toward rock 'n' roll, but Hayes's heart was not in it: he was a jazz man himself. Missing the beat of rock 'n' roll, he missed the dark nihilism and unreasoning hope that played through the lyrics of rock 'n' roll, and through rock 'n' roll into the sixties youth culture. *Esquire* should have paid more attention to rock 'n' roll, *Esquire* editor Tom Ferrell said later.

To Ferrell, who had left a Ph.D. program at Harvard in 1967 to run *Esquire*'s research department, the best years of the sixties *Esquire* had already passed by the time he became an editor in late 1968. In the earlier sixties, *Esquire* had invited readers into an inner circle of those who knew better with the promise: "We'll show you the foolishness in the culture around you." In the face of Vietnam, riots—the drama of the high six-ties—readers had lost their sense of humor. Instead of being detached, they had become "engagé."

Aware that magazines ride on the currents of time, Hayes had periodi-cally encouraged editors not to let their definition of the magazine become too fixed, their understanding of what it could do become overly narrow; he knew magazines had to change or be left behind. From the late 1950s, when he assigned Martin Mayer to write about the *Daily Worker,* he had wanted an *Esquire* that would always surprise.

Yet for all Hayes's efforts to encourage varied points of view—and *Esquire*'s range outstretched any other commercial magazine's—*Esquire* did have a satiric stance, announced every month in George Lois's covers and at the start of every year in the Dubious Achievement Awards. Read-ers expected *Esquire* to be, among other things, funny, in a twisted, intel-ligent way. When Michael Herr interviewed Westmoreland, the general asked him if he intended to write "humoristical" pieces on Vietnam. *Esquire* managed to be "serious, and at the same time jolly," Edward Grossman would write in a review of Hayes's collection of *Esquire* articles from the sixties, *Smiling Through the Apocalypse,* published in 1969. Without question *Esquire* preferred satire, loosely defined. And satire as a mode, locked in a symbiotic relationship with culture, required constant adjustments as the culture underwent change.

By 1968, Hayes himself would say a few years later, the *Esquire* atti-tude, born in the late 1950s, had run its useful course. "Against the aridity of the national landscape of the late Fifties we offered to our readers in our better moments the promise of outright laughter; by the end of the Sixties the best we could provide was a bleak grin." How could *Esquire* go on

being satirical when no one wanted to laugh? The Dubious Achievement
Awards for January 1969 laid out the lament:

Back in 1962, when we started this thing, there was Florence Aadland
(Mother of the Year), the comedy team of Ev and Charlie, stretch pants and a
whole lot of other stuff to break you up. What do we have now? Not one assassination this year, mind you, but two. Not just the good old air pollution of sweet-
smelling exhaust fumes; no, now we've got tear gas and Mace in the atmosphere.
Your minds are twisted with drugs, your bodies unbathed, your clothes indistin-
guishable by sex. America, you aren't funny anymore. Polack! Jap! Wop! Nigger!
See, you didn't laugh. The man below is right.

The man below was Spiro T. Agnew: "The Most Dubious Achievement
of 1968."

EIGHT

Ugly beyond Belief

HREE MONTHS after the 1968 Democratic Convention, William F. Buckley, Jr., called Harold Hayes with a proposal. During the convention, Gore Vidal and Buckley, set up as adversaries on ABC-TV, had called each other names that, as David Susskind said later, "we'd never heard on television before." Vidal called Buckley a "pro-crypto Nazi" and Buckley responded: "Now listen, you queer. Stop calling me a pro-crypto Nazi or I'll sock you in the goddam face. . . ." Since then, Buckley had been troubled by comments from friends and acquaintances. He proposed writing an article for *Esquire* explaining himself.

Although both men were contributors to *Esquire,* Hayes's relationship with Buckley was closer than his relationship with Vidal. Buckley was one of those writers, like Martin Mayer and Gay Talese, who seemed always willing to take on a subject Hayes wanted him to take on, from Joe Namath to Whittaker Chambers. Moreover, Buckley had sent Hayes a writer who became one of his favorites, Garry Wills. Hayes felt friendly enough with Buckley to use him as a reference a couple of times, once when Hayes wanted to get his daughter into a private school, and again when he bought a cooperative apartment.

Hayes's relationship with Vidal was more distant. Vidal had been a columnist for *Esquire* in the early sixties and later wrote other articles; Hayes valued him as a writer, but even at his most generous, Vidal seemed to Hayes faintly condescending. He had once accused Hayes of indulging Buckley, whose politics, Vidal said, were "dangerous."

Hayes supposed he liked Vidal's politics better than Buckley's but preferred Buckley as a person over Vidal. As an editor, Hayes saw himself as apolitical—"apersonal too, for that matter," he added, writing later about Buckley's call and what it led to. "I doubt either could have persuaded me to follow him to the other side of the street," he remarked, "though I would have listened closely to the arguments of both."

Back in 1964, in a staff memo, Hayes had said, quoting Gingrich, "We don't like to fight but we do like to start them and then stand aside and hold the guys' coats." Hayes had run combative pieces before—for instance, Gore Vidal's on the Kennedys, first on Robert Kennedy in March 1963 and then, in April 1967, on the entire "Holy Family." Showing no signs of his sometime preference for calm reasoning, he had encouraged Rust Hills to pump up a piece on Norman Podhoretz's confessional autobiography, *Making It,* from "a mild little piece" to a "huge, great, long malicious vicious piece," as Hills would recall. "Harold said, 'Get him on this.' So I'd write some more nasty stuff. Eventually it turned out to be what I think Mailer in *Partisan Review* called a 'dreadnought' of a piece. It was one of the things that annoyed Mailer again, because he was reasonably good friends with Podhoretz. But it was Harold who made it excessive. And he had a capacity for doing the excessive."

The brief exchange between Buckley and Vidal during the convention had been excessive. An extended exchange was unlikely to be less excessive. Yes, Hayes told Buckley, he would run Buckley's explanation if, in turn, Vidal would write a reply. Buckley agreed, so long as Vidal's article did not appear in the same issue as his.

Before Buckley could proceed, *Esquire*'s lawyers had to be satisfied that Buckley could repeat his allegation that Vidal was a homosexual. Hayes had not been much of a law student at Wake Forest, but his years at *Esquire* had given him a pretty good education in publishing law. He understood that, in 1969, calling someone a homosexual without good evidence was like labeling someone a Communist—libel *per se.* With homosexual behavior still outlawed in a number of states, labeling someone homosexual could have serious consequences. Had Vidal ever identified himself as a homosexual? *Esquire* turned up a statement in the London magazine *Queen* in which he had said,

In some ways, I was lucky to be brought up with no sense of sexual guilt. I was never told that masturbation was bad or that it was particularly wicked to go to bed with boys or girls. I also went into the Army a month after my 17th birthday, and there was very little one didn't do. That established a promiscuous pattern, which I am sure has had its limiting side. But there have been compensations.

That statement, in itself, was inconclusive, but *Esquire*'s lawyers thought it was strong enough to clear the way if Hayes himself thought there was reason to believe Vidal was homosexual. In 1964 the U.S. Supreme Court had ruled in the case of *The New York Times Co. vs. Sullivan* that in matters of public interest, a plaintiff has to prove actual malice, defined as reckless disregard of the truth, to win a libel judgment. *Did* Hayes believe that Vidal was a homosexual? *Esquire*'s lawyers asked. Hayes did not know for certain, he acknowledged, but he did say that—as he wrote later—"it was the general belief within the literary community . . . that he was." The lawyers told Buckley he could proceed—subject, of course, to further review.

Reading the fifty-two-page manuscript Buckley turned in, Hayes found much to delight: "a polemical thrust which responds instantly to the slightest pressure; breathtaking, often suicidal syntax; an extraordinary range of knowledge and experience; in all, a style which, countering the intensity, is as good humored and sometimes as breezy as Dwight Macdonald's." He called Buckley to say he had accomplished all he meant to except for his basic purpose: he had not offered a satisfactory explanation for the name he had called Vidal. Several days later, Buckley returned a revision. He had changed the last paragraph to include a backhand apology to Vidal. Commenting on what he saw as contradictory social attitudes, Buckley noted that "faggotry is countenanced, but the imputation of it—even to faggots—is not." Then he went on to say, "But the imputation of it in anger is not justified, which is why I herewith apologize to Gore Vidal."

On February 26, 1969, Hayes forwarded the manuscript to Vidal in Rome with the comment, "He's pretty rough on you, of course, but you would have expected that." Vidal had told Hayes on the phone that he would prefer only to correct Buckley's facts, but Hayes expressed the hope that he would "answer to whatever length" suited him, "and in whatever form." He added: "I think you will know that we are staying neutral in all this."

A few days later, Don Erickson, the managing editor, called Vidal to get his reaction. Vidal said he was coming back to New York City right away to consult his lawyers. Back in New York, he came to see Hayes. He wanted to call a halt to the whole thing—only Buckley would gain from it, by bringing attention to himself. *Esquire* would be put at risk because, Vidal insisted, he had never once identified himself as homosexual. Hayes heard him out, countering his points. Finally, Hayes put the question to him: Should he drop the project?

"To his credit," Hayes said later, "he answered: 'I wish you would, but if you decide to go ahead, I won't try to stop you. I'm not in the practice of censoring anyone. If you do go on, I will sue you only if you refuse to print my response.' "

Vidal hired a researcher and a private detective to prepare his response to Buckley. When it came in, Hayes thought it, too, had its moments but bogged down in "a seemingly endless series of not-so-instant replays." He passed a later draft of Vidal's piece to Gingrich with the comment, "While it is still mean and vitriolic, there is considerable improvement, and at least two-thirds less than the original in his dwelling on his own sexuality and Buckley's." In fact, Hayes went on, "he has so smoothly toned down his excesses of the original that this makes both pieces worth doing. Both men emerge looking petty and the smaller for the confrontation but the reader at least gets to make that judgment. . . ."

Esquire's lawyer, Harold R. Medina, Jr., reviewed Buckley's and Vidal's manuscripts in late March 1969 and talked the project over with Abe Blinder, Arnold Gingrich, Don Erickson, and Hayes. The project still seemed workable to the lawyer, so long as *Esquire* was satisfied that statements of fact were true and comments fair. If *Esquire* believed statements of fact were true and comments were fair, *Esquire*'s lawyers could mount a constitutional defense under the First Amendment. Offering the writers right of reply would strengthen *Esquire*'s defense under common law.

The drafts went on their heavily scrutinized way, as *Esquire*'s research department subjected the manuscripts to what Hayes said was the most thorough review Hayes had seen during his time at *Esquire,* although the chief of research, Kitty Krupat, had been on the job only a few days when these manuscripts came her way. She had had experience in research at the *Saturday Evening Post,* but the *Post* had folded only a few months after she was hired, and, besides, *Post* stories were never like this. When Vidal's piece went to Buckley for his scrutiny, Buckley returned it with forty-eight major exceptions, which Vidal then took exception to, and the research department tried to sort out the truth. Finally, Hayes wrote a memorandum, seventeen pages long, adjudicating the differences. Buckley shot back a six-page memorandum.

Since the research department was turning up errors in Vidal's manuscript, Hayes gave it a stiff edit. Then he made a last attempt at mutual consent: he sent both pieces to both men and asked if they would sign statements agreeing to the publication of both pieces and promising not to sue either the other writer or the magazine. If either refused to sign, Hayes reserved the option to publish the article by the other party anyway.

That idea went nowhere. Buckley, reviewing Vidal's last version, pronounced it unsatisfactory in a letter to Hayes on April 24, 1969: not factually true. Hayes asserted that it was indeed *"fair in comment and true in fact."* Hayes, Erickson, Blinder, and *Esquire*'s lawyer, Medina, conferred, and Medina assured the rest that Buckley's protests were both unfounded legally and inappropriate morally. He believed the article could be safely published. *Esquire* had by now given up on the original idea of getting each writer to agree to the other's version. *Esquire* would be the judge of what was accurate and fair.

On April 30, a cable from Vidal's lawyers arrived at *Esquire* advising *Esquire* that the Buckley article *Esquire* was about to publish was defamatory. Meanwhile, there was no word on whether Vidal wanted *Esquire* to run his edited reply to Buckley, and Hayes began to assume he was trying to publish a fuller version of his reply elsewhere; there were rumors (which turned out to be false) that Vidal had offered the reply to *Playboy* and the *New York Review of Books*. On the basis of those rumors, Buckley sent a letter to leading publishers letting them know that if they planned to publish Vidal's accusations they should give him a chance to refute them first.

Furthermore, on May 6, Buckley filed a $500,000 defamation suit against Vidal in connection with the remarks Vidal had made on television and was disseminating in the article he had written for *Esquire*. When Harvard professor John Kenneth Galbraith wrote to Buckley suggesting that such a suit "would be costly and most unwise," Buckley explained that Vidal had written "a piece of such filth and venom as would have persuaded the average reader that where I belonged was the dock at Nuremberg."

The same day Buckley filed his preemptive suit against Vidal, his lawyer sent *Esquire* a list of fifteen points that he deemed libelous in Vidal's last draft. The lawyer closed with a reminder that libelous remarks could affect Buckley's business as the writer of a column that appeared three times a week, the editor of a magazine, the host of a weekly television show, and a lecturer who commanded high fees. Medina responded: Publication of these articles was just the kind of free-flowing debate the Supreme Court had sanctioned.

Buckley's article was published in the August issue, which appeared in mid-July. Vidal's appeared in the September issue, which came out in mid-August with some of the cut passages restored after further investigation by the legal department and reinterpretation by the lawyers. Buckley promptly sued *Esquire* for $1 million; Vidal countersued Buckley for $1.5 million.

Despite Hayes's efforts to set up a fair process that would allow each man to speak his piece against the other, despite diligent fact-checking and complex pre-publication negotiation, the project had wound up in a legal tangle. When it was all over, Hayes would write (then cross out the statement—which he probably meant but preferred not to make), "Events now show we all would have gained had I simply called a halt to the affair."

Esquire lawyers and editorial staff members would spend many hours over the next three years preparing for trial. To Kitty Krupat, the researcher swept up in the case, Buckley's suit sometimes seemed a stunt, with Buckley in his favorite stance—very outraged, tongue in cheek. Both sides seemed to be playing games. Once when Krupat was in Hayes's office with several others to discuss the case, Vidal whipped out a little green book that somebody had published—an alphabetical listing of famous homosexuals: the last listing was "Zeus." As Krupat recalled, Vidal pointed out Buckley's name in the book, then when Vidal turned away to take a phone call, he handed the book to someone else, who opened it to the V's and found Vidal's own name there, and everybody laughed at this obviously ridiculous book, which nobody took as serious proof.

The very idea of having Vidal and Buckley face off was, in its way, a stunt, it seemed to Krupat. *Esquire* always seemed to be searching for some odd way of juxtaposing realities, she recalled. It was part of the atmosphere in the sixties: finding nontraditional ways to examine ideas and people, breaking down barriers in journalism. The intent was to thumb noses—to engage in iconoclasm. But everyone took the depositions seriously enough.

Indeed, for Hayes the deposition process was an ordeal that called into question his basic editorial philosophy. He had gone into the depositions convinced that he had behaved responsibly as an editor in the Buckley-Vidal project—"dispassionately and without prejudice." He had tried to afford each writer "as much freedom of expression as possible, to insist on accuracy and fair play, and, if possible, to avoid legal injury to either party or the magazine." In what seemed to him a bizarre twist of events, he had agreed to Buckley's own proposal to meditate on what it meant for him to have called Gore Vidal "queer." Now, defending against Buckley's suit, Hayes found himself explaining *Vidal's* allegation that *Buckley* resembled

Myra Breckinridge, the homosexual who became a woman in Vidal's novel of the same name, which Hayes admitted he had not even read.

Pressed to say in a deposition whether he himself believed when he published Vidal's article that Buckley resembled Myra Breckinridge, Hayes said he did not, but he argued that his personal beliefs did not and should not dictate the contents of the magazine. As an editor, he allowed writers writing under their own names to say whatever they felt was true, so long as what they said was "true in fact and fair in comment."

"I publish many things that I do not personally believe in. We publish people of widely varying opinions. These do not always reflect my opinions. It is necessary therefore for me to distinguish my opinion about a given episode, mine as a private citizen who has his own head, context and reference, as against material which I feel nevertheless is legitimate and of value to publish which may vary with the opinions different than my own."

"Do you make some distinction between 'I believe' and 'I personally believe'?"

"I believe as an editor and Harold Hayes as a private citizen believes. Those are the two distinctions I would make."

Buckley's lawyer, Charles Rembar, did not relent. Vidal had used an incident of vandalism involving three Buckley children as evidence that Buckley was anti-Semitic. Retracting the allegation he had made on television that Buckley was a "pro-crypto Nazi," he had gone on to say, "But in a larger sense his views are very much those of the founders of the Third Reich who regarded blacks as inferiors, undeclared war as legitimate foreign policy, and the Jews as sympathetic to international communism."

Now, the lawyer insisted on knowing if he, Harold Hayes, believed Buckley resembled Hitler's propaganda minister Josef Goebbels; Hayes said no, he did not, personally, believe Buckley resembled Goebbels. What about when Hayes published Vidal's piece—did he believe, then, that Buckley was anti-Semitic? There was no safe response, as Hayes saw his predicament. If he agreed with Vidal, then he would be guilty of contributing to the libel. If he said he disagreed with Vidal, he would be guilty of publishing out of malice what he believed to be false. Pinned by the lawyer, he could no longer say, let the reader decide. "The reader had come and gone," Hayes later observed. Alone on the spot, he did the best that he could.

"Did the submission of Vidal's article give you an occasion to think about whether he was an anti-Semite?" Buckley's lawyer asked.

"It certainly gave me a professional occasion to think about it," Hayes replied.

"What was the result of your thought?"

"The result of my thinking was that Vidal—it was permissible for Vidal to draw the conclusion that he put in his piece regarding Bill's anti-Semitism."

The cross-examination certainly did not leave room for neutrality, Hayes thought, but *Esquire*'s lawyer Bob Rifkind told him not to worry: after all, *Esquire* had a record of publishing divergent views. Hayes found himself worrying anyway. Now that the question was raised, what *did* he personally think about Vidal's allegations? Later on, he sat down to read the 570 pages of Rembar's deposition of Vidal, and found himself forced out of neutrality. The question for him as an editor, he could see now, was this: "What was *purely* personal, having to do only with the private life of William F. Buckley and not at all with his politics, and therefore entitled to some privilege?" Considering the article, Hayes concluded that "in nearly every case" Vidal had tried to relate whatever he said about Buckley's personal life to the basic political charge that he thought like a fascist.

Could the same be said of Buckley? Hayes found his answer in a long interrogation in which Rembar tried to get Vidal to agree that he was a homosexual. Vidal evaded his grasp. To the question, "Have you ever engaged in an act which you, yourself, would describe as homosexual," Vidal replied, "What you might describe as a heterosexual act I might view as a homosexual act. What you might view as a homosexual act I might see as a bisexual act. I don't think I can define every possible interpretation that I might have on anything."

Again and again Rembar thrust, and again and again Vidal parried. He stood his ground: his sexuality was private and he would keep it that way. Now, in Hayes's view, Buckley's and Vidal's mutual insults sorted themselves out into separate categories. "Both men employed personal references ruthlessly to establish characterization—an essentially political characterization of Buckley ('pro-crypto Nazi') by Vidal, but an essentially moral characterization of Vidal ('queer') by Buckley."

The complex picture came into focus for Hayes when he reviewed Rembar's brief to the court, arguing that the case should be allowed to go to trial. Hayes concluded his own written, unpublished analysis of the affair by quoting from Rembar's brief:

"We submit it is clear that the charges that Buckley is a homosexual and a sexual degenerate fall outside the constitutional privilege.

"To be sure, the sexual life of important public figures may be a favorite topic among gossip mongers and those who feed upon the intimate secrets of the famous. But such voyeurism does not make the sexual life of a public figure a matter of 'public or general concern' in the constitutional sense. . . . The public's interest must be substantial and legitimate. . . . The public has no legitimate interest in Buckley's sexual life. Further information on that subject cannot possibly help them to form opinions about needed social or political change or help them to cope with the exigencies of the period. . . .

"Thus the Supreme Court . . . has already made clear that the sexual life of even a public figure is outside the area of 'public or general concern' which is protected by the constitutional defense."

Applying the same standard to Gore Vidal, Hayes regretted giving Buckley a forum in which to discuss Vidal's sexual life, "which is why I now personally believe I, too, owe an apology to Gore Vidal," he wrote.

In the end, the court dismissed Vidal's countersuit but ruled that Buckley's suits against *Esquire* and Vidal had sufficient merit to go to trial. By this point, legal costs for all parties had mounted high. "Aware now that he had the advantage," Hayes wrote later, "Buckley proposed a settlement out of court, favorable to himself, which *Esquire* and Vidal accepted." The settlement—which the parties agreed not to disclose—actually cost *Esquire* very little but it saved face for Buckley. The agreement, filed away by Hayes in his papers, specified that Buckley would receive $115,000 from *Esquire* to reimburse him for legal expenses. That part Buckley would be allowed to make public. What neither party could make public was how the $115,000 would be paid: $15,000 in cash, and $100,000 in advertising space in *Esquire* to advertise the *National Review*.

Esquire was also to run a statement in its November 1972 issue that *Esquire* was "utterly convinced that Mr. Buckley is not 'anti-Black,' 'anti-Semitic,' a 'war-monger' or, in any respect whatsoever, 'pro-crypto Nazi'—all of which charges were made in the Vidal article. We published that article because we believed that Vidal had the right to assert *his* opinions, even though we did not share them."

Even then, the affair did not end: after Buckley gave his account of the dispute in the *National Review,* October 13, 1972, Hayes felt obliged to write a letter to the editor correcting Buckley's version; Buckley declined to publish the letter, saying it was time to let the matter rest.

For Hayes, Buckley's suit was deeply disappointing, a source of real personal grief; the decision to settle rankled for years. It proved nothing, he said later, "and satisfied only William Buckley's sense of his own righteousness." The pieces themselves, Edward Grossman wrote in *Commentary,* amounted to little more than "an interminable exchange of mutual bitchiness." Yet when Hayes edited *Smiling Through the Apocalypse,* published before the suit was settled, he closed the 981-page volume with Buckley on Vidal and Vidal on Buckley—"as appropriate a conclusion to the Sixties as any other, yielding as they do almost no direct information on the changing times other than by suggesting indirectly—through the bitterness, jealousy, ambition and despair of two of our most eloquent sensibilities—the character of America's collective confusion."

In August 1969, the issue in which William F. Buckley's article on Gore Vidal appeared, *Esquire* published another article that Hayes was worried about because he was afraid it would be seen as sensational. He went ahead and led the issue with it—how could he not, when it was so important?—but he underplayed it otherwise, using no illustrations and only the simple title "An American Atrocity," with a subhead and, in small italic type at the bottom of the first column, a note: "The facts of this report are available for public inspection in the office of the Judge Advocate General of the Navy in Washington, D.C."

A magazine writer named Normand Poirier told the story:

On September 23, 1966, a small Marine squad—nine men—had terrorized several Vietnamese families in a village in what was considered a pacified area. When they had raided nine huts and had found no weapons, no contraband, no information on the Vietcong, they descended on the tenth with a terrible fury. They pounded the lone man in the hut until he was almost unconscious and dragged his young wife to the side of the house.

She had heard her husband's protests of innocence and his cries as he was beaten and the cries of her mother-in-law and sister-in-law and the wailing of the children. But she could not even cry out because a man had a hand over her mouth and two others held her arms and legs and they had her on her back on the ground. When there were five men around her they forced open her legs and ripped her pajama pants away and tore open the top of her pajamas. . . . The hand cracked her face back and forth and she felt the blood trickle down her chin. Then the hand came down on her face again, ... She felt the first man go inside her and she prayed for her husband and baby. . . . All the men were talking and laughing and then a third man raped her. Tears streamed from her eyes. . . . And then a fifth man. Her husband's voice was loud, now. He was screaming for his wife. . . . He was hysterical with hatred because, he said, he knew what they had done to her. . . . But then she heard the first burst of gunfire. . . . And then another burst, two or three bursts together, and there were no voices. My baby, she thought. My baby! She got to her knees and heard bamboo snap and saw a blinding flash of light. . . .

The Marines killed a man, two women, and two children. One of the women, the one raped repeatedly, survived and made her way to a Marine base, where she told her story. Called in for interrogation, the Marines, one by one, abandoned the cover-up story they had concocted to explain these civilian deaths and told what had really happened. Returning to the hut to try to cover up what they had done—trying to make the deaths look more like the result of a Vietcong ambush—they had found a baby still alive; it was screaming.

Poirier presented one Marine's account of what happened next. One man, Potter, was standing over the baby.

"What did Potter do when you were looking at him while he was standing over the baby?"

"He had his rifle in his hands . . ." Vogel said.

"What did he do . . ."

"He said, 'Somebody count for me!' "

"Somebody count what?" Ellis asked.

"Count! Just count!"

"Count cadence?"

"No, just count for him. So I started counting. I turned around and started counting . . ."

"You *looked* at him and then you started counting! You can't make it any easier."

"I said one . . . two . . . three . . . And he was hitting the baby with the butt!"

"How was he doing it?"

"Dropping it down."

"Picking it up and smashing it down or just letting it fall down?"

"Picking it up and hitting it down," Vogel said, softly.

"Like a baseball bat or like he was chopping wood or straight up and down like a butt stroke? Did you ever see anyone churn butter?"

"It was straight up and down."

"Like someone churning butter," Ellis said in conclusion.

"Yeah," Vogel said. And after a long pause he said: "Then it was quiet and someone said to Potter, 'You sure got some balls to do that.' "

Hayes needn't have worried about public response. Although *Esquire* slipped early copies of the issue to the *New York Times,* the *Times* did not pick up the story. Although this was one of the earliest reports of atrocities in Vietnam, the public response, Tom Hedley recalled, was confusion.

Some readers even thought it might be an *Esquire* hoax. *Esquire* was going to have to be careful. Its collegiate, satiric voice was getting too familiar. "People don't really trust us," Hedley said to himself.

To Michael Herr, the war had laid a curse on America, like the curse that William Faulkner said slavery had laid on the country. The late sixties had turned "ugly beyond belief." Herr was in New York writing the Khesanh section of *Dispatches,* his book on Vietnam, and hearing, now, voices, real voices in his head, the voices that became the voices of the book, saying the things he had heard soldiers say and sometimes, though not often, saying things he had not heard anyone say. The book would be full of voices—the language of Americans in Vietnam. ("Mayhew, crazy fucker, he sleep bare-ass. He so tough, man, li'l fucker, the hawk is out, an' he's in here bare-ass." "What's that? About the hawk?" "That means it's a co-o-old Mother Fucker.")

Herr had always been able to re-create the conversation of other people utterly different from himself, and he did that now: re-creating the voices he had heard in Vietnam—all wound together in the long monologue the book became. "Were the voices real?" interviewers would ask him. "They were real," he said. But he wasn't writing dialogue from notes. He didn't remember, later, even taking notes on what people said—just on what he saw, the country, the people, and less and less of that as he went along. And the characters were not always exactly who he said they were. Day Tripper was a composite, Mayhew was mostly Mayhew but in real life he wasn't called Mayhew. Sometimes Herr thought of the book as a novel, sometimes the best description for it was a "distillation" of an extreme experience "in the most honest and truthful way which did not happen to always be the most factual way."

The narrator's voice held it all together—the scattered pieces of war: a voice deliberate, tense, holding hysteria back to give an account the narrator knows, knows without any question or doubt, must be given. It was urgently necessary that these things be told, said, understood. The Khesanh pieces were full of dread—death and dread and more death, that "laughing death-face" that hid behind the newsprint and lingered on the television screens after the news reports that denied its presence in the war. Death lingered on Herr's every page: bodies, stacked, shoved into body bags, torn apart—the object of jokes and anguish and casual disregard. Death and love: Herr had loved the Marines, who were pathetic and fucked up and forlorn and abandoned and lost, but who had real heart. They were an embarrassment to any historical sense of masculinity, but there was something going on there, something that was very moving.

Hayes read the Khesanh chapter overnight and called him the next morning: he would run it all, the whole Khesanh section, in two parts, in the September and October issues of 1969.

What meant most to Herr about going to Vietnam for *Esquire* had not been the accreditation but Hayes's support, the feeling Hayes gave him: "Nobody is going to touch a word of this kid's work." He kept on having that feeling, even after his work *was* touched—its rawest edges rubbed smooth, the "motherfuckers" and "fuckers" turned into "motherf---er" and "f---er," "Shit" into "S---." Herr negotiated word by word on the expletives, with Hayes or with Don Erickson. Once Herr and Erickson were going over the manuscript, and Erickson was saying, "Rather than say 'motherfucker' here, can't we say, 'mother-blank' or 'blank-blank-er' or—," and Herr looked up to see a window washer who had been listening to this entire conversation, amazement and contempt on his face.

Important as the language was in the piece, important as language was to Herr, it never occurred to him to publish the excerpts elsewhere—in *Playboy,* say, as Garry Wills did once when *Esquire* wanted to sanitize a piece. Herr had such strong feelings for *Esquire.*

Both Khesanh installments ran with full-page color photographs—for the second, a young Marine, bearded, face grimy, eyes blank like the eyes Herr described: eyes that "never had anything to do with what the rest of the face was doing," eyes that made young men old. The photograph with the first installment showed soldiers kneeling in a trench; all that was visible was their hunched backs and helmets and hands clutching their heads, braced for attack; the unprotected photographer taking the picture was implicit. The pictures were made by a young photographer working for *Newsweek,* Robert J. Ellison. Herr had been with him at Khesanh a couple of times and had seen him off at the Danang airfield on the day that he died, his plane blown up on landing at Khesanh. The word came that evening, when Herr was having dinner in Saigon with an editor from *Newsweek,* who was called to the telephone, and Herr could hear his voice from across the room, almost shouting: "Is he *dead?* Is he *dead? Is...he...dead?"*

Esquire announced the imminent publication of *Dispatches* in "Backstage," October 1969, when the second Khesanh installment ran, but *Dispatches* did not appear. Herr was living with Valerie Elliott, who worked for Herr's agent, Candida Donadio. Elliott would say to Donadio, "He doesn't write, he doesn't write anything." And Donadio would say,

"You must understand, writers spend *years* thinking. They just spend years thinking and thinking."

In fact, Herr was writing, but slowly. Elliott would come home and he would have the television on, and he would be lying on the sofa, and writing on a yellow pad: a few lines, dot-dot-dot, then a blank line, and a few more lines. He was trying to give the *Esquire* material a frame that would make *Dispatches* a book—a real book with a narrative that he could tell was there, even if no one else could. But the high that had carried him almost all the way had come to an end: he had come home from his adventure in Vietnam, virtually the only one of his New York set who had gone to Vietnam, and he had come home unhurt, full of energy and ego and vanity.

Then two colleagues from Vietnam, photographers Dana Stone and Sean Flynn, went off to Cambodia and never returned, and *Life* photographer Larry Burrows died in a helicopter accident over Cambodia. A breakdown that Herr would come to feel had been lurking for many years, at least ten, a breakdown he had avoided by moving fast through the sixties, descended on him. He had felt it coming during the summer of 1969: then a year later it hit him hard. He had seen things in Vietnam he really shouldn't have seen—things he had not been prepared to see. He had had pretensions, ambition, and he had gotten in over his head, gone to an extreme place where he was not prepared to go. He had begun to sense what was in store for him when someone in Vietnam asked him, "Are you a reporter?"

"And I said, 'No, I'm a writer.' And he said, 'Well, be careful, 'cause where you're going you can't use an eraser.'

"And I knew I was being told something of extreme profundity, it really made my blood run cold.

"You know, I was looking at bodies—but I didn't believe—I saw this guy shot across the aisle from me in a helicopter, and that didn't do it. Nothing that I was seeing did it, and then this guy said that to me and it was like—

"I've often wondered where that guy is and wished I could speak to him. Thank him."

The flower children were leaving Haight-Ashbury, the San Francisco home of the hippies, for rural communes, Berkeley, other places. Living in the Haight, said a runaway who was still living there, was "like living in a jungle," *Esquire* writer John Luce reported. Real criminals walked the streets—fighting, hustling, stealing, preferring heroin and speed to LSD. These weren't the refugees from the middle class the media had made famous: these were young toughs, lower-class kids with criminal records, seriously crazy, bent on maintaining "terminal euphoria"—drug use so intense that early death was inevitable. There was nothing—*nothing*—romantic about the scene, as *Esquire* presented it.

Esquire reported "The Final Decline and Total Collapse of the American Avant-Garde" in May 1969, assigning Andy Warhol to take photographs of New Theatre groups (he took one of his own scar, too) and getting Claes Oldenburg to stage his last happening, just for *Esquire.* Oldenburg got the *Esquire* crew thrown out of the insurance office where it was staged. Hayes was annoyed; he didn't like the Warhol crowd. "It's just art, Harold," Tom Hedley said. "We're doing art here."

The SDS disintegrated at its Chicago convention in June. When Nora Sayre went to Oakland, California, to report on a Black Panthers conference for *Esquire,* she found "a good eighty percent" of those present were white: it appeared to her that the Panthers (whom she regarded sympathetically) had lost the neighborhoods. Across the Bay in San Francisco, Tom Wolfe reported that some young Chinese had adopted the confrontational political style of militant blacks, while other young Chinese engaged in old-fashioned warfare. When Tom Hedley met with Daniel Boorstin, an academic historian who wanted to write an anonymous critique of SDS campus activity, Boorstin began to speak of the time when America had one hundred institutions of learning as good as any in the world. In twenty-five years, Boorstin predicted, because of the democratization movement on campus, America would be lucky to have two or three left. As he talked, Hedley saw tears in his eyes.

In mid-July, the weekend men went to the moon, Edward Kennedy, the last surviving Kennedy brother, drove a car off a narrow bridge on Chappaquiddick Island, and a young woman named Mary Jo Kopechne drowned. Woodstock, August 15–17, 1969, "was a nightmare, just a nightmare," Michael Herr thought, "a pseudo-event, all of those sweet liberating impulses had become completely co-opted by the media. . . ."

On the evening of December 6, 1969, at a Rolling Stones concert at the Altamont Raceway fifty miles east of Oakland, members of the Hells Angels killed a member of the audience, an eighteen-year-old black man, as, twenty feet away, Mick Jagger sang, "Under my thumb. . . ." In his

Esquire account, Ralph J. Gleason, the *San Francisco Chronicle* jazz critic who had done as much as any man to herald the music-based counterculture—not just at the *Chronicle,* but in *Ramparts* and *Rolling Stone*—
passed ambiguous judgment on the event, concluding with a quotation
from Ken Kesey, another architect of the counterculture: " 'There are
some things which aren't true even if they did happen,' Ken Kesey once
said. Altamont is like that." *Esquire* titled the piece "Aquarius Wept."

In late 1969, the editors came up with an idea that would capture the
feeling that these were latter days. The idea emerged when the editors
went on a Bermuda cruise in October, a welcome break from a major
renovation of the offices. The editors had approached the cruise as a
lark—managing editor Don Erickson, in a memo, called it the Ding-Dong
School. Hayes was headmaster, Erickson dean of women. Editors met
every few days to talk business—that is, all editors except Alice Glaser,
who was withdrawing more and more from her fellow editors and had not
come along. Talking about ideas for the magazine, they began to consider
California, which had come to seem an especially troubled place. In early
August, Sharon Tate and four companions had been murdered in Los
Angeles in what appeared to be a ritual killing; a couple named Leno and
Rosemary LaBianca died in similar circumstances. Spending time in California, Hedley had observed that someone on speed in New York would
just be a fast-talking character; in California you got the impression he
might be a mass murderer. There was a strange edge to California life.
Hedley thought it was sex and drugs, but the others said that was simplis-
tic—they would have to investigate.

After the staff returned from the cruise, Sherrill spotted a brief news
item that chilled him to the bone. Datelined Indo, California, October
30, 1969, the story described the ordeal of a small boy who had been
chained up in a packing crate in the farm-commune where he lived. Sherrill proposed running a feature section on evil.

California evil, said Hayes.

Hedley had contacts in California, and Hayes dispatched Jill Goldstein to Los Angeles to see what she could put together: Goldstein was the
editor Hayes most relied on to get things done, especially in a hurry—put
together group portraits, set up covers. Armed with little more than the
concept and a few contacts, Goldstein surveyed the field. She ac-
cumulated a set of fourteen theories explaining the Tate-LaBianca murders. She tracked down witches and warlocks. Once she had her subjects
lined up, photographer Bud Lee went into action.

Self-taught, Lee had come to *Esquire* right out of the army, with a portfolio of pictures that combined bad lighting and good composition. The wire services didn't like his work—it was too offbeat, too satirical, but *Life* magazine sent him to photograph the Newark riots of 1967. *Life* put one of his pictures on the cover, and his work earned him *Life*'s award for Photographer of the Year. By 1969, Lee had joined Carl Fischer, Diane Arbus, Art Kane, and Pete Turner as one of *Esquire*'s favorite photographers. Hedley thought of Lee as "Arbus in Technicolor." Both Lee and Arbus seemed to be telling stories, entire complex narratives implied by a single image. Lee wanted, really, to make movies—like Newman and Benton, he loved the European films of the early sixties—and his still photographs had the dramatic quality of movie stills. Bud Lee was just the photographer to capture the eerie zeitgeist of California at the end of the decade.

For the "California Evil" spread, Lee and writer Tom Burke spent hours in the company of Princess Leda, the acid goddess, who covered her body in feathers, performed sensuous dances, and served fruit laced with acid. When Burke and Lee showed up late in the afternoon, she asked them to drive her down to get the replacement for her black swan, which had just died. They agreed and, following her directions, wound up at a Los Angeles county wildlife preserve.

As weary mothers watched, aghast, with their children, Leda scooped up a black swan from a lake.

"*What is she doing to the swan?*" one mother protested. "Officer," she said to a park guide with a tour group, "they are *torturing* that swan!"

"*I am Leda!*" said Leda, bird in arms.

"I'm Frank," said an old gentleman.

"*I will conceive by this bird!*"

"They're uh, making a TV commercial," said the guide.

Sending the photographer and writer on ahead in the car, Leda met them at the gate, carrying the swan in a carpetbag. As they pulled out of the parking lot, she popped an acid cap and unzipped the bag. The swan's neck rose. A motorcycle patrolman, passing by, looked in but moved on.

Back at the Princess's castle, Bud Lee did what he had been warned not to do—he ate some of the fruit and set off on an acid trip. He pulled a fire alarm, and when the firemen came he thought they were devils. He wound up in jail (an event not covered in the *Esquire* story, although it was covered by the local press), where his cellmates turned into angels. Unpleasant as the acid trip was, even worse was taking photographs of a Black Mass, where strange things were being done to a naked girl hanging upside down. It was to him the saddest, most despicable thing he had seen.

And then an odd thing happened to Lee's film. He had it developed and put the slides into a carousel to check them out, and was running the carousel through in a men's room, while Goldstein waited outside, poised to take the slides back to New York. From within she heard sustained groans. All the slides were dark, as if, Lee thought, the film had been cursed (apparently his borrowed strobe light misfired). Goldstein had to get the witches and warlocks together again and restage the scenes.

Just days before the "California Evil" section was to go to press in the March 1970 issue, the Manson family was arrested for the Tate-LaBianca murders. Goldstein's theories of the murders were out; something else had to go in. Hayes sent Gay Talese to the Spahn Ranch, where the Manson family had lived. The other editors doubted that was going to work. Talese was not a quick writer and he had less than a week to do the story; it was impossible—he couldn't deliver. But Hayes said, No, he could. He had been a *New York Times* reporter. He could meet the deadline.

Talese found a blind man, George Spahn, who told him how the Manson women used to do things for him that his girlfriend had done and how he himself had come to this place. It was the perfect California piece, Talese thought: the man who was blind, the ranch that had been a movie set and now had become a settling place for murderers.

The "California Evil" issue had barely reached the newsstands when the wife and two daughters of a young army doctor named Jeffrey MacDonald were killed in their home at Fort Bragg, North Carolina. According to MacDonald, who had been wounded, his family had been killed by four intruders dressed like hippies: one had carried a candle and said, "Acid is groovy" and "Kill the pigs." The Fayetteville newspaper raised the question: "VICTIMS OF HIPPIE CULT?" Later, MacDonald was arrested on charges of killing his wife and two daughters. An acquaintance of Bob Sherrill's called him to tell him about the slayings. Why are you telling me? Sherrill asked. Because, his friend answered, authorities had found the "California Evil" issue of *Esquire* in MacDonald's house.

On February 19, 1970, Harold Hayes returned to his North Carolina alma mater, Wake Forest, to describe the lay of the American wasteland. He told some of America's more conservative students:

If you aren't blowing up buildings at the moment, you are out there somewhere in the land of Aquarius, stoned to sleep by the Creedence Clearwater Revival, and when you finally wake up—if you ever do—you'll come to where you think it's at. The occasion for your role is the dilemma we've passed on to you, which is just too much to cope with: your country is involved in a war you oppose; cities are decaying; minorities are oppressed; business is venal; education is irrelevant; and the air you breathe is polluted. The country is run by an establishment and that establishment is corrupt.

This role of yours makes it difficult for the rest of us to deny our complicity. Even as you turn on and drop out by the thousands, we stand to the side appalled not only by your rejection of our concern but by the hollow ring to our protests that society is worthy saving after all. Even if we did cause this mess, we *know* that Judeo-Christian civilization deserves a better ending than this—a grubby rock festival attended only by easy riders.

By this time there were those who thought *Esquire* was little better. When Hedley ran into Norman Mailer at a *Paris Review* party and floated the idea of sending Mailer to Cuba to interview Castro, Mailer brushed him off with contempt. Mailer had come back into *Esquire* with a December 1967 piece on a movie he made called *Wild 90,* which Hayes told Rust Hills was "one of the worst features in that issue," but as Hedley recalled, "He looked at me—he was a bit drunk—and he said, 'You punk, you're just a punk,' he says. 'Get outa here.' And he made some crack about Harold Hayes, which was derogatory, I don't remember what he said. And he says, 'Anyway, I wouldn't wanta do it, because I don't like the way this magazine is going, 'cause you wanta put my asshole over Fidel Castro's nose on the cover.' He says, 'I'm going to write something very serious, probably the best I've ever done, and you're gonna treat it frivolously.' He says, 'Forget it.' "

Mailer's fears were well-founded. In September 1971, *Esquire* would illustrate a Germaine Greer piece on Mailer with a photograph of performance artist Patricia Oleszko portraying Mailer as a werewolf.

In August 1970, Jean-Paul Goude, a Frenchman who had shared art direction for a while with Jean Lagarrigue after Sam Antupit left, illustrated an article called "Three Meanies"—"The New Indian," "Superjew," and "Weathermen"—with heads of angry men sticking their tongues out, and Dwight Macdonald, no longer writing his column but still wooed by Hayes for articles, protested: "so ugly, depressing." Sending a piece to *Esquire,* he said, was like committing a serious singer to a rock festival—it would get "lost in the three-ring circus."

Hayes replied, "I'd wish the illustrations didn't distress you quite so much—this is a three-ring circus time and short of turning everything over to David Levine, the problem for a magazine with a flexible format is to try and stay somewhere roughly within the range of current fashions and attitudes."

There had always been something of the hurly-burly about *Esquire* under Hayes. Once he actually sent photographer Pete Turner off on a Ripley's Believe It Or Not–style tour of the South Pacific to get photos of giant clams, a fire eater, a poisonous snake. "Step Right Up Folks, to Thirty Million Square Miles of the Greatest Show on Earth" read the title, and there was something of that spirit throughout *Esquire* in the sixties. Yet the vaudevillian spirit did seem to be intensifying at the turn of the decade, maybe because the *Esquire* attitude was running its course, maybe because Tom Hedley was there.

Hedley came up with ideas like getting celebrities to interview themselves, as in Rod Steiger's "Let Us Now Praise Famous Me" (November 1969). Bud Lee, who hung out with Hedley, was embarrassed, later on, by the sideshow quality of some of the spreads he and Hedley came up with. One of them—"Do Whites Make the Best Domestics? Ask de massah"— featured portraits of blacks with white servants, and when Lee had trouble finding real examples, he asked a couple of people he knew to fill in. (A lawyer for one of the subjects wrote Hayes complaining that because *Esquire* had portrayed his client as wealthy, his creditors were after him.)

Lee and Hedley would sit around the office, tossing ideas back and forth—"Bad Names," featuring relatives of notorious villains, or "Big Jocks," portraits of aging musclemen, still showing off. The cover photo Carl Fischer took for the "Big Jocks" issue presented Johnny Weissmuller and Maureen O'Sullivan as Tarzan and Jane looking seasoned but brave. It seemed to Bud Lee very cruel, although it was no more cruel than Diane Arbus's 1966 *Esquire* photograph of Diana Duff Frazier, "The Girl of the Year, 1938," smoking in bed, wasted by age.

Carolyn Cassady, wife of Neal Cassady, who had been Jack Kerouac's good friend, wept when she saw, in the March 1970 *Esquire,* accompanying an article by Jack McClintock, a Jean-Paul Goude painting of Jack Kerouac in his last days—beer-bellied, in a seedy room with a television and overflowing ashtray stand, and on the worn rug, scattered issues of the *National Review:* in its details of Americana, a perverse play on Norman Rockwell. She was crying, she wrote later, not so much for Kerouac, but for anyone who could derive "either satisfaction or income from such a disgusting display of callousness."

NINE

Joy Boys

*I*N THE SPRING of 1970, Hayes offered John Sack a story he had already offered to three other writers, so far without any success. Lieutenant William L. Calley, Jr., the Marine facing trial for killing more than a hundred villagers at Mylai, was willing to sell *Esquire* exclusive rights to his story, if Hayes could just find a writer. It was a big story—the Mylai massacre had become a symbol for many of what the war had done to Vietnam and America. Yet writer after writer turned Hayes down. He tried John Hersey and William Styron. He tried Garry Wills—really gave him a hard sell: told him it could count as two of the three stories due that year by his contract, but Wills held firm. He wasn't going to describe a killer, he told Hayes. It was the only time there were hard feelings between them. Then John Sack came along—stopped by the office to pay a call—and Hayes asked him to take Calley on.

Sack had read the *New York Times* front-page story reporting the charges and had sworn in disgust—not at Calley but at the press for being so slow to catch on to what was happening in Vietnam. Sack had seen soldiers feeling like they wanted to kill Vietnamese—*any* Vietnamese. In "When Demirgian Comes Marching Home Again" he had told the story of how Demirgian's sergeant came back to his station in Vietnam from a trip to Bangkok, and found two Vietnamese laundry boys sitting and looking at pictures of people having sex—and laughing. The sergeant got angry and picked up his rifle and killed them both. Sack did not approve of killing laundry boys, but he understood how it could happen.

Even though he was in the middle of writing another book, Sack was tempted to take up Calley's story. Was Calley the sicko all America thought he was? If he was, Sack would pass. But maybe he was a perfectly sane person, even a nice guy, who had found himself in the course of the war killing 109 people. If that was his story, then it was the quintessential story of Vietnam—nice, normal American guy killing Vietnamese civilians.

Hayes told Calley's agent, R. Smith Kiliper, that Sack wanted to meet Calley, and one evening Kiliper showed up at Sack's New York apartment with his client. Calley and Sack were mixing drinks in the kitchen while Kiliper was on the phone in the living room. As they talked, Sack found himself more and more astonished: Calley, the man accused of murdering more than one hundred villagers in a hamlet in Vietnam, was coming across as the most considerate, the most compassionate, the most caring soldier of any he had met in Vietnam. He didn't believe Calley was just trying to impress him. After a drink or two—*in vino veritas*—Calley was talking from the heart.

"Do you know what I think the American army is like?" Calley asked Sack.

"No," said Sack.

"It's like Dr. Frankenstein—the Frankenstein monster."

"What do you mean?" asked Sack.

"There's Dr. Frankenstein, and he decided that he was going to help humanity—he was a good guy, and he was going to create this creature, that was going to just go out and do good, and help people, and so he worked in his laboratory, and he worked day after day, year after year, and he finally put it together, this great culture that was going to help mankind. Then this thing gets up from the table and goes clomp clomp clomp across the land, killing peasants, destroying people. That's the American army. We all formed this to do something good, in the hope of doing something good, and all it's done is it clomps across Vietnam—"

Sack was stunned. He had never heard a soldier talk like that. The next day Sack called three friends, an editor and two reporters, and he asked them if he should take on the assignment Hayes had offered him—to write Calley's story for *Esquire* and then turn it into a book. The first two advisers he talked to (one was David Halberstam) said he shouldn't, the last one said he should. Sack didn't need that last vote in favor to make up his mind. When the first two said no, don't do it, he had thought, Oh my God, these intelligent people, they don't understand. They still don't understand what's going on in the war. They don't understand what's going on with the soldiers.

With Kiliper acting now as his agent, too (Kiliper got 10 percent from Sack, 10 percent from Calley), Sack made the deal with *Esquire*. *Esquire* would pay $30,000 for a series of three exclusive articles. Calley would get $20,000 and Sack would get $10,000. This was a much higher price than *Esquire* usually paid for material—up to $1,500 a piece. Only twice before had Hayes exceeded usual rates to make major purchases: once for an excerpt of Gay Talese's *The Kingdom and the Power*, and again for an excerpt from a novel by Gore Vidal.

While Kiliper started work on a book contract, Sack went down to Alabama to start interviewing Calley. Calley was living at Fort Benning, Georgia, and Sack stayed at a motel across the river in Phoenix City, Alabama. They decided to retreat to a cabin out at Lake Opelika to start the interviews. The tape recorder running, Calley began his story like a briefing officer, explaining the military situation—where Mylai was situated, what the Communist defenses were, what you had to do to take it. This was all wrong, Sack thought, for Calley to come on like the chairman of the Joint Chiefs of Staff. He was not the man who made United States policy. He was the man who was supposed to carry it out.

After about five minutes, Sack said, "Rusty, stop, don't tell me. When did *you* learn this? When were *you* told this military situation?"

They started over.

They talked for a while, then Calley told Sack he felt nervous at the lake, and they went back to Fort Benning and Calley called his girlfriend, and Sack called a girlfriend, and the four of them went back out and stayed for several days. They would tape in the morning, tape in the afternoon, and go water skiing and slalom skiing and ski jumping in between. Later, Sack did more interviews at Calley's house and at the motel. Once when they were both at the motel pool drinking, Calley tried to teach Sack how to dive. They alternated interviews and diving lessons and drinks until, between diving lessons, Calley paused—and it was a moment Sack would always remember—Calley paused, reflecting, thinking hard, and said, almost in a whisper, "I sometimes think—Did I really do that? Did I do what they said? Is that me, did I do it?"

The interviews went on for weeks, with Sack making trips down from New York and Calley coming up to New York. Always, the story stopped short of the events at Mylai: Calley's lawyer had put them off-limits until after the trial. Sack pushed to get the Mylai part of the story so that he could release the book right after the trial, but the lawyer wouldn't budge.

So Sack took what he had—about twenty-five hours of interviews—and began work on Calley's story.

Nobody, certainly not Hayes, had told him to write the story literally as Calley's story, with Calley speaking in the first person. The idea was for John Sack to write a story on Lieutenant Calley. Looking over his notes, Sack found Calley himself had said everything that needed to be said. Calley had seemed to him honest and forthcoming. Sack decided the natural way to tell the story was to let Calley tell it. When he made that decision, he didn't worry about what would happen to his byline or his reputation for writing an as-told-to book, making him into Calley's spokesman—a lower form of journalism. He didn't think about whether "Calley's confessions" would make a splashier story for *Esquire* than Sack writing on Calley. He just thought letting Calley tell his own story—the transcripts cut, shaped, and slimmed by John Sack—was the artistic way to do it.

He had to work fast—Hayes wanted the piece right away. So instead of writing his first draft out by longhand, as he usually did, he spoke it into a tape recorder, drawing sections from different parts of the transcripts, rearranging their order, making cuts. He added words here and there, too, to strengthen the impression that Calley was just talking. When Calley would replay conversations, Sack put in "he said" and "I said," because that's the way he thought people usually described conversations. And because he thought the reader would want to know whom Calley was talking to, every once in a while he'd have Calley drop in the word "John."

When he was done, Sack thought he had produced a marvelous piece of work. He gave it to Hayes, and, after a decent interval, called Hayes from Kiliper's office to hear Hayes tell him how good it was.

"I read the piece, can you come in and talk about it?" Hayes said.

"Oh, there's no need to talk about it," said Sack. "Any problems—tell me now."

"I'd really rather talk to you about it," replied Hayes.

"Harold," said Sack, "that's silly. I'm on the other side of town. It's okay—"

"John," said Hayes, "we really should talk about it."

Sack was getting annoyed but he trekked over to Hayes's office and sat down to talk. It did not take him long to realize that Hayes did not think the piece was as marvelous as he did. Patiently, Hayes went over and over the manuscript—for two hours, at least—encouraging Sack, telling him the same thing over and over, pointing out the problem places in the manuscript, until finally, *finally,* Sack stopped seeing with his own eyes, the eyes he had used to write the piece, and started seeing with Hayes's eyes.

Some of the problems were minor—Sack needed to make small cuts throughout the manuscript to clean it up. And Sack did not need to remind readers of his own presence; Calley should just speak to the reader, not to John Sack. But there was a bigger problem, too: Sack had taken too long to get into the story, to set the wheels of the plot turning—the charges leveled against Calley.

Sack liked to think he would have seen the problems if he could have put the article aside for a week and come back to it. As it was, it took Hayes going over it, never implying, as Sack recalled later, "I've got a crazy author here, he doesn't get what I'm saying, how can I drive this into this numbskull's head." No, nothing like that. While Sack protested, thinking about Hayes, "Why can't this idiot see it, it's clearly beautiful," trying to explain what he was doing, Hayes just patiently, genially, talked on until Sack saw.

Sack took the manuscript home and reorganized it in a few days. By the second paragraph of the new draft, Calley was being recalled from Vietnam to face charges on Mylai. Then Sack showed the manuscript to Calley. The story would appear with a joint byline—"by First Lieutenant William L. Calley Jr., interviewed by John Sack"—so Calley had a right to object to the form it took. He balked at the first line: "I liked it in South Vietnam." It wasn't true, Calley protested. True, there was a time when he did like South Vietnam, at the end, just before he was called back to the States to face charges. But he didn't like it all the time. Sack knew Calley was right, in a way: the reader might think that statement meant he had liked South Vietnam the whole time he was there, including, pre-sumably, the time when he was killing people. But the story had to start somewhere, and it had to catch the reader's attention. And after putting the piece through one major revision, Sack wasn't excited about plunging back in. Sack, Calley, and Hayes gathered in Hayes's office to argue it out, and Sack and Hayes convinced Calley to let it stand.

Next came the cover. John Sack would recall Hayes explaining the idea to him as an old-fashioned daguerreotype—a formal portrait of Calley and four Asian children, like a photograph from 1890. Calley would be seated and they would be standing around him, staring expressionless into the camera. Tom Hedley thought the idea came from Calley himself; Hedley had been standing in a coffee line at the office near Calley, and Calley had mentioned liking kids—said he sent money to Asian kids—and Hedley told Hayes what Calley had said. George Lois remembers the coffee-line story, but he thought that came later; Hedley's coffee-line conversation with Calley didn't have anything to do with the idea for the cover. Lois came up with the idea himself, and it never had anything to do with an old-fashioned daguerreotype. He just wanted to take Calley's picture with Asian children around him and let readers make of it what they would.

Calley agreed and showed up, with Sack along, at Carl Fischer's studio, a converted carriage house on East 83rd. As Lois describes the session, he thought Calley seemed nervous, so he told the makeup people to stay away while he and Calley talked informally, conversationally, on the ground floor. He told Calley he himself was a Korean veteran, and he told him some war stories, so that Calley would trust him. He said he wanted Calley to look at the camera, proud, not ashamed. Posed behind him would be the Asian kids. While Calley was being made up, Lois walked upstairs and cocked his thumb as a signal: Everything was set.

Lois did not share Sack's sympathy with Calley. Yes, he understood combat, he would say later; he had even killed a civilian once during the Korean War. He had been on guard duty when he spotted a man running away, with something in his hand. Lois was not going to fire on him, but as the man started climbing a fence, he turned around and looked at Lois and Lois looked at him. The man had a revolver and fired it at Lois. Lois shot back. But what was happening in Vietnam was very different, in Lois's mind. "They would go into the huts and they would beat up people. They did shit, they did shit. It was hit mentality—it was anti-communism," he said later.

After the photo session, as Hayes was looking at the Polaroid shots in his office, he called Jill Goldstein in to see them. She saw Calley with one Asian child, Calley with two. She started to gasp, but before she could say anything Hayes said, "By the way, I'd like to introduce Rusty Calley." She had not seen him sitting there.

Hayes asked her to fly to Salt Lake City to clear the story and cover with Judge George W. Latimer, Calley's lawyer. When she got there, Latimer's young colleague read the story and set to work eliminating passages in which Calley spoke too harshly of the army, which was trying him, or in which he appeared to be actually confessing his guilt.

THE LOOK OF
Esquire

Designer: Robert Benton   Photographer: Ben Somoroff

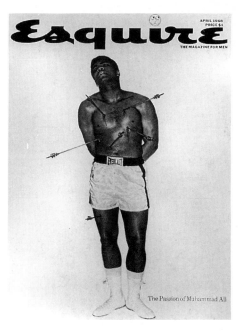

George Lois's *Esquire* covers, usually photographed by Carl Fischer, were powerful icons—among the most memorable in American magazine history. When Muhammad Ali was banned from boxing and ordered to jail for refusing to fight in Vietnam, Lois posed him as Saint Sebastian.

Weary of covers like the one on the left, Harold Hayes said to George Lois, "Do me a cover," and Lois did (*right*), accurately predicting defeat for boxer Floyd Patterson.

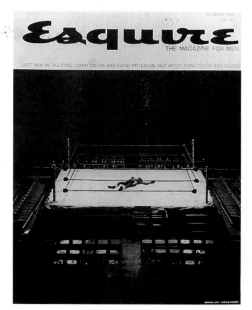

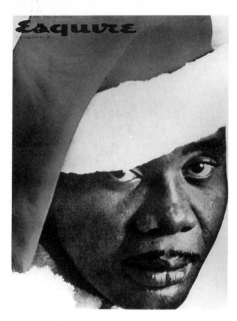

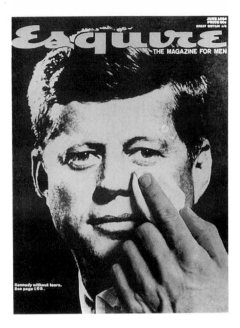

Every month Lois put a face on *Esquire*.

Above, left to right: Heavyweight champion Sonny Liston as Santa Claus, a cover that cost *Esquire* at least $750,000 in pulled advertising; President John F. Kennedy, after his death.

Below: The Vietnam War; Richard Nixon, running for office.

On the opposite page, at top: Andy Warhol, going under; young Asian models with Lieutenant William Calley, Jr., convicted of murdering civilians at Mylai.

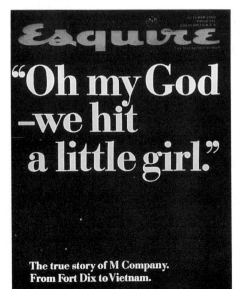

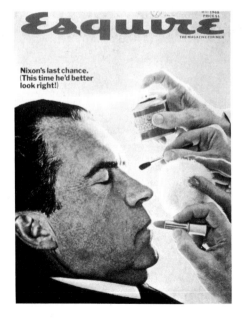

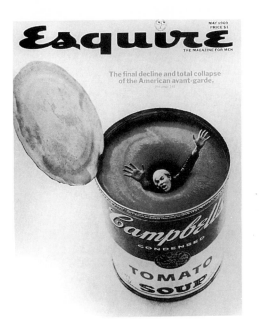

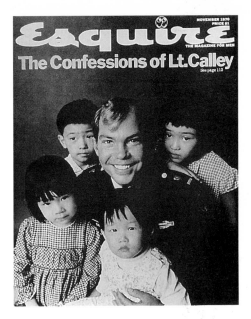

Overleaf: When Rust Hills put together a chart showing "The Structure of the Literary Establishment in America" (July 1963), a sweep of red designated the red-hot center. To *Esquire,* the center of the hot center was Candida Donadio, an Italian-American literary agent with a sexy telephone voice and some of the best writers around.

For the last cover of the old-sized *Esquire,* Lois featured Joe Bonanno (*below, left*), a Mafia figure from Gay Talese's *Honor Thy Father.* The smaller covers could still carry a sting (*below, right*)—Norman Mailer hated this one, pairing him with feminist Germaine Greer.

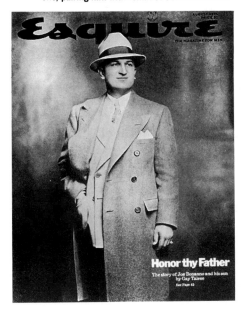

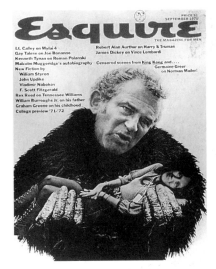

THE POETRY SITUATION

Two recent anthologies, both offering the "new" American poets, have not a single name in common in their tables of contents.

Some poets in Anthology "B" ("B" for Beat)

Donald M. Allen, editor
The New American Poetry

Charles Olson
Robert Duncan
Robert Creeley
Joel Oppenheimer
Jonathan Williams
Paul Carroll
Denise Levertov
Brother Antoninus
Jack Spicer
Lawrence Ferlinghetti
Bruce Boyd
Philip Lamantia
Kirby Doyle
Allen Ginsberg
Jack Kerouac
Gregory Corso
Gary Snyder
Philip Whalen
Peter Orlovsky
John Ashbery
Kenneth Koch
Frank O'Hara
LeRoi Jones

Some poets not involved in the War of the Anthologies:

John Crowe Ransom
Ezra Pound
Carl Sandburg
W. H. Auden
Conrad Aiken
R. P. Warren
Archibald MacLeish
John Berryman
Yvor Winters
J. V. Cunningham
Theodore Roethke
Randall Jarrell
Stanley Kunitz
Marianne Moore
Richmond Lattimore
Muriel Rukeyser
Richard Eberhart
William Stafford
John Updike
Elizabeth Bishop
Allen Tate
Leonie Adams
Karl Shapiro
Louise Bogan
Cecil Hemley
John Ciardi
Paul Engle
Sandra Hochman
Jean Garrigue
Galway Kinnell
Kenneth Rexroth
Kenneth Patchen
Kenneth Koch
Norman Mailer

Some poets in Anthology "A" ("A" for Academic)

Pack, Hall & Simpson
New Poets of England & America

Robert Pack
Robert Bly
Philip Booth
Catherine Davis
Donald Finkel
Donald Hall
Anthony Hecht
Donald Justice
Melvin La Follette
William Meredith
W. S. Merwin
Howard Moss
Adrienne Cecile Rich
William Jay Smith
W. D. Snodgrass
May Swenson
Reed Whittemore
Richard Wilbur
James Wright
Elizabeth Harrod
John Hollander
Robert Lowell
James Merrill
Robert Mezey
Howard Nemerov
Louis Simpson

CAMPUSES

Some campuses have a distinguished writer or two, and occasional courses in creative writing:

Penn State: John Barth
Alabama: Hudson Strode
Denison: Paul Bennett
Auburn: Madison Jones
Brown: John Hawkes
Rutgers: Ralph Ellison
Amherst: Rolfe Humphries
St. Mary's: George P. Elliott
U. of Mass.: Jos. Langland
Western Reserve:
Mac Hammond
Wayne State:
W. D. Snodgrass
Nevada: Walter V. T. Clark
New Hampshire:
Thomas Williams
Dartmouth:
Richard Eberhart
Russell Sage: George Abbe
Wagner: Willard Maas
Washington:
Theodore Roethke
Oregon: James B. Hall
Minnesota: Allen Tate
Ohio State: Peter Taylor
Montana: Leslie Fiedler
Jesse Bier
Duke: Reynolds Price
William Blackburn
Missouri: William Peden
Tom McAfee
Bard: Paris Leary
Theodore Weiss
Chicago: Richard G. Stern

Also in Chicago:
1) Nelson Algren lives in Chicago
2) Poetry is still edited there—now, gently, by Henry Rago
3) Big Table was a little magazine featuring Beat Writers

Many campuses have several distinguished writers, or a little magazine, or a major writing program:

Carleton College
The Carleton Miscellany
Reed Whittemore
Wayne Carver
Erling Larsen

University of Illinois
Accent (suspended)
J. Kerker Quinn
Daniel Curley
John Frederick Nims

University of Michigan
Hopwood Awards in Creative Writing
Allan Seager
Donald Hall

Antioch College
The Antioch Review
Nolan Miller
Judson Jerome

University of Nebraska
The Prairie Schooner
Karl Shapiro

University of the South
The Sewanee Review
Andrew Lytle
Francis Fergusson

Kenyon College
The Kenyon Review
Robie Macauley
George Lanning

Cornell University
Epoch
Baxter Hathaway
David Ray
Arthur Mizener

Princeton University
Philip Roth
Edmund Keeley

Barnard
Marcus Klein
Robert Pack

Rollins College
Louis D. Rubin

Writers In Residence:
Golding
Nemerov
Warren, etc.

Brandeis University
Philip Rahv
Mark Harris

Bennington
Warren Carrier
Bernard Malamud
Stanley Edgar Hyman
Howard Nemerov

Sarah Lawrence
Curtis Harnack
Muriel Rukeyser
Joseph Papeleo
Hallie Burnett
Harvey Swados
Jane Cooper

University of California
(Berkeley)
Thom Gunn
Jackson Burgess
Mark Schorer
Josephine Miles

Harvard University
Richard Poirier
Theodore Morrison
Monroe Engel

Several campuses are important because of advanced degrees, fellowships, or adult courses:

The Writers Workshop at the State University of Iowa is the most important, having a graduate program that has produced teachers now teaching elsewhere; some of the people who have taught there:
Paul Engle (director)
Donald Justice
R. V. Cassill
Vance Bourjaily
George P. Elliott
Philip Roth (now Princeton)
Edmund Keeley
(ex-Princeton)
James B. Hall (now Oregon)
Karl Shapiro (Nebraska)
Herbert Gold
Harvey Swados
(Sarah Lawrence)
Curt Harnack
(Sarah Lawrence)
Hortense Calisher
Walter Clark (Nevada)
Ray B. West (SF State)
Calvin Kentfield (SF State)
Herbert Wilner (SF State)
Robert Penn Warren
Robie Macauley (Kenyon)
W. D. Snodgrass
Andrew Lytle (U. of South)

The New School faculty:
Charles Glicksberg
Don Wolfe
Gorham Munson
Louis Vaczek
Herbert Kubly
Marguerite Young
Hayes B. Jacobs
Anatole Broyard
Kay Boyle
LeRoi Jones
Bernice Kavinoky
Kenneth Koch
Frank O'Hara
and by proxy:
Hiram Haydn
Simon Michael Bessie

Columbia General Studies
John Richard Humphreys
Martha Foley
Sylvia Shirley
Anatole Broyard
Caroline Gordon
Leonie Adams
Stanley Kunitz
Alice Morris

The Stanford Writing Center (offers 6 fellowships in writing each year)
Teaching at Stanford:
Wallace Stegner
Richard Skowcroft
Yvor Winters
Janet Lewis Winters
Albert Guerard Jr.
Blair Fuller

Some fellowship winners:
William Wiegand
Dan Jacobson
Robert Gutwillig
Peter Beagle
Robin White
Tillie Olsen
Ed McClanahan

San Francisco State College has a huge writing program with a large staff of literary writers hired by Caroline Shrodes:
Herbert Wilner
Mark Harris
Ray B. West
Wright Morris
Herb Blau

SF State has connections with Contact, a little magazine in Sausalito.

LITTLE MAGAZI[NES]

Partisan Review
William Phillips
Philip Rahv
Steven Marcus
John Hollander
Roger Straus
Harvey Breit
Jason Epstein
Sidney Hook
Gore Vidal
William Barrett
James Johnson S[?]
Saul Bellow
Leslie A. Fiedler
Dwight Macdona[ld]
Mary McCarthy
Lionel Abel
Alfred Kazin
Diana Trilling
Lionel Trilling
Robert Lowell
Stephen Spender
Karl Shapiro

The Paris Review
George Plimpton
Robert B. Silvers
Peter Matthiessen
Donald Hall
Thomas H. Guinzb[urg]
William Styron
John Phillips
Harold L. Humes
Max Steele
Blair Fuller
Eugene Walter
Terry Southern
Philip Roth
Hughes Rudd
Frederick Seidel
Olga Carlisle
Jonathan Miller
Kenneth & Elaine[?]
Evan S. Connell
Jill Fox
Rose Styron
X. J. Kennedy
James Leo Herlihy
Jean vanden Heuve[l]
Jack Gelber
James Jones
Robert Bly
Mac Hyman
John P. C. Train
Norman Mailer

Commentary
Norman Podhoretz
Ted Solotaroff
Alfred Kazin
Norman Mailer
Wallace Markfield
Benjamin De Mott
Lionel Trilling
Philip Roth
Alfred Chester
Marion Magid
Paul Goodman
Midge Decter
Bernard Malamud
I. B. Singer

The Hudson Review
Fred Morgan
Joseph Bennett
Mary Emma Elliott
William Arrowsmit[h]
Herbert Gold
Louis Simpson
George P. Elliott
W. D. Snodgrass
John Simon
Gerald Weales
Marius Bewley
Anne Sexton
Anthony Hecht
W. S. Merwin
Richard Lattimore
William Stafford

Story
Whit Burnett
Hallie Burnett

Contact
Bill Ryan
Calvin Kentfield
Evan S. Connell
Kenneth LaMott

THE COOL WORLD

Three Beat Saints:
Henry Miller
Edward Dahlberg
William Burroughs

Three who carried the word:
Jack Kerouac
John Clellon Holmes
George Mandel

Some intellectual hipsters:
Chandler Brossard
H. L. Humes
Terry Southern
Norman Mailer
Paul Goodman
Ned Polsky
Allen Ginsberg
Seymour Krim
Paul Krassner
Nat Hentoff
Kenneth Rexroth
Karl Shapiro
Jack Gelber
Milton Klonsky
Mason Hoffenberg
Alexander Trocchi

Grove Press (& Evergreen Review)
Barney Rosset
Donald Seaver
Fred Jordan
Donald Allen

Grove, most avant-garde U. S. publisher, has published many new French and German novelists and playwrights, the British "Angries," and American "Beats."
Jack Kerouac
Charles Olson
Henry Miller
William Burroughs
Kenneth Koch
Robert Gover
John Rechy
Jack Gelber
Michael McClure
Arnold Weinstein
Robert Duncan

Three important bookstores:
Gotham Book Mart:
Frances Steloff
City Lights:
Lawrence Ferlinghetti
8th Street:
the Wilentz brothers

The Village Voice
Edwin Fancher
Dan Wolf
Bill Manville
Jules Feiffer

The Provincetown Review
William Ward

The Chelsea Review
Ursule Molinaro
Venable Herndon

Mutiny: Jane Esty; Paul Lett

newspaper: Jack Green

Yugen: LeRoi Jones

The Realist:
Paul Krassner

Monocle: Vic Navasky

Trace
in Southern California:
James Boyer May
Curtis Zahn
Gil Orlovitz
Lawrence Spingarn

THE DRAMA SITUATION

Off-Broadway Playwrights:
Jack Gelber
Arthur Kopit
Arnold Weinstein
Kenneth Koch
Prime movers:
Julian Beck
Judith Molina
Alan Kapprow
("happenings")

On and Off Broadway Playwrights:
Edward Albee
Jack Richardson
Prime movers:
Richard Barr
José Quintero
Molly Kazan
Jerome Robbins

On Broadway Playwrights:
Arthur Miller
Tennessee Williams
Paddy Chayefsky
William Gibson
William Inge
Robert Anderson
Gore Vidal
Lillian Hellman
Arthur Laurents
Prime movers:
Elia Kazan
Audrey Wood
Cheryl Crawford

Some critics who pronounce on the state of the theatre in America:
Eric Bentley
John Gassner
John Simon
Kenneth Tynan
John Mason Brown
Martin Esslin
George Steiner
Harold Clurman
Joseph Wood Krutch
Robert Brustein

The Academic Critics

Shifting from their usual work on the classic texts to the learned journals, they frequently apply their techniques to contemporary writing.

John Crowe Ransom (Kenyon)
Harry Levin (Harvard)
Walter Bate (Harvard)
Robert Penn Warren (Yale)
Henri Peyre (Yale)
Martin Price (Yale)
Louis Martz (Yale)
Walter Schorer (Berkeley)
Leslie Fiedler (Montana)
Richard Ellmann (Northwestern)
Leon Edel (NYU)
Lionel Trilling (Columbia)
Jacques Barzun (Columbia)
F. W. Dupee (Columbia)
Eric Bentley (Columbia)
Robert Guerard (Stanford)
Carlos Baker (Princeton)
Warren Beck (Lawrence)
Allen Tate (Minnesota)
Hugh Kenner (Berkeley)

The Theoreticians

Their conception of the nature of literary value ultimately shapes the structure of the literary establishment.

William K. Wimsatt (Yale)
Austin Warren (Michigan)
René Wellek (Yale)
Northrop Frye (Toronto)
Ronald Crane (Chicago)
I. A. Richards (Harvard)
Philip Wheelwright (Smith)
R. P. Blackmur (Princeton)
Mike Abrams (Cornell)
Yvor Winters (Stanford)
Kenneth Burke (Bennington)
Richard McKeon (Chicago)
Wayne C. Booth (Chicago)

The Working Critics

They frequently elevate book reviewing to the level of criticism.

Alfred Kazin
Granville Hicks
Robert Gorham Davis
Malcolm Cowley
Edmund Wilson
Anthony West
Paul Pickrel
Arthur Mizener
John Aldridge
Mary McCarthy
Elizabeth Hardwick
Steven Marcus
Norman Podhoretz
Ted Solotaroff
Dwight Macdonald
George Steiner
Ihab Hassan
Stanley Edgar Hyman
John Simon

Writers Who Get in Columns:

Gore Vidal
Paddy Chayefsky
Truman Capote
William Saroyan
Tennessee Williams
Edward Albee
Norman Mailer
Romain Gary
Carl Sandburg
James Jones
Joseph Heller
James Baldwin

Random House (and Knopf and Pantheon)

With the acquisition of Knopf, Bennett Cerf secured Random's position as the most important literary publisher.

Random:

Jason Epstein*
Joseph Fox*

William Styron
John O'Hara
Robert Penn Warren
Dwight Macdonald
Anthony West
Ralph Ellison
Irwin Shaw
Philip Roth
George P. Elliott
Terry Southern
H. L. Humes
George Mandel
Calvin Kentfield
Truman Capote
W. H. Auden
Paul Goodman
Stanley Elkin
Richard Bankowsky
Burt Blechman

Knopf:

John Hersey
Shirley Ann Grau
John Updike
Kay Boyle
William Maxwell
Walker Percy
William Humphrey
George Steiner
W. D. Snodgrass
John Crowe Ransom

Viking

Thomas Guinzburg*
Malcolm Cowley*
Pascal Covici*
Helen Taylor*
Corlies Smith*
Catherine Carver*
Denver Lindley*

Arthur Miller
Saul Bellow
Jack Kerouac
Evan S. Connell Jr.
Wallace Stegner
Ken Kesey
Ivan Gold
H. E. F. Donohue
Oakley Hall
John Steinbeck
Hannah Arendt
Shirley Jackson

Houghton Mifflin

Dorothy de Santillana*
Robert Lescher*

Archibald MacLeish
John Kenneth Galbraith
Arthur Schlesinger Jr.
John Dos Passos
Louis Auchincloss
Carson McCullers
Maxwell Geismar
Arthur Mizener
Dorothy Baker
Clancy Sigal
Alan Marcus
Ellen Douglas
Charles Bell
Charles Bracelen Flood

Lippincott
Stewart Richardson*

With Keystone Books and a reactivated New World Writing Lippincott attracted some good new writers:
Tillie Olsen
Arno Karlen
Thomas Pynchon
Harper Lee
Barbara Solomon

Atheneum

Hiram Haydn*
Simon Michael Bessie*

Joan Williams
Edward Albee
Wright Morris
Reynolds Price
Gina Berriault
William Gibson
Randall Jarrell

Farrar, Straus
John Farrar*
Robert Giroux*
Cecil Hemley*

I. B. Singer
Bernard Malamud
James Purdy
Flannery O'Connor
Edmund Wilson
Robert Lowell
T. S. Eliot

G. P. Putnam's Sons
Walter Minton ("As a publisher he's a great general," says Norman Mailer) publishes strong literary books others won't do:
Norman Mailer
Vladimir Nabokov

Little, Brown
J. D. Salinger
Hortense Calisher
George Garrett
Peter de Vries
Nancy Hale
Edmund Keeley
Gore Vidal

Atlantic
Seymour Lawrence*
Peter Davison*

Edwin O'Connor
Brian Moore
Paul Adrian Brodeur
Ved Mehta
John Malcolm Brinnin
Dan Jacobson
Alfred Kazin
Katherine Anne Porter
Richard Yates

Macmillan
A. L. Hart*
Steve Zoll*

Mark Harris
Jack Gelber
Paul Goodman
A. J. Liebling
John Knowles
Albert Guerard

Simon and Schuster
Robert Gottlieb*

devoted to big-deal commercial books except for:
Joseph Heller
Bruce Jay Friedman
Lillian Ross
Niccolo Tucci
R. V. Cassill
S. J. Perelman
William Eastlake

Scribner's
Burroughs Mitchell*
Donald Hutter*
Harry Brague*

Still has a few tough writers:
James Jones
Davis Grubb
Bernard Wolfe
Michael Rumaker

McGraw-Hill
Robert Gutwillig*

Mark Schorer
Warren Miller
Richard G. Stern
Elizabeth Spencer
Allan Seager

Doubleday
Tim Seldes*
Sam Vaughan*

America's largest publishing house is not a factor in the structure of the literary establishment.

J. F. Powers

Harper & Row
Founded in 1817, Harper is now without a literary writer except for:
John Cheever

Holt, Rinehart & Winston
Founded in 1866, Holt is without a literary writer.

The Dial Press
James Silberman*

James Baldwin
Vance Bourjaily
Harold Brodkey
Thomas Berger
Herb Gold
Thomas Williams
Ed McClanahan

New Directions
James Laughlin used to do what Grove Press does today. Now N.D. publishes unsensational books by older writers:
Kenneth Patchen
Henry Miller
William Carlos Williams
Lawrence Ferlinghetti
Kenneth Rexroth
Edward Dahlberg
Tennessee Williams
Vladimir Nabokov
Ezra Pound

Also new writers:
Gregory Corso
John Hawkes

World Publishing Company
Aaron Asher*

Harvey Swados
Stanley Edgar Hyman
Burton Bernstein
William Gaddis
Peter Feibleman
James Baker Hall
Harvey Breit

Harcourt, Brace & World
Dan Wickenden*
Margaret Marshall*

Eudora Welty
Richard Rovere
Jessamyn West
Mary McCarthy
James Gould Cozzens

The New Yorker
Editor: William Shawn
Fiction Editors:
Roger Angell
Robert Henderson
William Maxwell
Rachel McKenzie
plus innumerable checkers and "editors" (of copy) and staff writers and persons on "drawing account" and other sorts of semi-staff basis.
Some Old Hands:
Joe Mitchell
A. J. Liebling
E. J. Kahn
S. J. Perelman
Geoffrey Hellman
Lillian Ross
Dwight Macdonald
Robert Coates
Edmund Wilson
Anthony West
St. Clair McKelway
Brendan Gill
Philip Hamburger
Peter De Vries
J. D. Salinger
John Cheever
John Updike
Nancy Hale
Mavis Gallant
Sylvia Townsend Warner
Jessamyn West
Maeve Brennan

Some Newer Hands:
Paul Adrian Brodeur Jr.
Burton Bernstein
Tom Meehan
Anthony Bailey
Bernard Taper
Roy Bongartz
Harold Brodkey
Donald Malcolm
Ved Mehta

Ladies' fashion magazines:
Rita Smith (ex-Mlle)
Eleanor Perényi (ex-Mlle)
Cyrilly Abels (ex-Mlle)
Tracy Brigden (Mlle)
Alice Morris (Bazaar)
Allene Talmey (Vogue)

Harper's Magazine
John Fischer (editor)
Robert Silvers
Katherine Gauss Jackson
Eric Larrabee
Russell Lynes
David Boroff

THE HOT CENTER

AGENTS

McIntosh, McKee & Dodds
William Styron
Jackson Burgess
Curtis Harnack
L. Humes
Russell Lynes
Warren Miller
Flannery O'Connor
Ed McClanahan
Evan S. Connell
Daniel Dodson
Cecil Hemley
Willard Motley
Jay Putnam

Ashley Steiner
Alan Harrington
Arthur Miller
L. C. Spectorsky
Thomas Kopit
Martha Gellhorn
E. S. Mathews
Mona Jaffe
Grace Paley
Niccolò Tucci

Curtis Brown
Has many important English writers via Curtis Brown Ltd. but only one American literary figure:
John Knowles

Georges Borchardt
Ursule Molinaro
George Steiner

Russell and Volkening
Diarmuid Russell
Henry Volkening
Candida Donadio

Saul Bellow
Keith Botsford
Vance Bourjaily
George Plimpton
Blair Fuller
Peter Mathiessen
Richard Scowcroft
John R. Humphreys
Granville Hicks
Robie Macauley
Peter Davison
Bernard Malamud
Mavis Gallant
Eudora Welty
Jessamyn West
Wallace Markfield
Josephine Herbst
Reynolds Price
Tillie Olsen
Pati Hill
Dan Jacobson
Christine Weston
Philip Roth
Nelson Algren
Richard G. Stern
Chandler Brossard
Robt Gutwillig
Emile Capouya
R. V. Cassill
George P. Elliott
Brock Brower
Alfred Chester
William Gaddis
H. E. F. Donohue
Harvey Swados
Joseph Heller
Hayes B. Jacobs
Hughes Rudd
Sylvia Shirley
Elise Sanguinetti
George Garrett
Bruce Jay Friedman
Joyce Engelson
Thomas Meehan
Anthony Bailey
Burt Bernstein
George Mandel
Thomas Pynchon
E. L. Doctorow
Burt Raffel
Peter Sourian

Sterling Lord
Jack Kerouac
Terry Southern
George Bluestone
John Clellon Holmes
Hubert Selby
Aubrey Goodman
Robert O. Bowen
Arno Karlen
Ken Kesey
Edmund Keeley
LeRoi Jones
Donald Barthelme

James Brown
Louis Auchincloss
Leo Litwak
A. J. Liebling
Jean Stafford
Herbert Gold
Herbert Wilner

Brandt & Brandt
Harold Brodkey
Dawn Powell
Frank Rooney
Herbert Kubly
Wallace Stegner
Hortense Calisher
Shirley Ann Grau
Mark Schorer
James Gould Cozzens

Watkins Agency
Kay Boyle
Glendon Swarthout
Peter DeVries
Allan Seager

McIntosh & Otis
John Steinbeck
Walker Percy
Dennis Murphy
Ved Mehta
Erskine Caldwell
Peter Beagle
Marguerite Young

Harold Matson Co.
Bernard Wolfe
Richard Condon
Davis Grubb
William Eastlake
Ray Bradbury
Morley Callaghan

*Most active literary editors

SQUARESVILLE

The NY Times Book Review
editors:
Francis Brown
Ray Walters
Eliot Fremont-Smith
Lewis Nichols
Charles Simmons
William Du Bois

Some book reviewers:
Martin Levin
David Dempsey
William Peden
David Boroff
Wilbur Frohock
Harry T. Moore

Daily reviewers:
Charles Poore
Orville Prescott

Herald Tribune Book Review
Irita Van Doren
Maurice Dolbier

All "out of town" book page editors, featuring:
Lon Tinkle: Dallas News
Alice Bond: Boston Herald
Robt. Cromie: Chicago Trib
Hudson Grunewald: DC Star
Stan Peckham: Denver Post
Rex Barley: LA Mirror
Bill Hogan: SF Chronicle
John Hutchens: NY Tribune

The Saturday Review
Norman Cousins
John Ciardi

Editorial Board of Book of the Month Club:
John Mason Brown
Basil Davenport
Clifton Fadiman
Gilbert Highet

All Drama Critics
Brooks Atkinson (dean)
Howard Taubman (Times)
Walter Kerr (Tribune)
Richard Watts (Post)
Norman Nadel (Telegram)
John Chapman (News)
Robert Coleman (Mirror)
John McClain (Journal)

Independent Squares
Howard Mumford Jones
All the Fadiman Brothers
John Mason Brown
Bergen Evans
Maxwell Geismar

In a square by themselves:
J. Donald Adams
Whitney Balliett

All anthologists, featuring:
Oscar Williams
Louis Untermeyer

All writers' conferences, featuring:
Bread Loaf

All writers' magazines, featuring: The Writer and Writer's Digest

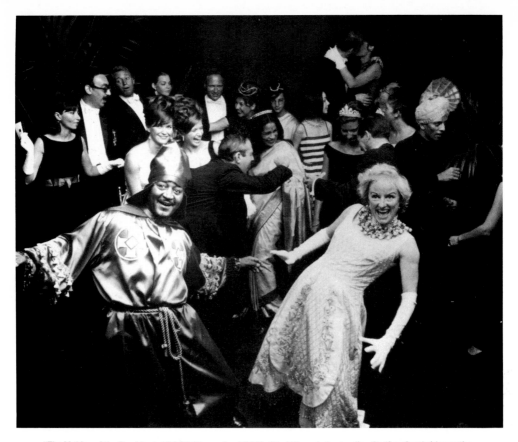

"The Making of the President, 1968!" (December 1965) pitted Klan-clad comedian Godfrey Cambridge as the Democratic candidate against comedienne Phyllis Diller as the Republican candidate. (Cambridge could not make the photo session, so the photograph was shot with a model, shown here, and Cambridge's head was stripped in.) *Esquire* staff members joined professional models in the photo. Art director Sam Antupit danced in the center while Bob Brown and Jill Goldstein kissed in the background. *Carl Fischer photo*

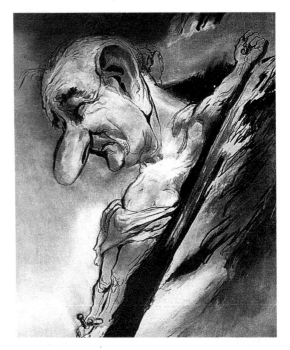

David Levine was drawing small caricatures for *Esquire's* front-of-the-book columns until Samuel Antupit became art director and gave him full pages for his satiric art, like his rendition of President Lyndon B. Johnson as Christ.

When young editor Lee Eisenberg had trouble writing a head for this Black Panther spread (November 1970), Harold Hayes came up with a characteristically improvisational solution: he wrote a head for a photograph *Esquire* didn't have, and then took the picture.

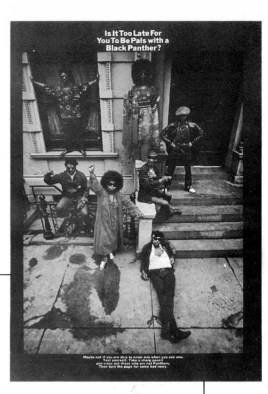

Is It Too Late For You To Be Pals with a Black Panther?

Maybe not if you are able to know one when you see one.
Test yourself. Take a sharp pencil
and cross out those who are not Panthers.
Then turn the page for some bad news.

You lose

There are no Black Panthers on the previous page. The friendly and respectable seven are: (1) Jean Pace, singer and dancer; (2) Oscar Brown Jr., songwriter; (3) Charles Gordone, playwright; (4) Les McCann, jazz pianist; (5) Roberta Flack, singer; (6) Montego Joe, one of America's greatest conga-drum players; (7) Samuel Overton, ad salesman for *The Village Voice*.

This is closer to the real Panther
It ought to be. A Panther posed for it

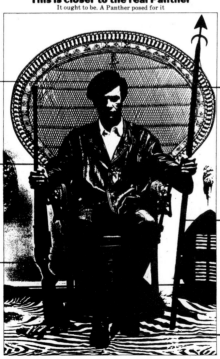

The Official Beret
The Black Panthers wear berets because berets are the prominent trademarks of military elitists — hotshot British Commandos, Nazi tank gunners, etc. Ché Guevara also wore one. The beret may be colored for camouflage in alien environments. American Special Forces wear green ones over in the jungles of Southeast Asia while the Panthers wear black ones in the streets of America.

The Official Leathers
Leather is primeval. To a flabby suburbanite like you, it means a tough outer skin. That's why the Panther wears leather. What would you think of a Panther in a jacket made out of permanent-press polyester?

The Official Gun
An unarmed Black Panther is not as newsy to newsmen as an armed one. As Minister of Defense, Newton recommends these guns for the neighborhood arsenal: an Army 45; the dependable M-16; a 12-gauge High Standard Magnum shotgun with an 18-inch barrel; the P-38. An unarmed Panther is not as groovy on a poster either.

The Official Afro
Long hair is now on everyone, of course, but when you started to let yours grow it didn't have anything to do with racial pride. Letting it all hang out is, to black psychiatrists Grier and Cobbs, "psychologically redemptive." In other words, the Afro is good for the Panther's head. What's your excuse?

The Official Shades
Although Huey doesn't need them, a Panther wears shades to scare you. They hide what he's thinking and make him look cool and mean. A cool, mean, scary black can give even the best of liberals, even you, sleepless nights.

The Official Roots
African trappings—spear, shields, a zebra rug, and throne—underline the Panther's identification with The Great Worldwide Revolutionary Struggle Against Oppression and Colonialism. So what if the throne looks like Hong Kong wicker?

The Official Shoes
Many Panthers prefer combat boots but the sharper ones can be seen tearing down the walls in knobs, footwear defined by Bobby Seale as "soft, alligator, and expensive."

Now that you've seen what a Panther should look like, you are in a better position to be his friend. However, to stop here would be to leave you with a few ambiguities.

Photograph on preceding page by Carl Fischer

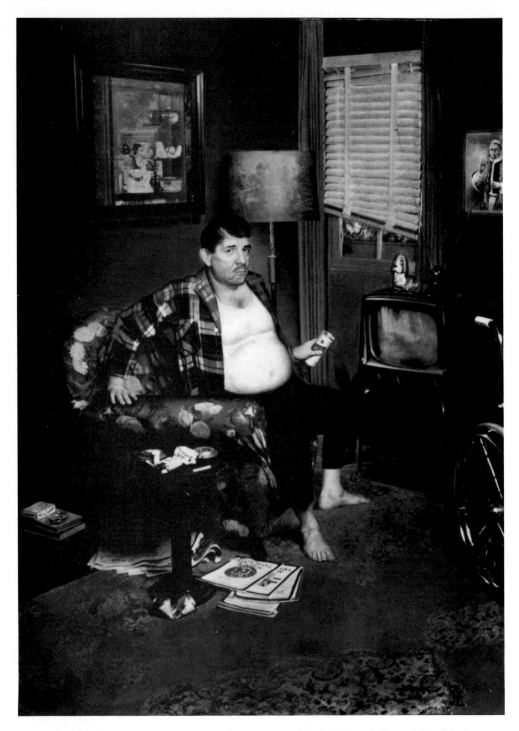

Jean-Paul Goude's painting of Jack Kerouac in his last days (March 1970) made Kerouac's friend Carolyn Cassady weep. The painting seemed to her "a disgusting display of callousness."

I'm sorry, I'm not myself today. I didn't think that I'd be uptight about it, talking about it. I thought, *I've gone to Vietnam and I've done the job the best I could. I shouldn't have any hang-up about it.* But after talking about it yesterday, I don't know. I thought about it. I couldn't sleep. I lay there and I asked myself, *My god. Did you really hack up all those damned people? Did you really pull a machete out and—kkk! Chop into all those people and do all those horrors? Did you,* and I got the answer back, *Yes. I hacked up those people, I hacked up millions of people*—not millions. But yes, I killed plenty of people, I killed lots of NVA, I killed lots of VC with weapons on, I killed lots of—people. I asked myself why did I do it? Why didn't I stand on a corner like everyone else and say, *"It's wrong."*

After the lawyer reworked the passage with Goldstein, Calley no longer confessed:

I'm sorry, I'm not myself today. I didn't think that I'd be uptight about it, talking about it. I thought, *I've gone to Vietnam and I've come back. I shouldn't have any hang-up about it.* But after talking about it yesterday, I don't know. I thought about it. I couldn't sleep. My country accuses me of slaughtering innocent people. Even the President calls it a massacre. I lay there and I asked myself, *My god, who are they talking about? I only know, I went to Vietnam and I did my job there the best I could.* I even asked myself why did I do it? Why didn't I stand on a corner like everyone else and say, "I won't go. It's wrong."

The change wiped out the coverline *Esquire* had planned—a condensed version of Calley's question: *"Did you really pull a machete out and—kkk! Chop into all those people and do all those horrors?"* Would the lawyers eliminate the cover image as well? Goldstein showed Judge Latimer several pictures of Calley with the Asian kids—all possibilities for the cover. She was casual about it, bringing the pictures out almost as an afterthought, but she knew the importance of getting Latimer's tacit approval. The magazine was already past its cover deadline. What if Latimer objected?

He looked at the pictures of Calley and the children. "Don't you think that's gilding the lily?" he asked. He raised no objections.

While Goldstein was in Latimer's office, a call came from Hayes: How were things going? Okay, she said, feigning nonchalance. There were no objections to the cover. She would catch a plane out of Salt Lake City that afternoon.

The cover of the November 1970 *Esquire* showed a smiling, friendly Rusty Calley, blond hairline receding, blue eyes crinkling with cheer, surrounded by somber Asian children. One leaned on his shoulder, the youngest—a toddler—sat in his lap, and a young girl stood comfortably in the crook of his arm. A blue background picked up the blue of his uniform. Yellow letters floated above his head: "The Confessions of Lt. Calley."

It was the first picture Sack had ever seen that looked like the Rusty Calley he knew, but he couldn't understand the point of the cover—what was it supposed to say? He thought the original idea was more powerful. He looked at this cover and thought, Yeah, there's Rusty, good picture of Rusty. Lois didn't see it that way, or at least as he told the story years later, he didn't. He thought anyone who saw Calley as guilty would think, You slimeball, the idea you could pose with children. At the same time, he knew the cover was ambiguous, as he thought a great cover should be.

Anyone who went beyond the cover to "Backstage" would find John Sack's view of Calley prevailing over George Lois's. Comparing Calley to Sirhan Sirhan, who killed Robert Kennedy, "Backstage" called Sirhan "his own creation, but Lieutenant Calley had all the guidance an ungrateful nation, which includes you and us, could lend him in arriving at the crossroads of destiny. Therefore, we reason, nothing in Calley is alien to us and if he feels moved to talk it behooves us to listen and heed."

The Calley cover stirred up more controversy than any Lois cover since Sonny Liston as Santa Claus. The furor began in the *Esquire* offices. The staff read the cover as a statement favoring Calley's side of the case. *Esquire*'s new fiction editor, Gordon Lish, recalled it as "an absolute insult to decency, as an effort by *Esquire* to be playful about something which was in no wise susceptible of playfulness. We all felt Harold had gone too far." Connie Wood, Hayes's secretary, who vigorously opposed the war, was so enraged by the cover that she threatened to resign. Described by Lish as "the kind of person whose moral center was never in doubt," she was scandalized. "And I must tell you that I don't think there was an editor in that office who wasn't on her side," said Lish.

Hayes told Wood that deciding what was to go on the cover was not her province, it was his. He did not try to explain to her, or to anyone on the staff, what the cover meant. You either got it or you didn't. He did not try to justify it. Recalling the controversy as the most intense during his time at the magazine, Lish said, "Harold had been a Marine, had he not? And he understood these things. We didn't understand them at all. We took the common and easy view that this man was a villain, and I think such a view is an entirely superficial view, too little knowing what it is to be in combat, too little informed of the actuality of such an experience; our view was childlike and stupid, obtuse, and Harold was the only editor in publishing who sought to say . . . that there's another side to this story."

After the issue was published, *Newsweek* featured it in a critical report. Describing Calley's return to Vietnam to gather evidence for his trial, *Newsweek* said journalists could not get near him. Perhaps *Esquire* was to blame, said *Newsweek:* perhaps the army was protecting Calley's $150,000 exclusive contract with the Viking Press and *Esquire* magazine—a hypothesis *Newsweek* supported with a quotation from John Sack: "I don't hang out with Army brass. But I suppose they might think the *Esquire* articles and the book were useful to them. Like most career soldiers, Rusty believes that the people of the U.S. have ordered the soldiers to fight this war . . . and the soldiers are doing as best they can." Commercial arrangements with murderers were not without precedent, *Newsweek* noted, citing books by Caryl Chessman and Dr. Sam Sheppard, and Sirhan Sirhan's $15,000 for an interview with CBS, but Calley was getting a good deal more—$50,000 from *Esquire* alone, *Newsweek* reported erroneously.

In London, Helen Lawrenson read the *Newsweek* article and "was stunned—and appalled." She wrote Gingrich,

I will reserve judgement until I see the issue, but however it is presented, I am shocked at the immorality of paying Calley. Christ, it's like paying Ilse Koch to write an article on "How to Make Lampshades." To all the English I know, making Calley rich—rewarding him—is incomprehensible, especially for a magazine of *Esquire*'s prestige. I'd love to know the thinking behind it—and, as I say, I haven't yet seen the issue.

Seeing the issue didn't change her views, which she laid down for Gingrich at length in a letter about a month later, but she had no objection to the cover, she said; in fact, the cover was "brilliant."

I can even understand running the articles to show what the American mind is like—or what this particular mind is like—and those of the people who praise Calley—as an example of a type of thinking—very real, very revealing. . . . I do think, however, that the commentary in the front of the book about the article should have made it clear that *Esquire* does not really believe Calley is just any good-natured, innocent all-American Boy—to say, as it did, that he could have been "all the adult males of sound health in the United States," is certainly not true—as 70,000 adult males have deserted from the army rather than go to Vietnam, and many others have deserted *in* Vietnam, and many more than that number have refused to go—either by leaving the country or otherwise evading the draft or just plain risking prison rather than go. Even some of those at Mylai refused to join in the massacre. Anyway, it is not a matter of "good taste" or "bad taste." It is a matter of moral principle—and even if, as I say, you ran the pieces as an important and revealing bit of Americana—which they certainly are—I don't think that Calley should be *rewarded* for what he did. (And so munificently, too.)

But enough. You will no doubt continue to get letters. The English I know are uniformly appalled. And one American woman I know—in her forties—said she felt like taking her American passport and burning it on the steps of the Embassy. This is a woman who loathes "hippies," student rebels, etc. etc.—so I was surprised at the vehemence of her reaction. . . .

A couple of advertisers were upset enough about the cover to withdraw their ads from upcoming issues of *Esquire*—$200,000 worth of them, Hayes told Sack. Jerry Jontry, the former advertising director who was by now a vice-president of the company, reported to Hayes that neither Volkswagen nor Porsche, which had together bought nine advertising pages in 1970, would advertise in *Esquire* again. Jontry understood Volkswagen thought the Calley cover was "like showing 'Hitler talking in a synagogue.'" Jontry arranged a luncheon meeting with the advertising director and the marketing director from Volkswagen. Jontry would go, along with two other members of the *Esquire* business staff. "We will need you as a key member of the salvage squad," he said to Hayes.

Possibly in preparation for the meeting, Hayes made notes outlining his justification for the Calley cover and, for that matter, the Calley confessions. His notes provide the most complete and reasoned account of Hayes's thoughts about the Calley story and the way *Esquire* played it.

As Hayes saw it, the public had missed an essential point in the Calley affair, "not who had *killed* all those people but who was *responsible*. Calley was a servant of the people."

The question was: "How to force this point?

"If he was not a mad, bestial killer, how could the public be challenged to reconsider its attitude?

"If he alone was guilty, the cover was cruel and savage.

"But if he were no more guilty than any other soldier carrying out an act of war, *what next possibility does that cover lead to?*"

Telford Taylor, chief prosecutor at the Nuremberg trials (*"NO RADI-CAL,"* Hayes wrote in the margin), "has publicly implied we are trying the wrong man. On precedent of Nuremberg and the Japanese War Trials, General Westmoreland—his subordinates and superiors—bear the guilt." If the military was on trial, the military ought not to be acting as judge. Instead, a presidential commission ought to investigate U.S. war atrocities, although Hayes doubted President Nixon would take such an action.

Was showing Calley with the Asian children like showing Hitler in a synagogue? "If there had been such a cover at that time, perhaps we would never have had a Buchenwald," Hayes wrote.

At no point did *Esquire* back down from its decision to run the cover. When readers wrote in accusing *Esquire* of bad taste, *Esquire* replied to the letters with an "Editor's Note" quoting Sack on Calley: "He's kind, he's considerate, he's compassionate, and when he sees little children, he wants to hug them." Sack hoped readers would study the cover photo and say, "He isn't a murderer. *And ask,* Well, who is the murderer then? *And answer,* It's us."

Arnold Gingrich responded to criticism of the cover—specifically to *Newsweek*'s description of it as "gleefully tasteless"—with uncharacteristic sharpness. In his publisher's column for the issue containing the second installment of Calley's story, February 1971, Gingrich accused readers of demonstrating prejudice when they assumed Calley's guilt before he had even gone to trial. "People wrote in likening the portrayal of Lieutenant Calley, surrounded by Vietnamese children, to a depiction of Hitler, kissing Jewish babies on their way to the gas chambers, and to Himmler, fondling little Poles and Czechs, before handing them over to waiting S.S. officers." Yet, said Gingrich, the cover appeared and the letters were penned before the trial had even started.

Readers were not even listening to what Calley said in the story, said Gingrich. In the first installment he had spoken against the war, yet hawks still hailed him as a hero and doves still maligned him as a monster. The cover had given them all a chance to sound off on their tightly held views.

All *Esquire* was trying to do with that cover, Gingrich explained, was what it always tried to do with its cover—"present an unexpected aspect of any subject that is currently in the national consciousness." Often, he said, that simply meant presenting subjects with an open mind, and that was why *Esquire* liked George Lois—"his is the openest mind we've encountered, in a long spell of dealing with artists and designers."

The furor over the Calley cover had reminded Gingrich "that just as there is no puritan more austere than a reformed rake, there is nobody more bigoted than an outraged liberal." He closed with a suggestion that readers of the second installment ask themselves, "in the light of as much

as you may know about the case, what you would have done, if you had
been there, and in this man's shoes."

Calley's trial by an army court-martial jury began on November 12,
1970, in Fort Benning, Georgia. A couple of days into the trial, Sack got a
call from Hayes. The press coverage was making Calley look like such a
monster that Hayes was worried about how the next two *Esquire* articles
would be received. Not to worry, said Sack. The rest of the press could
make Calley out to be a monster and then *Esquire* would come in and let
everyone know he was an average American guy.

No, said Hayes, the coverage was so negative that when *Esquire*'s
version came out no one was going to believe it. He suggested that Sack
try to get other reporters close to Calley so they could get to know Calley
as Sack and Hayes knew him.

With the consent of Viking, Hayes was abandoning *Esquire*'s exclusive rights to Calley's story. The problem was, Calley did not really want
to talk to the press. He thought the press was out to hang him. When
reporters approached him in the hall during breaks in the trial, he would
speak briefly and then walk away. And not everyone in the press wanted to
meet Calley. According to Sack, Homer Bigart, reporting the trial for the
New York Times, believed that talking to Calley might bias his coverage
of the trial—that knowledge of Calley himself, gained outside the trial
setting, might contaminate his objectivity. To Sack, that was a clear example of the difference between Old and New Journalism. Sack felt the only
way to know the truth was to surrender to it, to become part of it, to get as
close to it as possible.

Sack was not trying to be objective. He had a clear view of the trial as a
hypocritical act. He figured if the United Nations wanted to try Lieutenant Calley for war crimes, that was fine, let the United Nations try him
and convict him. If the North Vietnamese won the war and put him on
trial for war crimes, that, too, would be absolutely appropriate. If Jane
Fonda and other peaceniks wanted to have a mock trial and try him and
convict him, that would be absolutely right.

But when the very people who sent Calley to Vietnam, the very people
who gave him the order, the very people who had already destroyed 85
percent of the villages in Quang Ngai province when Calley arrived—
when the United States Army prosecuted him, it was not the injustice, it
was the hypocrisy that infuriated Sack.

One day Sack was sitting in the defense room during a recess when he received word that Captain Aubrey M. Daniel III, the prosecutor, wanted to see him. Daniel had a subpoena for all of Sack's interview tapes and files on Calley.

Sack had an apartment in New York, but he had also rented a house in Aspen with the idea that he would go there to write the Calley book when the trial was over. He had friends living in both of his residences. A playful man, almost boyish, Sack started teasing Daniel.

"Gee, Captain," he later recalled saying, "this winter I'm living in Aspen, Colorado. If my files are in Aspen, Colorado, are you going to pay me to go to Aspen, Colorado, to get my files?"

Daniel said that he would.

"The United States of America is going to *pay* me to go to Aspen, Colorado, and to come back here?"

Yes it would.

"Gee," said Sack, "can I go skiing while I'm there?"

Back in the defense office, he showed the subpoena to one of Calley's lawyers, and he also called Harold Hayes. At no point in the discussion with *Esquire*, that Sack could recall later, had the possibility arisen that Sack's tapes and transcripts might be subpoenaed, although Calley's lawyer probably considered the possibility—hence the precaution of putting the Mylai episode off-limits to Sack until after the trial.

Hayes passed Sack on to *Esquire*'s lawyer, who broke the bad news that in his judgment Sack would not be protected by reporter's privilege. Shield laws, he said, protected reporters who did not want to reveal their sources. But what Sack had was an alleged murderer who had told him his story, maybe even confessed, and under the law, he had to turn over what he had.

"Listen, listen," said Sack, "let's get this straight. I'm *not* going to turn it over. I did not become friends with Calley, I did not make this deal with Calley, I did not ask Calley all these questions, in order to help the United States government hang him, and I'm not going to do it. And if you can find a legal reason to get me out of jail, great, otherwise, I'm going to jail."

At some point, someone suggested that if Calley himself had the tapes, they could not be subpoenaed because he would be incriminating himself if he turned them over.

At lunchtime, Sack went to a pay phone nearby and called the friend who was staying at the house in Aspen.

"Hello, how are you, how's the weather, everything's fine, yeah, great," said Sack. "You know, I just want to make sure that you remember what I told you when I left. You know those boxes I have in the closet?"

And Sack's friend, a smart woman, replied, "Oh, yeah, sure, the boxes in the closet in your bedroom."

"You remember those boxes in the bedroom, I pointed them out."

"Yeah, you pointed them out—"

"With all my files on Lieutenant Calley."

"Yeah, sure, what about them?"

"I just want to make sure you remember that I told you they're not my property. They're Lieutenant Calley's."

"Sure, you told me that."

"And I said, And if Rusty wants anything with them, that they're his property, and you're to do whatever he says."

"Sure you told me that, why are you mentioning it again?"

"I just wanted to make sure you remembered."

Later on Calley called her and asked for the tapes. She boxed them up, not too carefully, and mailed them off. A few days later the box arrived, and as Calley was carrying it across a parking lot at the post office—all these tapes and multiple copies of transcripts—the bottom of the box fell out. The subpoenaed papers started flying around the parking lot, and other people in the parking lot started running around picking them up. With most of the papers retrieved, he put everything in a safe deposit box.

Sack ultimately got off the hook on what might most succinctly be called a technicality. But meanwhile, the subpoena earned *Esquire* more publicity. *Newsweek* began a February 1, 1971, report with the unlikely claim that "the editors of *Esquire* had worked out a seemingly sure-fire device for promoting interest in their 'Continuing Confessions' of First Lt. William L. Calley." The device was withholding Calley's account of Mylai until part three appeared after the trial. Now, *Newsweek* said, the prosecutor was foiling the plan by subpoenaing the taped conversations— *Esquire*'s exclusive confession. Sack had reveled in his distinction from other journalists covering the trial, *Newsweek* reported—he saw himself, said *Newsweek*, "as a sort of Dutch uncle to the accused." *Newsweek* underlined the friendly relationship with a picture of Sack and Calley grinning at each other like the good buddies they were. In *Newsweek*'s eyes, Sack was a man who had boasted of leaving journalism because of its space limitations and now was trying to return to the fold to avoid the subpoena. With something that sounded like triumph, *Newsweek* reported the trial judge's ruling that Sack could not claim journalistic immunity because the Calley story was a commercial transaction.

Hayes drafted a letter of protest to *Newsweek,* although he may not actually have sent it. He noted *Newsweek*'s error, made in the earlier *Newsweek* story as well: the confessions cost *Esquire* $30,000, not $50,000 as *Newsweek* was reporting. Then he laid to rest the idea that Sack had Calley on tape describing Mylai. On the contrary, Hayes said, *Esquire,* Sack, and Calley had agreed in August 1970 that possession of information about Mylai would make Sack vulnerable to a subpoena requiring him to testify against Calley.

"Sack has refused to testify"—wrote Hayes—"not because he is in possession of a hot 'exclusive' for *Esquire,* but because he is unwilling to assist the government in its prosecution." Hayes rebuked *Newsweek* for denying Sack status as a journalist. "Is CBS News to be denied such privilege because it paid $10,000 for an interview with Paul Meadlo? Is Richard Hammer of the *Times* disqualified because he paid Varnardo Simpson $500? Has *Newsweek* ever paid a source for what it considered news information?" Hayes concluded: ". . . We all lose if precedent is established enabling the government to decide who is, and who is not, a member of the press."

On March 29, the jury found Calley guilty of murdering twenty-two South Vietnamese civilians at Mylai. While Calley's attorneys set their appeals in motion, Sack was able, finally, to interview Calley on the events at Mylai. Then he settled down to write the third and final article for *Esquire.* He thought of the book as having five segments. *Esquire* already had the first two; he would write the third and let that be his last installment for *Esquire.* Then he would write the last two segments, including the trial, for book publication. That seemed the only way to get a third installment done for *Esquire* without undue delay.

Sack was working as fast as he could. He got up in the morning around eight, sat in his chair writing by hand until six that night, went to the Greek restaurant at the corner of 63rd and Madison, came back and wrote until ten o'clock that night, took a hot bath, went to bed, got up, and started over. He turned the manuscript in, Hayes read it, Hayes asked: Why had Sack not included the trial?

Sack explained: He and his agent had promised to deliver to Viking a book manuscript that was at least 40 percent unpublished in *Esquire*—a promise made without consulting *Esquire,* Hayes said in a memo to Blinder and Gingrich. The way Sack was writing the manuscript that fresh 40 percent included the trial. Since *Esquire*'s agreement with Sack predated his agreement with Viking, Hayes thought his first responsibility was to *Esquire*. If Hayes had to, he had told Sack, he would refer the matter to *Esquire*'s lawyer.

Viking asked for a meeting; Hayes, Sack, and Calley's and Sack's agent, Kiliper, met with Viking's lawyer and editors over a conference table at Viking. While Sack looked on, Hayes and Tom Guinzburg, president of Viking Press, went back and forth: Viking wanted fresh material, Hayes wanted the trial in *Esquire*. Sack, feeling like a squash ball, said he was working as hard as he could, he couldn't write any faster. They paid no attention.

The solution they came up with left Sack panting for air. Sack would simply have to write the rest of the book—the final two sections—in approximately two weeks, and deliver that manuscript to *Esquire*. *Esquire* would trim the manuscript down to a 10,000-word article.

Out of the meeting, Sack, shaken, called his secretary. He arranged to meet her by the seal enclosure in the Central Park Zoo. He told her what he had to do. She put him on an airplane to Fire Island for a day's rest, and when he came back he went to work.

When Sack's manuscript for the rest of the book came in, Hayes gave it to his new young editor Aaron Latham, who had won an in-house cutting contest on an earlier manuscript, and Latham prepared the excerpt. He was very opposed to the war, and, he said later, he tried to undermine Calley with his cuts.

This final installment contained Calley's comments on Captain Ernest L. Medina, who Calley said had ordered the killings at Mylai (Medina himself faced a court-martial but was found not guilty). Medina was represented by an aggressive lawyer, F. Lee Bailey. To be on the safe side, *Esquire*'s lawyer recommended that *Esquire* put forth Calley's account as clearly *his* version, without *Esquire*'s endorsement, even though *Esquire* believed his account to be true. The article ran in the September 1971 issue with a head, "The Concluding Confessions of Lieutenant Calley," and underneath that a deck: "The lieutenant's account of the day at Mylai Four, the aftermath, the trial."

After Calley was found guilty and sentenced to life imprisonment, President Nixon was deluged with phone calls and telegrams asking for clemency. Even some who opposed the war saw Calley as a scapegoat, used to deflect guilt from the powerful men who had made national policy. More condemnations of the verdict came from congressmen, leaders of veterans associations, radio stations, and Governor George C. Wallace of Alabama, who asked the director of the state's Selective Service System to find out if Alabama could suspend the draft.

Calley's sentence was reduced by the military; then, in September 1974, the U.S. district court in Columbus, Georgia, overturned his conviction. The judge, J. Robert Elliott, said "massive adverse pretrial publicity" had prevented Calley from getting a fair trial. "Never in the history of the military justice system, and perhaps in the history of American courts, has any accused ever encountered such intense and continuous prejudicial publicity," he said. Elliott also ruled that the army was wrong in refusing Calley's request to subpoena as witnesses Melvin R. Laird, then secretary of defense, and General William C. Westmoreland, commander of U.S. forces in South Vietnam. Perhaps, he suggested, Calley's superiors "could well have been worried about their own possible criminal responsibility as a result of the Mylai incident."

Elliott's judgment was overturned by a U.S. circuit court of appeals, but by that time Calley had been approved for parole.

John Sack never stopped liking Rusty Calley. They had come to be comrades—Sack thought of Calley as his best friend that year. Once after they had worked late the night before, they came into Hayes's office linked arm in arm and singing, "We are the joy boys of radio, hello, hello, hello, hello-o-o." Hayes looked up, incredulous, at his star reporter and the man accused of mass murder. Sack thought Hayes liked having Calley around the office, and when the first article came out, and *Esquire* described Calley in the "Backstage" column as merely "much like the rest of us," Sack was surprised by the cautious wording.

After Sack's book on Calley appeared, Sack went on a sixteen-week promotion tour, doing radio, television, lectures. When it was over and he went to Aspen, he felt all wrong that winter. A girlfriend, an actress, said no wonder—he had been on a bus and truck tour. In the spring, when he still had not recovered, Sack went into primal therapy and stayed in therapy for ten years.

In December 1971, Harold Hayes received a Christmas card from Lieutenant Calley:

> MAY YOU AND ALL WHOM YOU HOLD DEAR
> BE GRACED WITH THE BLESSINGS OF GOOD HEALTH AND HAPPINESS
> PEACE, FREEDOM AND SECURITY AT THIS HOLIDAY TIME
> AND IN THE COMING NEW YEAR.

Hayes saved the card and wrote on the envelope a note, dated October 17, 1985: "As good as any way to start a book on *Esquire* in the sixties—"

Part Three

Smiles come easily; never trust them. Far more difficult it is to cry well, and much more revealing.

"Giants," *Esquire,* July 1968

TEN

Stand-up Guys

*H*AROLD HAYES was fearless, *fearless,* it seemed to Gordon Lish, who had taken over as fiction editor. Bob Brown had left in early 1969 and Rust Hills had come in three days a week for a while; then, tired of the arrangement, he passed the job on to Lish. Of all the editors who came to work at *Esquire,* Lish could claim the most checkered past. He had grown up on Long Island much impressed by the life of Edgar Allan Poe and the power of Dylan Thomas; if he could have been both a southern drunk and a Welsh polymath, he said later, he would have been happy. He passed through years of a miserable childhood subjected to one treatment after another for a severe and intractable case of psoriasis. He was kicked out of prep school for fighting—it was the first time in his life he had been called a dirty Jew— and was making his own way in the world by his mid-teens. He worked as a radio announcer in New York and Texas, a wrangler in Arizona. By the time Jack Kerouac's *On the Road* came out, he had acquired a wife and a couple of kids; he packed them up and headed to San Francisco's North Beach, looking for Dean Moriarty. Settling in the Bay Area, he joined the crowd that hung around with Ken Kesey and the real Dean Moriarty, Neal Cassady.

Lish taught English in high school, then, after a much publicized dispute with the school administration, turned to writing textbooks for a living and editing a literary magazine on the side until, passing through New York on his way to Vermont, he got the fiction job at *Esquire;* Hayes gave it to him because he wrote such a great letter saying why he wanted the job—and because he wanted it so very much. He was, Tom Wolfe later wrote, "a very dapper and presentable fellow in the Litchfield briar-thistle tweedmore squire manner and at the same time just the sort of maniac who is capable of perpetuating *Esquire*'s carnival of contrariness."

In Harold Hayes, Lish met, if not his match, at least a man he could respect, as he discovered just a few weeks after he started work. Lish was having lunch with a well-known writer at a fancy restaurant, and after lunch, the waiter refused to accept a credit card.

"Can't you bill me at my office, at *Esquire?*" Lish had asked.

"You work for *Esquire?* They're a bunch of four flushers—they're a bunch of crooks."

"Can we discuss this in a more private place?" asked Lish, still dressed in his California clothes—tweed jacket, corduroy trousers, desert boots— and still inhibited by Bay Area politesse.

The waiter took that as an invitation to fight and started calling the other waiters. Out on the street, there was some pushing, then Lish and the writer fled, running six blocks or so back to the office. There Lish began thinking: Oh my God, a call is going to come to Hayes declaring that one of his people was in a near rumpus in an elegant French restaurant, and I'll be fired. He worried for a while, then decided he had better go in and confess.

"Tell them to go fuck themselves," said Hayes.

Hayes was afraid of nothing and no one, Lish thought. "He never paid court to anybody, he didn't kowtow to anybody—he stood up to everybody in sight, those persons senior to him at *Esquire*—everybody." Yet, Lish thought, too, he was always the gentleman—courtly, even "deep in his cups," incapable of meanness.

He liked the man, and Hayes seemed to like him. After work sometimes, the editors would go across the street to the Berkshire Hotel to drink and talk, staying until deep into the evening while Hayes told Marine stories. They would be sitting around a table, about eight of them, and Hayes would say, "You can't believe what Gordo showed me today—," and he would press Lish to explain why he liked the stories he liked. Hayes spoke in the character he liked to wear—the guise of a hick— but he also wanted to know; he genuinely wanted to understand. It seemed to Hayes and Gingrich that Lish liked some very peculiar things. *Esquire* had favored familiar writers: Philip Roth, Saul Bellow, William Styron. Lish had a different plan. He would publish writers whose work he liked, whether anyone had heard about them or not: Donald Newlove, Robert Ullian, Hilma Wolitzer. Hayes was astonished, Lish said later—"*stunned*"—to see what Lish came up with.

There was, for instance, Alma Stone, "virtually unpublished, an utter original," as Lish said in a little note dated March 13, 1970, attached to a manuscript passed up the line to Don Erickson, who passed it on to Hayes with a note: "I'll swear I just cannot get on this woman's wavelength. I've tried because of Gordon's admiration for her, but her prose seems like a bouillon cube of writing to me, waiting to be dropped into water, there to expand into a Carson McCullers novella."

Hayes turned the story down.

Lish tried a couple of stories by an old acquaintance from Palo Alto, Raymond Carver, and Hayes turned those down too. Lish passed them on to other magazines—one, "Fat," appeared in *Harper's Bazaar.* Carver expressed polite concern that Lish's advocacy of his work might be hurting his standing at the office, but he kept trying, sending Lish a story called "Neighbors" on August 20. Lish sent it on to Erickson with the comment, "just as effectively eerie as FAT, I think, but not as instantly forgettable, I hope." Erickson was more likely than Hayes to appreciate Lish's selections, but he was not enthusiastic about this one. Still, *Esquire* took the story.

The "Neighbors" that ran in the magazine the next year was considerably different from the manuscript Lish had received. At *Esquire* editors did not usually line-edit much, unless a story or article flirted with legal danger or violated *Esquire*'s restrictions on four-letter words or ran too long for the space available. There was none of that heavy interlining of manuscripts common at some other magazines. Lish was, in contrast, an aggressive editor; he went after manuscripts with firm confidence in his editorial hand. On several pages of the twelve-page manuscript, fewer than half of Carver's words were left standing. Close to half were cut on several other pages. (See facsimile copy of a sample page, p. 242) Lish's cuts gave the story a dry, minimalist feel. Uncut, Carver's manuscript read a good deal more like an ordinary realistically rendered story, although the plot was strange no matter how many words it took to unfold it.

For instance, one passage in manuscript read:

"Bill! God, you scared me. What're you doing home so early?"

He shrugged. "Nothing to do at work. And I kept thinking about last night. I've been horny all day."

"You're just saying that," she answered, but her eyes brightened. She let him use her key to open the door. He eyed the door across the hall before following her inside.

"Let's screw," he said.

"Bill! ·God, you scared me. What're you doing home so early?"

He shrugged. "Nothing to do at work, ~~And I kept thinking~~ he said. ~~about last night--I've been horny all day."~~

~~"You're just saying that," she answered, but her eyes brightened.~~ She let him use her key to open the door. He eyed the door across the hall before following her inside.

"Let's ~~screw~~ go to bed," he said.

"Now? Are you crazy?" She laughed. "What's gotten into you, honey?"

"Nothing. ~~I just told you I was turned on. Let's make it here in the living room, okay? Right here, standing up. Just~~ okay, take your dress off, ~~and nothing else~~." He grabbed for her playfully, and she said, "~~I don't know what's happened to you.~~ Are you serious?"

~~"Watch me," he said as he unfastened his belt.~~

~~"At least let me pull the shades first."~~

Later they ~~splurged and~~ sent out for Chinese food, and when it arrived they ate hungrily, without speaking, and listened to ~~a clamorous Jefferson Airplane~~ records.

"Let's not forget to feed Kitty," ~~Bill~~ she said, ~~"I was just thinking about that.~~ "I'll go over right now," he said ~~"You don't have to do it. You went over last night."~~ ~~"That's all right. I'm glad to. Be back shortly."~~

~~As he fumbled with the lock he heard Kitty on the other side of the door, mewing.~~ He selected a can of ~~ocean~~ fish for the cat, then filled the pitcher and went to water. When he returned to the kitchen ~~Kitty was scratching in her box. She looked at him steadily for a minute before she turned back to the litter. This time~~ he opened all

"Now? Are you crazy?" She laughed. "What's gotten into you, honey?"

"Nothing. I just told you I was turned on. Let's make it here in the living room, okay? Right here, standing up. Just take your dress off, and nothing else." He grabbed for her playfully, and she said, "I don't know what's happened to you. Are you serious?"

"Watch me," he said as he unfastened his belt.

"At least let me pull the shades first."

Later they splurged and sent out for Chinese food, and when it arrived they ate hungrily, without speaking, and listened to a clamorous Jefferson Airplane record.

Here is Lish's edited version, which would run in June 1971:

"Bill! God, you scared me. You're early," she said.

He shrugged. "Nothing to do at work," he said.

She let him use her key to open the door. He looked at the door across the hall before following her inside.

"Let's go to bed," he said.

"Now?" She laughed. "What's gotten into you?"

"Nothing. Take your dress off." He grabbed for her awkwardly, and she said, "Good God, Bill."

He unfastened his belt.

Later they sent out for Chinese food, and when it arrived they ate hungrily, without speaking, and listened to records.

In this case, Lish threaded out phrases and sentences. On some pages he took out entire paragraphs, giving the story a flat ironic style characteristic of a writer he particularly liked, James Purdy.

Carver accepted Lish's changes—publication in *Esquire* was, after all, a big break for him—and Lish would always get credit for discovering his work. Other writers were not so submissive. Doris Betts went through a lengthy analysis of his changes in one of her stories before she said she did not think they would do. For a story to be serious, she said, "the reverberations have to be there so that each note struck goes humming off along several other octaves." Rather than let Lish make the changes, she sold the story elsewhere for $25 instead of the $400 she might have reasonably expected from *Esquire*.

Paul Bowles was more blunt:

. . .I fail completely to understand the meaning of the suggestions, or of the story as it incorporates them. Instead of being about Hercules, it becomes a story about someone named Paul; instead of taking place twenty-five centuries or more ago, it apparently takes place in the present; instead of Tangier's being the locale, the

action passes in an unidentifiable no-man's-land; and Antaeus, instead of revealing himself as a typical Moroccan guide and thief, becomes a mysterious sort of
guru. What does it mean? Why should Hercules be called Paul? (Because when
someone whose name is actually Paul gives it to one of his characters, there arises
the question of his motivation, naturally. It's not exactly as if he had chosen
another name,—no?)

Bowles had decided to publish the story elsewhere.

Gingrich and Hayes were just as puzzled as Bowles by Lish's predilec-
tions. Hayes returned one story to Lish with a note expressing their mutual
confusion about what Lish was doing. Without making grand claims for
the literary worth of Hemingway, James Jones, or Zelda Fitzgerald, Hayes
did have to wonder if there was a happier medium—fiction that was not
quite so akin to abstract art.

Lish responded in a note attached to a manuscript, explaining that
writers were just not writing the kind of story Hayes wanted—"that is, a
piece strong in both character and event and cast in an orderly narrative
fiction. . . . The major stuff is getting pretty oblique in manner." But,
gamely, he was sending on to Hayes an old-fashioned story even though
Erickson hadn't liked it—or rather, said he liked it more the first times he
had read it, in various versions, back in the early 1950s.

". . .This isn't what I had in mind, exactly," Hayes replied.

Hayes himself was negotiating for rights to excerpts from new fiction
by James Jones and Philip Roth. He explained to Abe Blinder why he
wanted to publish an excerpt from an unfinished novel by Philip Roth, *My
Life as a Man*, which was "dull in places, deliberately slow going, and
sometimes laboriously plodding in its efforts"—and pay $10,000 or more
for the privilege. Gingrich wanted to pass on it—he didn't think much of
its literary value and he disliked "the joyless and perverse rendering" of a
sexual act that, in his memo to Blinder, Hayes tactfully left undescribed.
Hayes wanted the Roth excerpt, he explained, to strengthen *Esquire*'s
standing as a literary medium. *Esquire* had gone too long without major
literary events. This was November 1970, and Mailer and Roth had not
appeared since 1967; Bellow since 1965; Arthur Miller since 1966; Styron
since 1968. Within the last year, Hayes had purchased rights to work by
Gore Vidal, Ernest Hemingway (his last, unfinished novel), and James
Jones as part of an attempt to strengthen *Esquire*'s literary visibility.

Hayes had paid $30,000 for the Hemingway excerpt, and felt obliged
to feature it on the cover. "Harold," Tom Hedley said, "dead writers will

not sell magazines. It's a disaster, believe me." It was one of *Esquire*'s worst-selling issues that year, but Hayes was determined to keep *Esquire* in what he saw as the center ring of fiction. *Playboy, The Atlantic Monthly,* and *Harper's* were giving *Esquire* stiff competition for big-name writers, and seemed to be able to meet the writers' demands for money and freedom from taste restrictions. Would it matter if *Esquire* pulled out of the competition? Hayes thought so. Readers were fickle these days— they would go where the action was, Hayes wrote to Blinder. "My own guess is that the national interest in politics and cultural shifts is diminishing; and should this be so, a stronger effort in literary representation can be a valuable element until the reader's mood settles down."

Hayes was no aesthete, Lish thought, but while Hayes pursued the big writers he thought *Esquire* ought to have, he also defended Lish's right to publish the fiction he liked, even in the face of Gingrich's utter befuddlement. When Lish sent up a story by David Ohle, Hayes jotted a note to Gingrich in the corner of Gordon's: "AG Weird & truly frightening. HH." Gingrich jotted his own note at the bottom: "The only parts of this I could understand were 6, 7, 9, 13, 15, 17, 19, 22, 24, 27, 29 & 31. No objection to them. In fact, if another person than Gordon can understand the other sections, I have no objection to them either. AG"

Perhaps feeling that other readers besides Gingrich needed a clue as to where *Esquire* fiction was tending, Hayes asked Lish to write down his thoughts for Hayes to pass on in his "Editor's Notes" for January 1971. He prefaced Lish's remarks with a column of his own commentary on the difference between, say, James Jones, whose novel on the Paris youth revolt *Esquire* was excerpting, and Robert Ullian, whose story "A Snag in the Harp" would appear in the next issue. "If there is a contemporary mode to fiction these days, the drift is clearly toward Ullian and his generation and away from Jones and his." But why, he asked Lish to explain, "are their metaphors so unbelievably abstruse?"

Lish offered an explanation reminiscent of Marshall McLuhan: writers had discarded meaning for feeling; to convey feeling, writers arranged images not in a linear, logical way but in a circle, aiming for "spontaneity—flashes, everything at once." Interest in narrative had died out; tone, atmosphere was all. Writers were after *effect,* not elaboration on theme "or otherwise perceivable meaning BECAUSE NOTHING MEANS ANYTHING."

John Gardner, a poet and fiction writer who had just published *The*

Wreckage of Agathon, had something to say to Lish about that. "It seems to me—no offense old man—that your theory of fiction is ridiculous. 'NOTHING MEANS ANYTHING' has been the slogan of half-wits for centuries. The truth is (and has always been) MOST OF THE THINGS PEOPLE TELL YOU MEAN SOMETHING DON'T MEAN ANYTHING, BUT THE ONLY HUMAN ACTIVITY IS THE DISCOVERY OF WHAT *DOES* MEAN."

Gordon Lish was not *Esquire*'s only man on fiction: following Lish's suggestion, Hayes had employed a fiction writer named Barton Midwood to write a column on fiction that began December 1970. Midwood was, Lish recalled, "quite a piece of work," one of the few people whose presence in the office could provoke Hayes to close his door, even though he was, Lish also said, Hayes's own "invention." *Esquire* had published several short stories by Midwood before Lish got to *Esquire,* and Hayes even tried to turn him into a reporter, inviting him to write a profile of the actor Douglas Fairbanks because, Hayes explained when he told the story later, "he was a skillful writer with a deep interest in moral ambiguity." When Midwood agreed, Hayes gave him $500 to go to California.

Seven weeks after he took the assignment, Midwood appeared before Hayes and handed him a check for $500, with the request that Hayes not cash it until the end of the month. He couldn't do the story, Midwood said; to write about someone living was to "create a character who is frozen in time." Midwood had liked Fairbanks, and Fairbanks had told Midwood enough to bring him down, and Fairbanks knew that he had. When Midwood had first showed up, Fairbanks had said, "I want you to know that *I* know you observed the fact that I'm wearing a carnation in my lapel. And I want you to know *I* know there are a thousand different meanings you can attach to this. . . ."

Midwood told Hayes, "I don't want to be responsible for this sort of thing, I don't want to do this kind of writing. . . ."

Still, Midwood did accept an assignment to pay visits to several writers and write about them. Among them were James Purdy and Grace Paley, both writers who had published in *Esquire,* both writers Lish would have liked to see publish in *Esquire* again. Midwood's article—"Short Visits with Five Writers and One Friend" (November 1970)—was a sharp piece of work, written in a style much like Paley's own: small clear sentences and dialogue sets. Midwood was not especially unkind to Paley, who came off like a Grace Paley character, but Purdy came off as a surly simpleton.

Lish tried to soften the blow in a letter of October 12, 1970, explaining to Purdy that *Esquire* had a policy of letting writers say what they would, and not editing out opinions the editors didn't like. *Esquire*'s aim, Lish wrote, was "to promote a free forum of ideas," even if, as in this case, that sometimes led to discomfort for individual editors. Lish had found that out the hard way just a few months before. When Midwood had turned in his first fiction column, one of the books he took on was the poet James Dickey's new novel, *Deliverance*. Dickey was chiefly a poet, and Lish had only recently talked Hayes into making him *Esquire*'s poetry editor—a new position (poetry was replacing cartoons as space filler). When Midwood's first column arrived, Lish was aghast.

Midwood, so tenderhearted toward Douglas Fairbanks, was, toward James Dickey, a man of cold steel. Dickey's characters were "idiots," and "the most disappointing thing about the book is that only one of them is killed." *Deliverance* was a "metaphor for the homosexual psyche," the main character "a latent homosexual," threatened with rape "by way of the mouth"—a suspenseful moment, Midwood observed, since "the question before my mind at the time was: How is he going to keep narrating with that thing in his mouth?"

Appalled by what he saw as a personal attack, Lish went to Hayes with the column. Dickey was on the verge of making his debut as *Esquire*'s poetry editor in the January issue; now here was Midwood attacking him in the issue before. What, Lish asked Hayes, were they going to do?

"We're going to run it," said Hayes.

"But we can't consider it—we must protect our friends," Lish replied.

No, Hayes explained, *Esquire* was not in the business of protecting its friends. *Esquire* had no friends. *Esquire* was an open forum and most exciting when it was seen as the dog biting its own tail. *Esquire* would run Midwood's column.

Lish had hit on a touchy point: Wilfrid Sheed, *Esquire*'s movie critic from 1967 to 1969, then theater columnist for a couple of issues, had told Hayes he wouldn't write for *Esquire* again after—as Hayes put it—"some free-lance writer mentioned his name in our pages with something less than reverence." Hayes wrote Sheed back sharply:

"Right on! I've sure learned my lesson. The next time somebody writing in these pages says anything about somebody I know personally, or have published in the past, and says it without consulting me as to whether I agree with him—you know, just puts it down in black and white, his own unfounded opinion, even though it may not be libelous or an invasion of privacy—you can be sure I will be prepared to make him *cut it out* or else be prepared to lose a friend and contributor.

"Thanks a lot for setting me straight."

Hayes's refusal to protect *Esquire* contributors from other *Esquire* contributors left a deep impression on Lish. "He was concerned to make this magazine an entirely open forum, and a place of supreme energy—if there were any kind of journalistic principle, that was it. . . . There was never anything shadowy, anything at the edges, anything that one might be suspicious of acting on his judgment."

Dickey did not back out as poetry editor. After Lish gave him advance warning, and before he saw the piece, Dickey wrote back cheerfully. Not to worry; he would just avoid reading it. He did read it, though, and sent Lish a reaction he declined to have reprinted here.

The debate over Lish's taste in fiction subsided—maybe under the force of Lish's persistence (for a while as "Captain Fiction," he wrote detailed monthly reports on what was coming out)—but from time to time Hayes would express concern over not getting enough fiction by big-name writers into the magazine or suggest Lish try harder to widen his range. What was to Lish remarkable about Hayes was that "over his own instincts in the matter, and over Gingrich's continuing rejection of the kind of thing I wanted to do, he nevertheless let it happen."

Lish heard Jean-Paul Goude complain that Hayes's ideas about art were retrograde—yet the staff held him in high esteem and thought of him with affection, Lish believed. "He was our boss, and we might have felt that he was not as up-to-date in certain ways as were we, and was not as given to invention as were we, but he after all had hired us for the very qualities that had made us take that position. He admired that in us, and he was, I suppose, a kind of leveling and centering influence at all times."

Once, Lish recalled, a man from a radical group in California came to the office after hours with a carton and a woman he said was an agent and offered Lish his life story. The man said he had gotten Lish's name from Neal Cassady, the charismatic member of, first, Jack Kerouac's circle and, later, Ken Kesey's. As Lish told the tale later, the man said,

"I hear you're a stand-up guy. I understand from Neal you're a stand-up guy. And I want to show you my life story, in which I talk about seven people I offed. I confess to my murders. Do you want to look at it?"

"Oh, absolutely, absolutely, an *Esquire* coup, are you kidding? You just leave it here, and I'll look at it and let you know Monday because I'm the fastest gun in the West when it comes to editing—there's no faster gun in New York City."

"Well, go ahead."

"What are you talking about?"

"Go ahead and look at it."

"What do you mean, 'look at it'?"

"Well, there it is."

It was in a big corrugated carton.

"I will, I will."

"Now. I'm not going to leave that here. That's— I confess to murders in there. I'm not going to leave it with you."

"Well, you know I can't look at it now. I gotta get home. It's the end of the workday and that's an enormous manuscript. I can't possibly go through all of that."

"Well, you're not going to leave here unless you do."

Lish was terrified.

"I'm giving it to you now," the man said, and, "Neal says you're a stand-up guy."

"You can't be serious. This is not the way you do these things."

There was nobody in the office by then except Lish and the man and the woman he had brought with him—and Hayes, in his office.

"Can you excuse me for a minute," said Lish, "my boss is down there, the editor of the magazine, and maybe we can work this thing out."

Lish filled Hayes in on what was happening, and Hayes said, "Well, look, Lish. You got yourself into this by being a good guy—you're the one who's so accessible. Get yourself out of it. I can't get you out of it."

"Well how? This guy could really hurt me. Can you call the police?"

"I'm not going to call the police. You want to call the police? Here's the phone, call the police."

It was a characteristic response. "He probably knew I wasn't in any danger. The man was playful in the crunch," Lish said later. "He was never not playful. He never stopped enjoying himself."

Not everyone shared Lish's sunny assessment of Hayes. To Aaron Latham, the new editor, who came to *Esquire* from the *Washington Post*, there was a formality about Hayes. Latham might look into Hayes's office and if Hayes was there, he might go in to talk, but the conversations never lasted long; Latham could feel Hayes willing him to leave. Sheila Berger, who had been an art associate for several years (she would marry Tom Wolfe later on), recalled everyone having a lot of fun in the office—and yet everyone seemed terrified of Hayes: he was so demanding.

One old acquaintance who did not share anyone's favorable impression of Harold Hayes was Gloria Steinem, and on April 12, 1971, she wrote him a letter. Rex Reed had asked to interview her for *Esquire* and she had turned him down. She wanted to explain why.

Dear Harold,
    Ever since I had lunch with Rex Reed and promised him that I would explain to you why I had declined to have an interview done (Rex didn't want you to think him a bad reporter), I've been wanting to ask you out for lunch or a drink or a hotdog so we could talk.
    But it's hard to call someone who, since our first meeting thirteen years ago (jesus!), various well-meaning people have been telling me didn't like me at all. Or at least, it's hard for me; which is my problem, not yours. Someone even told me you might hang up if I called.

Now, several things had come up to make her think she had been wrong not to call. For one thing, a young Time-Life correspondent named Leonard Levitt had been writing an article on her for the Sunday *New York Times Magazine*—which had turned it down, she was relieved to learn—and he had been to see Hayes. Levitt had told her (she said years later) that he was having a hard time finding enemies to interview for the story, and she had suggested Hayes. Afterward, Levitt had passed on to Steinem some of the reasons he gathered Hayes might not like her. "They turned out to be the kind of crazy rumors we all get saddled with in New York," she wrote Hayes. Then, too, she had read Helen Lawrenson's piece, "The Feminine Mistake," an attack on the women's liberation movement that had appeared in *Esquire*. No wonder Hayes had a distorted impression of the women's movement. "God knows, the press ridicule and distortion have been extreme enough to bring all sorts of misunderstandings."
    Finally, she had realized that she could not trust personal relationships to intermediaries. She had known Harold and Susan longer than anyone in New York—"So how about lunch Friday or Saturday?" She suggested a chili place they used to go to—she thought it was on Times Square.
    They did talk, and made lunch plans. Hayes asked her if she would return the Fred Astaire album he had lent her years before in Cambridge.

She wrote back on May 21, before they had lunch, that she had lost so many records in various moves that she had had to look for a replacement. The best that she could do was three new re-recordings, which she was sending him; record specialists had assured her they had most of the songs from the old album.

Then she got down to business: Len Levitt had told her that the article the *New York Times* had turned down was now going to run in *Esquire*. Steinem expressed reservations about the Levitt piece and asked Hayes for a favor.

It's ironic that I should seem dimly newsworthy just at the time that I've figured out how destructive the American publicity mystique is for a person; especially for me. And for the Woman's Movement, which should have no stars. As Len will tell you, our problem has been that he did the *New York Times* article without help from me, and therefore—through no fault of his—had to rely on peripheral interviews. I checked facts afterward, but felt strongly that the result (again, through no fault of his) was much more an image than a real life person with habits like great self-doubt and picking up the laundry.

She had resigned herself to reading about someone she didn't know, but she did hope the piece would touch lightly on one area of her life: her childhood in Toledo. It was an extremely difficult childhood, as she described it later in an essay, "Ruth's Song (Because She Could Not Sing It)." Her mother had been mentally ill and, during her teen years, Steinem had cared for the two of them in a dilapidated house. She asked Hayes that the article not be tough on her mother, who had finally managed, after years of treatment in a mental hospital, to put the Toledo memories behind her. As long as her mother lived, Steinem wanted to keep her childhood to herself—one reason she did not welcome profiles.

Esquire had toyed with the idea of doing a piece on Steinem for some time. At one point after he left *Esquire*, John Berendt had suggested he might write a piece on Steinem. Hayes had laid out for him what he would want:

Please bear in mind we don't want yet another testimonial to the canon of her true greatness but rather an article on her *manufactured* greatness. I raise this now because you mentioned you felt the piece should be fair (it should) including both the "good and bad" about her (this too, maybe). . . . Her accomplishments and public positions, including in the "good" department, are a matter of record (an inexhaustible one!). . . . If you should move from these primary considerations you would, I fear, wind up with a conventional profile rather than holding to the force of context suggested by Ferrell and Sherrill ("Gloria in Excelsis": a short history of fashionable liberalism, from the CIA to Women's Lib).

Also on record is her acuity, charm, and intelligence, but what is *not* on record is how she uses this equipment to further her own ends. Apart from the background information on her rise to prominence—which is absolutely fascinating stuff and central to the piece—there is a real challenge in trying to decipher her subterranean art in spotting a trend early enough to get cosy with the driver of the bandwagon.

The private record—and the singular point of view suggested by title and subtitle—is what makes this an *Esquire* piece. . . .

Hayes's outline of the piece he would like to see on Steinem was in keeping with *Esquire*'s usual approach to celebrities. About the same time Levitt's piece on Steinem was in process, Hayes encouraged Gore Vidal to write a piece on Norman Mailer along a similar line—how Mailer made himself famous (or "Advertisements for Himself"): "Certainly he is a creature of the mass media, magazines more specifically," Hayes wrote Vidal, "and it's hard to imagine where he would be today had he not conformed so precisely to the needs of modern-day magazine journalism, manipulating the appetites and interests of editors more skillfully than any other part of his constituency."

So *Esquire* was not singling Steinem out for special treatment. What did distinguish the Steinem piece from most *Esquire* profiles was the depth of Hayes's personal knowledge of "the private record" that would make the piece right for *Esquire*. He had watched Steinem's progress toward celebrity ever since those months in 1959 when they were both in Cambridge together. And, the fact is, he did not like her. Those who knew him could imagine several reasons why. Steinem had encouraged his wife, Susan—without much success—to have a life outside her home. Steinem had ditched his friend Walt Friedenberg; Steinem had gone from one man to another. Steinem was a powerful woman who did not, apparently, find Harold Hayes appealing.

Whatever the reasons Hayes felt as he did toward her, Steinem knew he did not like her. She thought the encouragement she gave to Susan had the most to do with his animosity, but she also saw Hayes as a repressed authoritarian who resented people, like his wife Susan, who were freer in spirit than he could be.

She watched uneasily as the piece moved through fact-checking. She was particularly concerned about the way *Esquire* would present her activ-

ities years before at a 1962 Youth Festival in Helsinki, where (along with
Clay Felker and Sam Antupit) she had helped Finnish student organiza-
tions run anti-Soviet newspapers in different languages to counter the
official Soviet festival newspaper. Steinem's plane fare to the festival was
paid by the Independent Research Service, her employer in Cambridge
in 1959–1960, which was getting funds from the Central Intelligence
Agency. The CIA had made a practice of secretly supporting liberal anti-
Soviet cultural enterprises like the National Student Association and *Encounter* magazine, as *Ramparts* magazine and the *New York Times* had
by this time revealed. To Steinem, the issue of CIA funding was more
complex than she thought Levitt and Hayes understood. For one thing,
she told *Esquire*'s fact-checker, the CIA money came to the Independent
Research Service indirectly, through foundations. Although she knew the
CIA was involved, she thought taking money from the CIA was simply a
matter of using CIA money for a good cause.

"I don't mean to get carried away," she wrote *Esquire*'s fact-checker,

—the whole thing was too long ago and boring to be of real interest. But it
concerns me for the obvious legal reasons, plus the fact that Leonard Levitt told
me Harold didn't understand it. (Harold actually told him to try to find who my
case officer had been. Do you think we're all suffering from the Mata Hari myth,
on top of everything else?) And it makes me mad as hell that something we
believed in and did at some personal expense (and risk of encounter with HUAC)
should now be described as a "job" that we were ordered to do by some sinister
force.

Steinem had lawyers send *Esquire* a letter stating her understanding
that the magazine intended to publish material that was "flagrantly false"
and "defamatory." Meanwhile, Blair Chotzinoff, one of her earlier boy-
friends and a source for the article, wrote *Esquire* twice in July expressing
concern about the accuracy of his quotations and the way the information
he had given Levitt would be used. He had told Levitt from the start, he
said, that he wanted nothing he said to be used to embarrass Steinem.

It was too late to retreat: the article was well on its way into the
October 1971 issue, where it appeared under the title "She," named after
H. Rider Haggard's all-powerful white African queen. Levitt did use Steinem's work at Helsinki as evidence that she changed politics as the wind
blew, transforming herself from Cold Warrior at the start of the sixties
into a champion of Left causes at the start of the seventies. According to
the fact-checker's report, Steinem had said she was not anti-Communist

at the time of the festival but was, on the contrary, in a Marxist period. Years later, she said she had actually been anti-Communist at the time of the festival as a result of her experiences in India, where the Communists had supported the British during World War II and earned the enmity of the independence movement they had once been a part of. Whatever the nuances of her political belief, there was no necessary inconsistency between Steinem's earlier anti-Soviet stance and her later support for migrant workers and women—the point Levitt was making; the American Left was full of Cold Warriors.

Levitt did pass lightly over her childhood experience, but framed what he did say in supercilious terms: "One gets the impression talking to Gloria that she was born in the Toledo equivalent of the manger." That was the tone of the piece—not ironic, in the mode of Gay Talese, but simply snide. Levitt set up his theme near the start:

No man who seeks to know how the wind blows can afford to ignore Gloria, the intellectuals' pinup, but no man can claim her undivided attention. And no man can ever know just where she stands, as Hugh Hefner was the first to discover. Gloria launched her variegated career by donning a Playboy Bunny costume. She masqueraded as a Bunny in 1963 and then wrote about her experience for *Show* magazine. Since then she has been out of uniform, putting on, instead of long ears and a tail, one movement after another. She discards movements— and the leaders of movements—as once she laid aside the rolled athletic socks with which, she reported, she stuffed her bosoms during the Bunny days. Most recently, this woman, who advanced in public favor by appealing to powerful men, has moved to the front ranks of women's liberation, appealing now to women who do not like powerful men.

For his sources, Levitt drew heavily on members of the *Esquire* circle who were not always identified in the piece as such: Tom Morgan, the unnamed mayor's aide who figures in the beginning; Sam Antupit, identified several times by name but not as a former *Esquire* art director; and Tom Wolfe, who worked with her at *New York*. (Aaron Latham, the editor of the piece, interviewed Wolfe for the story.) Harvey Kurtzman, who had given Steinem her first New York job, supplied some of the more damaging remarks. John Kenneth Galbraith, who had published several articles in *Esquire*, apparently meant to speak kindly of Steinem but he, too, helped Levitt build up the image of a woman using her feminine attractions to amass political power: "He says that she owes her rise to 'brains, comic perception, and extremely good looks.' He knows his subject well enough to add that she might say that her looks had nothing to do with it, but he disagrees. 'I have to be honest,' he says."

Then there was an unidentified source, "a friend of some years back," who said, "She had the uncanny ability of adapting herself to the romantic image most appropriate for the boyfriend of the moment. In the late J. D. Salinger Fifties, just back from two years in India, she dressed Peck & Peck, fit to kill—everything a friend of mine, a country-boy journalist, could have envisaged as the perfect mate."

That, of course, likely came from Harold Hayes, the editor of the magazine running this piece, whose country-boy journalist friend had sent Steinem his way. The comment did not provide any key facts and could have easily been omitted. Its presence, set among all those other *Esquire* personages providing ammunition against Steinem, was another link in the personal relationship between the subject and the magazine and the magazine's editor—a relationship acknowledged only minimally, with a reference to her relationship with Robert Benton and a little section on her first article in a national magazine, "The Moral Disarmament of Betty Coed," in *Esquire*'s 1962 college issue.

Aaron Latham, the editor of Levitt's article, did not recall later having any idea that the unnamed source of the country-boy comment was Harold Hayes. So far as he knew, Levitt did not interview Hayes after the piece reached *Esquire.* What Latham did recall clearly was that Hayes himself kept a close eye on the piece, supervising draft after draft after draft. Hayes had not particularly liked the article when it came in, Latham thought, and Hayes knew that it would get a lot of attention when *Esquire* published it. He wanted it really focused, everything nailed down. "He wanted to make a splash, but he didn't want to get wet when the splash happened."

The piece ran with a three-page color comic spread, "Superwoman," which pressed Levitt's point home: With the word "CHAZOB" Steinem as Superwoman could transform herself into "a lithesome Lolita at Smith College," "a helpful humanitarian" in India, "a fearless agent of the free world fighting communism in Helsinki"—"TAKE *THAT,* @**! YOU RABID, RAUNCHY, RADICAL RED!"—"A BELLIGERENT BUNNY," "A FEMME FATALE," "A PRETTY POLITICIAN," until finally, in the last three panels, she proclaims:

"I AM *SUPER WOMAN,* PROTECTOR OF THE WEAK, THE MEEK, THE UGLY . . . THE UGLY? . . . THE PLUMP, THE

SHORT, THE PIANO LEGGED . . . UP AGAINST THE WALL,
MALE CHAUVINIST PIGS! OUR BLACK BROTHERS *ARE* OUR
SISTERS."

A corner closing line asked, "WHAT NEXT?"

Steinem didn't sue, but the article wiped her out for months, she said
later. She felt "totally betrayed." To Robert Benton, "printing that article
about her was really unnecessary, it really was."

Whatever personal animosity lay behind the Steinem piece, Hayes felt
a marked ambivalence toward the women's movement. In a speech, he
portrayed it as a fad that could become something more, since women
were raising serious issues: abortion, equal wages, day care "so that they
might escape the tedium of housework." But he thought women involved
in the movement had not demonstrated personal commitment to the
cause. And they resorted to "rhetoric and media-baiting techniques" instead of doing the hard political work of organizing votes. Demonstrating
again his distaste for unconventional politics, he said, "In my book, 'con-
sciousness-level raising' is less effective than a letter to your congressman.
A sit-in less effective than block parties to organize the vote. . . ."

Certainly, after the July 1962 issue on women, *Esquire* had given
women short shrift as serious subjects. They appeared in the magazine, of
course, but most often as pretty girls, wrestlers, lady bosses, strippers,
movie stars. Occasionally a writer would cast a feminist frame around one
of these subjects. Gina Berriault turned her profile of San Francisco's
Carol Doda, a topless dancer, into a moving portrait of female exploita-
tion, and Garry Wills did something similar with the women of Jack
Ruby's club world. Yet *Esquire* lapsed easily into coy appreciation, in the
girl stories, or outright contempt, as in George Lois's February 1967 cover:
"The New American Woman: Through at 21," a woman stuffed in a trash
can.

In the case of women, *Esquire*'s attitude had not caught up with its
practice. *Esquire* not only ran work by women writers, but ran it without
apparent regard to whether the topic was a woman's topic. Helen Lawrenson did make her name at *Esquire* in the thirties with "Latins Are Lousy
Lovers" (and went on to write more articles than any other *Esquire*
writer), but more of the time *Esquire* ran women writers not because they
had something to say as women but because they were good. A number of
women made quick appearances—among them, Simone de Beauvoir, Isak

Dinesen, Rebecca West, Midge Decter, M. F. K. Fisher, Susan Brown-miller, Susan Sontag.

Hayes sought out Dorothy Parker to be *Esquire*'s book reviewer in the early sixties and spoke of her with special kindness, in spite of her difficult ways, and he put Elaine Dundy and Sally Kempton on contract as contributing editors in the mid-sixties. Several other women writers contributed articles often enough to seem, for a while, almost like regulars—Sybille Bedford, Gina Berriault, Candice Bergen, and Nora Ephron, whose May 1972 article on breasts ran into and overcame one obstacle, Gingrich's reservations about her last word: "shit." A month later, a column by Ephron began appearing in *Esquire*. At a time when male dominance of fiction was extreme, *Esquire* did publish fiction by Joyce Carol Oates, Flannery O'Connor, and Grace Paley, and Gordon Lish pushed hard to publish the work of several women writers who were not widely known.

Hayes himself never took up a woman writer in the way he took up Talese or Wills, but he gave Diane Arbus encouragement and support and used her work often, and Jill Goldstein recalled his admiration and support for Helen Lawrenson. Goldstein would go to him and say, "Helen Lawrenson wants more money."

"Put it through, put it through," he would say. Then he would give Goldstein a little lecture on Lawrenson. She was, he would say "not only talented—she's a very courageous woman, you know, married to Jack Long, who died very young and left two children, and she's done the best for them. It's not easy raising two children on your own, and having a career like Helen Lawrenson."

One of Hayes's closest working friendships was with Candida Donadio; he said that another friend, Laura Bergquist, the editor at *Look* who introduced him to Arnold Gingrich, was the first feminist he ever met. Ann Zane Shanks, the photographer who had known him before he ever got to *Esquire,* was another close personal friend. She recalled that after the death of her first husband left her a young widow with two small children, Hayes, at Harvard on his Nieman, had invited her for a visit with him and Susan in Cambridge. Hayes always seemed to her to be buoyant and generous, open, eager, fun. Whenever she saw him, he made her feel very welcome. He would say something like, "Gosh, oh golly Ann, how is my girl?"

Yet Hayes's friendship with talented women did not translate into support for the women's liberation movement. He was himself, in at least one respect, something of a Victorian, with a wife at home and mistresses elsewhere, including the office. He kept the two spheres of his life neatly divided, with his wife eventually living off in the country with their children. Given his complicated personal relationships and the generation to which he belonged, his ambivalence toward the women's movement is not surprising. In the speech he prepared on women, he put the issues the women were raising "127th on my list of priorities—somewhere down there below prison reform and smog control."

It would be July 1973 before *Esquire* gave the women's movement the honor of an establishment chart in a special issue on women that included articles by Sara Davidson and Germaine Greer and a spread of *Esquire* cartoons illustrating the magazine's "perfectly *rotten* attitude toward women"—in the past "a long time ago, under a different set of editors." But *Esquire* did give feminists a forum earlier from time to time, for instance running Sally Kempton's frank expression of feminist rage in a piece called "Cutting Loose" (July 1970).

Craig Karpel, a bright young writer Hayes had taken on to supply ideas from the West Coast, wrote in a memo that Kempton's piece was the sort of thing *Esquire* ought to be doing—*Esquire* could take advantage here of *Playboy*'s weakness as a crusader against women's lib. Karpel further advised *Esquire* editors to keep out gratuitous remarks about women as "chicks" and irrelevant tags indicating their marital status. After first reference, Bella Abzug should be "Abzug" instead of "Mrs. Abzug"; Gloria Steinem should be "Steinem," not "Miss Steinem." Who cared whether either was married? Movement publications had already made these style changes—why not make *Esquire* the first on its block?

The very month before savaging Steinem, *Esquire* had featured Germaine Greer on the September 1971 cover, clutched, Fay Wray style, in the hairy arms of Norman Mailer. Mailer had debated Greer and had also attacked the women's movement in a major *Harper's* piece, "The Prisoner of Sex," which, for a while, Willie Morris thought cost him his job at *Harper's*. Now, in *Esquire,* Greer took on Mailer.

"Whether Mailer gets Greer or she gets his goat seems to us a matter of considerably less than cosmic significance," Gingrich wrote in his publisher's column. "This whole Women's Lib fracas bores us blind and one thing that sets Germaine Greer apart from the rest of the embattled sisterhood is that she appears to be the only one of the lot who actually enjoys being a woman." In fact, when Greer came to lunch at *Esquire,*

Gingrich had fallen asleep; like the dormouse in *Alice in Wonderland,* he always fell asleep at *Esquire* lunches, still holding his lighted Camel between his fingers.

Hayes reported to the readers only that Greer had lunched with the editors and had "charmed them silly." There had been no need to talk of *Esquire*'s "inequities toward womanhood," because twenty-three of the names of forty-seven on *Esquire*'s masthead were women's. Acknowledging that many of those women were not out having lunch with famous authors, Hayes maintained that they did have a lot to say about what went into the magazine and whether it got to press. He then introduced eleven of them—mostly in subordinate positions, like the research department.

There would have been fewer of them even there if Hayes had had his way. Back in 1968, when Hayes was anticipating hiring a new researcher, he argued for upgrading the salary so that he could hire someone like his current research chief Tom Ferrell—that is, someone male, to back up Ferrell and take his place if Hayes promoted him to an editorial position. To hire a man like Ferrell rather than "an inexperienced girl," Hayes observed, he would need to start the salary in the range of $100 a week rather than $80. The company president, Abe Blinder, explained to Hayes in response why women made better researchers than men: they were more content not to get raises.

There *had* been women editors on the staff in the sixties, although one of them was no longer on the masthead: associate editor Alice Glaser. The year before, Glaser had died in a fall. Nobody said openly then that the death was a suicide, but nobody, later, doubted that it was. She had been troubled for a long time; Gordon Lish would recall her standing in the back of editorial meetings in Hayes's office, muttering while he spoke, watching the others compete for Hayes's approval. Her death shook Hayes deeply.

Jill Goldstein, now the only woman associate editor, had always been less of an assignment editor than a producer, collecting people for group portraits, for instance. For a couple of her years as an editor, she did not even have a room of her own; she had a desk in the research department. She had gotten an office only after she raised a fuss with Hayes—one of the few times she confronted him. (Once she protested the disappearance of a bare-breasted model's nipples—airbrushed out so her breasts looked like balloons; he conceded the point and the art department drew the nipples back in on the plate.)

A couple of other women had already left *Esquire* for more powerful positions: after several years as art associate, Sheila Berger had become art director at *Harper's,* and Pat Rotter, editorial coordinator at *Esquire* and a close friend of Hayes's, had gone to *Harper's,* too, to handle fiction; stories Lish didn't use sometimes wound up in her hands. There seemed to be a glass ceiling at *Esquire,* and at least some of the women noticed it. Kitty Krupat, chief researcher, could not help thinking from time to time about the male editors, just a few years older than she was, doing all that interesting editorial work while she was out slogging around a Queens cemetery in the pouring rain looking for a headstone to check the spelling of a name in a piece by Gay Talese.

In late July 1971, Diane Arbus, one of the more important women in Harold Hayes's professional life, was found dead, her wrists cut, in an empty bathtub. She had lent her strange sense of humor to *Esquire* throughout the sixties; it was fresh, but it was mordant, too. Shadows played around the edges of her pictures: Blaze Starr in her bank-lobby living room, posed like a wind-up doll; Mae West, befrilled and ravaged. Arbus tinged even innocence with a hint of guilt, courage with a hint of eccentricity: Madeline Murray, the militantly atheist mother who got formal prayers banned from public schools, stood defiant in her bedroom, with a girdle supplied by Arbus dangling from her dresser.

While other photographers explored color effects—Hayes wrote in his "Editor's Notes" for November 1971—"Diane was more interested in the people she studied, the expression in their eyes; and black and white was good enough." She placed subjects in natural settings, straight in front of the center of her lens—"always with the same curious expression, as though seeking from the beholder some special understanding."

Hayes had used her work whenever he could; they had been close. Yet years later, at the opening of a museum exhibition of her photographs, when Hayes gave a talk on Arbus his presentation was oddly impersonal, based almost entirely on the records in his file. Perhaps he thought the audience would learn more about how she worked from the words of the time than from his memories of their conversations. Or perhaps his reticence derived from a respect for the dividing line between their editorial relationship and their friendship, of which he said only, at the start, that she was to him more than a contributor—she was "a personal friend." Reticence about his personal life was characteristic of Hayes. Only at the end of the speech did he go beyond the record and speak of her in personal terms, in an attempt to counter the way her death had bent the shape of her life:

"She was a genuinely wonderful woman. . . . I think she has been sort of mythologized into a romantic, haunted woman who was somewhat ahead of her time by leaving her home and making a career for herself and dying, and leaving a body of work that was extraordinary but incomplete. And this sort of gloomy, quite melodramatic image hovers around her. And she wasn't that way, she was genuinely warm, and had a marvelous sense of humor, a fresh, almost naive manner about her."

Connie Wood, Hayes's secretary, could remember Arbus calling him up to say, "I've got some sandwiches—let's go picnic in the park." And they would go to Central Park together. Or she would come by his office to talk. Or they would eat supper at a Chinese restaurant. "They were very close, Harold and Diane—they were very close." He was devastated by her death.

These years were proving hard for some members of the *Esquire* circle. After Rust Hills left *Esquire* a second time, turning the magazine's fiction over to Lish, he watched himself come apart in Connecticut. Bud Lee spent time in a mental ward, the consequence, he thought, of taking acid at Princess Leda's and maybe, too, of all the things he had seen as a photographer—the New Jersey riots and that craziness in California. John Sack went into primal therapy and Michael Herr passed through a period of deep and unsettling depression. When he came out of it finally with *Dispatches,* he would think of that book not as a book about Vietnam, but, as Hunter Thompson once observed, a book about America in the sixties. "And it was very personal, and I know, man, I know how many people got wiped out, how many people are dead, who never saw forty, never saw thirty."

By 1971, two of the people Hayes was closest to at *Esquire* had left the magazine—Bob Sherrill and Hayes's secretary, Connie Wood, who had worked for him since 1961. Wood had threatened to leave several times, and she really did leave in 1970, to move to the West Coast. Bob Sherrill left a few months later, after he came back from a trip and simply no longer wanted to be in New York. He stayed on the masthead as a contributing editor and kept on sending story ideas but he was no longer handy, in his office down the hall. The three of them—Hayes, Wood, and Sherrill—had been buddies, "the three musketeers." Hayes had been Wood's best friend in New York. And Bob Sherrill knew Hayes as nobody else quite did: he had known him so long, had known him in his home country, before he ever came north. Hayes loved Sherrill, Wood recalled. "He loved him. He loved him. Harold tried very hard to keep him in New York but he couldn't do it."

With the August 1971 issue, *Esquire,* as America had known it for almost forty years, ceased to exist. After months of batting the decision around, management downsized the magazine—reducing it from *Life*-size to the smaller size that had become standard for magazines. The proposal had surfaced in late 1970, when the economy was in a slump and *Esquire*'s advertising revenue had risen only 1 percent over the past year. The Publishers Information Bureau reported advertising revenue in monthly magazines, across the board, at a standstill that year. A smaller magazine would save on postal and paper costs and would suit advertisers better. *Holiday* and *McCall's*—both with declining revenue—had made the change already.

Hayes had fought the idea; he had thought he had defeated it. When he and the rest of the editorial staff learned the decision had been made, they learned the news the hard way, from the *New York Times.* Management had apparently planned to tell Hayes before making the decision public, but the *Times* had gotten the story and published it before management told him.

"It was a very ugly scene," Tom Hedley recalled.

The cover for the final big issue featured an old-fashioned sepia photograph of Joe Bonanno, a central character in Gay Talese's new book on a Mafia family, *Honor Thy Father:* a man in a great suit, dignified, smooth, a distinguished old-fashioned *Esquire* man, who happened also to be a Mafioso. It was a stylish, beautiful cover, out of the 1930s, when *Esquire* began.

ELEVEN

An Uproarious Affair

O N MARCH 13, 1972, Harold Hayes sent Gingrich a memorandum describing a job offer from Dan Melnick, the new production head of MGM. Melnick had taken Hayes to lunch the Friday before and invited him to come to MGM as executive story editor. Melnick was offering $60,000 salary plus stock options and the chance to produce his own films. Hayes was to let him know Wednesday if he wanted to move to the next stage—having his lawyer handle negotiations on terms. Hayes was giving "more than passing consideration" to the offer, he told Gingrich, because of his weak financial position at *Esquire.*

This was not the first time Hayes had complained about his level of income. None of the *Esquire* editors was handsomely paid, and although Hayes made a good deal more than the rest, he had not been content. Five years earlier, he had written a three-page memorandum to Gingrich outlining his financial circumstances—he was making $30,000 a year at that point, and living in a two-bedroom apartment on Riverside Drive at 100th Street, an area he considered "pretty seedy." His situation had improved in the years since then. His salary had gone up, although it was not high by New York magazine standards, and he had moved into a fourteen-room apartment at 89th Street and Riverside.

He was forty-five—would be forty-six the next month, he told Gingrich in his memo. "My salary is $48,500. After taxes, insurance and an installment-plan stock purchase, my take-home pay is $26,000. $15,000 of this goes to housing and tuition for my children. My co-op maintenance has gone up 40% over the past three years and tuition roughly 20%. This leaves a balance of $11,000 for everything else."

He had managed well enough for two years because he had gotten a bonus from *Esquire* and had earned money on the college lecture circuit. For several years, he had pulled in an average of $40,000 to $50,000 a year from his lectures. But this year the bonus had been canceled and college lectures had all but evaporated. His need for more income was "urgent and immediate."

Hayes dwelled on his financial motivation, but he was also really interested in making movies. For several years he had watched talent move from *Esquire* to Hollywood. Robert Benton and David Newman had written *Bonnie and Clyde*. Peter Bogdanovich had directed first *Targets*, then *The Last Picture Show*, and fresh from that triumph was writing a column on Hollywood for *Esquire*. Bogdanovich, Benton, and Newman had teamed up on a picture called *What's Up, Doc*, and Howard Zieff, who had worked with Benton and Newman on photo pieces, had started directing his first movie. Hayes had brought Thomas Berger on at *Esquire* as movie reviewer after Berger's novel, *Little Big Man*, was made into a blockbuster movie, and Berger discovered doing the column opened new doors for *him* in the movie world.

Susan Hayes liked the idea of Hayes going to Hollywood; she had grown up in Hollywood and wouldn't mind going back. She thought the boy she had married was now a "mature man" who could handle the bigger challenges of Hollywood. But Hayes knew people came and went in Hollywood. He told her he would rather stay at *Esquire*, but he needed to nail down his position there. In his March 13 memorandum, Hayes reminded Gingrich of an understanding that they had had for a long time:

Several years ago, when I received an offer to go with George Lois, Abe said the company had always seen me as the person eventually to succeed you, and you have said this, too, from the early days of our relationship. I have welcomed these assurances with gratitude and confidence, but this is a first-generation magazine whose top management is, by its own rules and regulations, approaching retirement, and as time has gone on, I have wondered what provisions are being made in this respect.

Would it not be possible for management to define these lines of succession?

Although phrased politely enough, this memorandum was a hardball: Hayes was threatening to leave if the company did not promise him Gingrich's job when Gingrich reached seventy and retired as publisher the following year. *Esquire* management responded quickly. On March 28, Hayes outlined the terms as he understood them in a memorandum to Gingrich (labeled, as few of his memos were, *CONFIDENTIAL*). Hayes would have a new title of editor and assistant publisher, but the title would not yet appear on the masthead. It would be publicized only within the *Esquire* company. It was, with the announcement taking effect April 3.

The understanding, as laid out by Hayes in his March 28 memorandum, was that managing editor Don Erickson would take on day-to-day direction of the magazine. If Erickson demonstrated "ability to move the magazine forward," in a minimum of six months he could become executive editor, and both men's title changes would be announced publicly. If Erickson did not "move the magazine forward," he would remain in his current position, and Hayes would name an executive editor from outside the magazine.

Twice Hayes mentioned a point that would become key in his negotiations with management over his changing position at *Esquire:* that he would continue to oversee the editorial department. He devoted the last, short paragraph of the two-paragraph memo to Gingrich entirely to the point, as if to make sure it was not overlooked: "Throughout the course of these changes and beyond whatever managerial assignments I may undertake, our understanding is that my central responsibility and concern will continue with the editorial department."

Perhaps no time at a magazine is an utterly safe time to make a move toward the top, but this time was more perilous than some. A recession in 1970–1971 had hurt magazines; Jerry Jontry, president of the Esquire Publishing Group, had referred in April 1971 to "these days of survival." The *New York Times* reported on April 20, 1971, that *"Esquire,* with five years of gains behind it, finally got caught up in the recession and dropped 12 per cent in pages." Although *Esquire's* revenue rose 5 percent in 1972, that compared weakly to much steeper increases at some magazines; the revenue total for monthlies rose 14 percent. In spring 1972, Jontry was reporting newsstand sales down to 148,000 from an average of 165,000 the year before; subscription renewals had slipped to 24.5 percent from 27.8 percent the year before.

For six years, in a bid for more advertising revenue, *Esquire,* like other magazines, had used subscription deals to push up its circulation, from just under a million in 1966 to just over a million and a quarter in 1972. The strategy worked so long as ad revenue kept coming in to cover the cost of selling cut-rate subscriptions. But ultimately the strategy failed, both for medium-sized magazines like *Esquire* and for the mass-circulation general-interest magazines, *Look, Life,* and *Saturday Evening Post.* Cut-rate

subscriptions reduced newsstand sales, undermined advertisers' confidence in the identity of the audience, and cost more in direct-mail and
production costs than advertisers were willing to pay. Too late, the big
magazines tried cutting their circulations back to more efficient levels.
The *Saturday Evening Post* went under in 1969; *Look* magazine folded
in 1971; *Life* in 1972. At *Esquire,* management watched nervously as
Esquire's newsstand sales—the industry's barometer of a magazine's
health—softened. Following the example of other magazines, *Esquire* was
cutting back on costly cut-rate subscriptions. Jontry was expecting a loss of
450,000 subscriptions in 1973, with additional losses in both subscriptions
and newsstand sales in subsequent years—signals to advertisers that *Esquire* was in trouble.

Could *Esquire* recoup some of this lost circulation by broadening the
magazine's appeal? The business side of the magazine had always wanted
more of a service magazine than Harold Hayes was delivering. Back in
1967, *Print* magazine had reported a challenge faced by *Esquire*'s promotion design department: the sophisticated content of the magazine, meant
to appeal to liberal readers, was less likely to appeal to the more conservative advertising community. Wouldn't a magazine more thoroughly devoted to service—to lifestyle and leisure—be easier to sell to a broad
readership, and to advertisers?

Hayes had always fought the definition of *Esquire* as a service magazine. He had never denied the advertising department its fashion spreads,
travel pieces, and Christmas guides, and he had tried to make them match
the quality and tone of the rest of the magazine. But they were peripheral
to his idea of *Esquire.* It had been hard for management to quibble with
that idea when ad money and subscriptions were coming in, but the times
had changed. Now, with the magazine's commercial position weakened,
the push for service was on. With revenues stagnating, the move Hayes
himself had made—his bid for the office of publisher—intensified the
vulnerability of his own position and his concept of the magazine.

In March 1972, the same month that he made his bid for the publisher's chair, he responded at length to a request by Jerry Jontry to explore
ways that *Esquire* could broaden its appeal. *Esquire* was a "topical magazine," he said, that tried "to keep in step with its times." But public
moods were changing so rapidly that they were difficult to predict. Hayes
had done some informal research, talking with recording and movie people, and had found "a pattern of drift." No trends were dominant. Good,

successful movies were being made—*Clockwork Orange, The Last Picture Show*—but they were original; they did not follow predictable patterns.

The record industry was wandering in confusion. Teenagers were no longer buying on command, although rock music had done better than any other entertainment form in holding on to its appeal. Hayes had had a long talk about the record industry over the weekend with Joe Raposo, songwriter for Sinatra and Barbra Streisand and musical director of *Sesame Street* and *The Electric Company.* "Raposo says the apprehension is greater behind the scenes than, thus far, is known outside the medium. Their problem is similar to everyone else's in the entertainment business: taste is changing and no one as yet knows where it is going to settle down." As for television—who would have guessed that *All in the Family* and *Flip Wilson* would be two of the three top shows of the season? Hayes was amazed to find a situation comedy about a hard-hat bigot America's number-one show, and no less surprised to find Flip Wilson so popular, "given the fact that the American black, as a type, is considerably less popular than he was six years ago."

The political world was no more predictable than the world of entertainment: "no one knows whether the wind blows on the right, left or in the middle . . . the settling process after recent years of nervous hysteria is still going on."

Hayes turned, then, to magazines, examining the ones building circulation: *Playboy, Penthouse, Cosmopolitan,* women's service magazines. *Esquire* was not about to follow the example of *Playboy* and *Penthouse:* nobody at *Esquire* wanted it to become a skin magazine. How about service, then, as an option? Although *Esquire* editors had several months ago agreed to increase service pieces in each issue, Hayes did not think increasing the emphasis on service alone would bring circulation gains.

Having gone through the motions of considering new options, he came around in the end to a pitch for going on doing what *Esquire* had been doing. "Our uniqueness is what we have to sell, what gives us appeal and the only basis visible for extending that appeal. You can't expect a poodle to turn into a collie by letting his hair grow long." He listed *Esquire*'s unique characteristics, among them, offering "a distinctive form of personalized journalism—a tradition marked in recent years by the work of Mailer, Talese, Wolfe, Sack, Garry Wills and others." *Esquire* was a literary magazine, a humor magazine, a magazine of graphic illustration, a magazine "that gives full measure." It was a magazine "of informed comment" for *educated* men, literate men. He listed cover subjects of recent months: Talese's *Honor Thy Father,* Calley's "Confessions," the 1,000 days of Teddy Kennedy, Galbraith on the decline of power.

"Is this enough to create a demand for 1,250,000 people? Given the fact that this country is the most educated mass society in history, you would think so."

He would not take responsibility for replacing the 450,000 subscriptions that would be lost when the company abandoned cut-rate subscription sales. And he was ready to try to find better ways to do what *Esquire* had been known for doing well. But, as he neared the end of his statement, he placed himself firmly in a defensive position: ". . . I would tend to resist the notion of bending any one of our various elements to a point that it begins to lose its shape . . . I feel very strongly that random change—in hopes of discovering a panacea—can be dangerous in the extreme."

Looking back on this moment of time, Sam Ferber, who had moved into Jerry Jontry's job as advertising director when Jontry moved up, saw Hayes justifiably rising up in his own defense. In a sense, Hayes had been victimized by *Esquire*'s circulation policies, which had given him a readership far larger than the core of readers who really wanted *Esquire.* "The fact is we were up to 1,250,000 at one point, and that simply was not all natural audience for *Esquire,* " Ferber said later.

Beyond that, Hayes had another problem, Ferber thought—the magazine was losing its most powerful subjects: the Vietnam War, the civil rights movement, and the sexual revolution on campus. The war was ending—a cease-fire would be declared on January 27, 1973. The civil rights movement had waned; the sexual revolution had triumphed. Watergate was about to seize the media spotlight, and the newsmagazines would profit greatly on the newsstand, but *Esquire*'s lead time was too long to cope with that fast-moving scandal. What Ferber called *Esquire*'s "ten golden years" were ending, and management was not going to stand idly by and watch it happen.

As newsstand sales slipped, Jontry, a rising power in the company, found a clear point of conflict in *Esquire*'s covers, which carried the ball on the newsstand. Ever since George Lois had started doing the covers in 1962, *Esquire* had become ever more prosperous—until lately. Now times had changed: maybe *Esquire* needed to change, too—to a new look, a new *Esquire* identity, new covers.

"If any icons of American graphic design are worth preserving," Steven Heller, then senior art director of the *New York Times,* would write in 1990, "George Lois's *Esquire* covers from the mid-1960s to the very early '70s are. Most were collaborations with photographer Carl Fischer that took an average of three days to produce; they are considered among the most powerful propaganda imagery in any medium and certainly the most memorable magazine covers ever."

The Lois covers had turned icons upside down, transforming Muhammad Ali into Saint Sebastian and St. Patrick's Cathedral into a movie theater. Lois drew a mustache on Svetlana Stalin (to Arnold Gingrich's and many readers' distress) and sent Andy Warhol swirling down in a can of his own Campbell's soup. Lois presented a profile of Nixon, eyes closed, submitting to a bevy of hands applying lipstick, powder, eye shadow, and spray. "Nixon's last chance. (This time he'd better look right)," read the coverline.

Lois was having fun, but he was not oblivious to how the covers played. He would pull back sometimes—he tried not to give Hayes "twelve killer covers." And he paid attention to newsstand figures, trying to figure out why, say, the portrait of the Native American who sat for the Indian nickel sent newsstand figures plummeting ("Son of a bitch, I guess it was just too intellectual").

Still, Lois came up with a lot of covers he and Hayes both knew were on the edge. "We were muckraking. We were lobbing grenades."

Hayes did not usually tell Lois how the advertising department felt about the covers; he spared him the aggravation. If he did pass on discontent—for instance, over the July 1965 cover for the teen issue: Ed Sullivan in a Beatles wig—he wouldn't say there'd been a problem, exactly; he'd just say something like "Can you believe it, George? Schmucks."

In the face of softening newsstand sales, the discontent that had rumbled around for years was rising. The month after Hayes's memo reaffirming his concept of *Esquire,* Jontry reported in a memo to John Smart, chairman of the board, the results of a decisive meeting on covers. Smart had always wanted several covers to choose from; he had always wanted Lois to give him more than one choice, illogically, Sam Ferber thought, since Lois could have given him one great cover and four duds—stacking the deck. Now Smart was getting his wish: from then on, for each issue, cover alternatives to the Lois covers would be developed in-house and tested, apparently as an experiment to see if Lois could be dropped. Following Blinder's suggestion, the alternate covers would be "less subtle" and "less clever," "to meet the changing times."

Reading that memo twenty years later, Lois exploded. "Isn't that great? Isn't that incredible. See what's going on. The 'changing times' is this: We're successful now. We're big. That's changing times. He's not talking about the changing mood. Young people and people who read are always interested in excitement and drama and revolution, etcetera. Trust me. To this day I'm on top of or maybe a week ahead of what's going on in the culture. That's my job. That's what I'm good at. So that's a code word for 'Hey, we're almost at 2 million. We were 700,000 or whatever it was all these years, and we're at 2 million. We don't need nobody. We don't need Harold—or maybe not we don't need him, but let's cut him down, let's bring in some new guys.' I'm sure Harold was plenty shnarky with them in many ways. I'm sure that Harold fought for everything that went into that book. His fight for the covers was very simple. His fight was—'George Lois covers got us newsstands. You don't like that? You think that's wrong? If I tell George that cover's dead, he's going to stop doing them.' But when you get almost 2 million, who needs them? I'm puttin' words in their mouths, but I betcha that's what's going on."

All the years he was doing the covers, Lois had known the advertising staff was sometimes uneasy, but when he saw some of Jontry's correspondence, the picture darkened: "This is enemy stuff," he said, reading the letter Jontry had written Hayes in 1981 about what that Sonny Liston cover cost *Esquire*. "They were walking around getting rich and meanwhile they're saying, 'We got two dangerous guys. Hayes is dangerous and that son of a bitch across town is dangerous—that Lois is dangerous.' And every month there'd be a package and they'd open it up and it would be a time bomb. And when it wasn't a time bomb they'd go, 'Ahh.' "

Hayes was losing ground rapidly on the covers; in fact, he was having to fight hard for editorial control of the front of the magazine. Not only were alternate covers being developed; they were actually being tested against the Lois covers with something called a "psychogalvanometer," which measured sweat in the palms to determine the degree to which individuals were aroused by the images in front of them. The idea of applying psychogalvanometer tests to the covers had been Jerry Jontry's. He was using psychogalvanometer tests on direct-mail pieces, and the man running the tests was throwing in tests of the covers without additional charge.

Although thus far the tests were to have no effect on cover decisions, Hayes could see the writing on the wall. When he found himself sitting next to an expert at a conference, he came back with the report that because of the many variables affecting audience response to covers on a newsstand, the psychogalvanometer tests were meaningless. He sent a detailed report of what he had been told to Smart, Blinder, Gingrich, and Jontry, along with a report from the editorial research department. Surveying academic research on the psychogalvanometer, the research department came up with a big vote of no confidence. Triumphantly, on May 9, 1972, Hayes pointed to the conclusion of one researcher that individual editorial judgment was both more effective and more direct than psychogalvanometer tests.

Meanwhile, he mounted a defense on another issue involving the covers. Back in February, at Smart's and Blinder's suggestion, he had agreed to add coverlines to the cover: not the single coverline Lois used to give punch to the cover image, but coverlines down the side promoting several pieces in the issue—"selling" the issue to subscribers at home, just like cover stickers sold it on the newsstand. If the coverlines were good enough, the stickers could even be dispensed with. After three issues bearing coverlines—June, July, and August—Jerry Jontry was not satisfied; the coverlines were not provocative enough. He suggested producing them at group meetings, with both editorial and business side represented, the way sticker lines were already produced.

Hayes resisted: The coverlines ought to be written by the people who had worked and lived with the features—not people who might not even have read them, he told Jontry in a memorandum on June 7. He had watched editorial changes being made in response to committee rule, and he didn't like it: committee rule undermined creativity and *Esquire*'s own tradition.

The very next day, June 8, 1972, Jontry responded in a memo directed to Smart, Blinder, Gingrich, Hayes, Erickson, and a couple of business staff members, and he did not retreat. Forwarding the results of the first psychogalvanometer tests on the covers, he used the very fact that they favored the Lois cover as evidence of their usefulness. A committee selecting the covers could easily make the wrong choice, he pointed out, but the psychogalvanometer tests would help the committee make the right choice. He looked forward to the day—which he hoped and apparently believed might come soon—when the alternate cover became an actual candidate for the cover, and a committee, aided by psychogalvanometer tests, would indeed make the decision.

To Hayes, the whole dispute must have seemed like a nightmare. It would have been funny, if it had not been so awful. His mood was bleak in a memo to the staff on July 13, 1972, when he reported on the applications he had had for an editorial position that had opened up when Clay Felker hired away associate editor Aaron Latham for *New York* magazine. Latham had agonized over the decision to leave *Esquire* after only a year. He was in awe of Hayes—thought he was brilliant: he had such a gift for imagining the magazine. "He could *think* through the prism of the magazine." Later, working with Felker, Latham would see that they were both great editors, but nobody he ever met could match Harold Hayes for envisioning, from the start, what an idea could become in the magazine: "He just saw the world in terms of *Esquire.*"

Still, Latham had heard so many good things about *New York* magazine, and Felker had said he could both write and edit, while Hayes had told him, "Our editors edit, our writers write." Latham lay awake at nights trying to make a decision. He talked with Hayes about it, and Hayes was understanding. He told him, Latham recalled, "You have to look at this as a gamble. You have to figure, in a few years, would you have a better chance at being the editor of *Esquire* or the editor of *New York?*" Latham did not want to be editor of either; he wanted to be a writer, so he left Hayes and *Esquire* for Felker's *New York.* He wrote Hayes an apologetic note explaining that *Esquire* was the best place he ever worked and Hayes the best editor he ever worked for, but he left anyway, and Hayes retired his softball shirt.

The letters from young applicants eager to take his place were wonderful—"the overwhelming, thrilling, frightening impression the very many good letters give is that *there are readers out there who are as smart as we are. Maybe smarter!*" Hayes reported to the staff. Reading the letters had left him feeling as though he'd "been living in Elaine's for a hundred years." He could see now that *Esquire* had been too interested in people everyone already knows about; he could see, too, "how rigid and self-conscious we have become in trying to extend the so-called *Esquire* approach."

He had found himself coming back to the office, after a weekend of reading applicants' letters, "feeling tired, grumpy and old, wondering as one reader wonders 'where the fire has gone' for all of us."

If the fire was gone, the world had not yet noticed. *Esquire* received a 1972 National Magazine Award for visual excellence that spring, and in his *Atlantic Monthly* magazine column a year later L. E. Sissman wrote of *Esquire*,

Now *there's* a magazine that appears to have waxed fat and prosperous on a formula—those Fischer/Lois covers in calculated bad taste, those painfully unfunny Dubious Achievement Awards, for all the world like a *Laugh-In* script anesthetized and stretched out on a timeless table, those awfully in, and awfully thin, little cues to with-it-ness—but really hides a great deal more in almost every issue. Not out on the sizzling million-bulb marquee but down in the engine room, the oily, muscular power of *Esquire* is the consistently good and interesting writing by both its regulars and its discoveries. Bogdanovich, in his little diaries of film-making life, is giving us a view of Hollywood we've never had before. Ron Rosenbaum, following his own nose, is turning up all sorts of contemporary Americana, my favorite being his exposition of the phone phreaks. Others are reporting otherwhere; still others are trying, and sometimes bringing off, new things in fiction. Mr. Hayes is some kind of alchemist who has gone pop with his left hand and serious with his right—and somehow made it work.

In-house, the mood was more uncertain. The spirit of the sixties *Esquire* seemed to be dissolving before everyone's eyes. The smaller page size had shrunk the interior out of all recognition. They couldn't just take the large format and make it smaller: those first smaller issues just looked wrong. A new look would evolve, under a new art director, Richard Weigand, who gave the inside a rawer finish, with more black-and-white pictures here and there, but there was no doubt about it: *Esquire*, a magazine defined from the start as an elegant magazine, looked cheaper, downscaled.

Familiar writers were still there: Tom Wolfe, Malcolm Muggeridge, Garry Wills—even James Baldwin, who returned to the magazine with a piece on Martin Luther King and Malcolm X. Tom Burke profiled Pat Boone; Bruce Jay Friedman wrote "Requiem for a Heavy: Sonny Liston, 1932–1971." Roger Kahn wrote a column on sports. But Hayes remarked in a memorandum to the staff that Wolfe, Talese, Mailer, Vidal, and Sack were no longer regularly available to *Esquire*.

Mailer was not simply unavailable to *Esquire;* Mailer was hostile to *Esquire.* In spring 1972, Mailer had his lawyer complain to *Esquire's* lawyer about his inclusion in a list of *Esquire* writers sent to prospective subscribers. Not only did he not want *Esquire* to promise readers future contributions by Mailer; he wanted all references to past Mailer contributions omitted as well, plus $1,000 in compensation for the use *Esquire* had already made of his name. Hayes wrote to Mailer promising not to identify him again in subscription solicitations as an *Esquire* contributor and acknowledging, further, Mailer's intention not to write for the magazine again as long as Hayes and Gingrich were associated with the magazine. He had begun the letter "Dear Norman," but on second thought struck out "Norman" and replaced it with "Mr. Mailer."

Reflecting on the absence of so many writers who had made the sixties *Esquire* what it was, Hayes took a philosophical stance: "they are not fresh anymore," he told his editors. The *Esquire* attitude was still holding up, he thought—"smart-assedness founded on a rational base," and maybe was even more suited to these times, which, like the magazine, had become "quieter."

For December 1972 Rita Hayworth, an actress from another era, wrapped her arms around a plastic model of Esky, the gentleman symbol of the old *Esquire,* in a Santa Claus suit. The main coverline asked, "Remember when Christmas was really Christmas?" Instead of letting a single powerful image and coverline carry the cover, a set of smaller coverlines advertised other contents: a novella by Vladimir Nabokov, "an exclusive interview" by Jean-Paul Sartre, a short story by Tennessee Williams, Tom Wolfe on "journalism vs. the novel," plus "a diet for gourmets" and "William Randolph Hearst's unpublished photo album."

Wolfe's piece, which would appear the next year in an introduction to a collection of New Journalism, summed up the journalistic experiments of the last ten years—backtracking to 1965, that luminous year when he and Capote burst into celebrity, then moving up to the present, through the work of that "marvelous maniac" John Sack, *M;* George Plimpton's *Paper Lion;* Hunter Thompson's *Hell's Angels;* Joan Didion's articles on California; Rex Reed's celebrity interviews; James Mills's pieces for *Life;* Garry Wills and Ovid Demaris's pieces for *Esquire;* and to top it all off, Norman Mailer's report on the Pentagon march, *The Armies of the Night.* While novelists were off writing fables, journalists were nailing down the exuberant reality of 1960s America, and using the techniques of realistic fiction to do it. Detecting the note of eulogy in his voice, Wolfe backed off at the end from his own definition: "With any luck at all the new genre will never be sanctified, never be exalted, never given a theology. I probably shouldn't even go around talking it up the way I have in this piece . . . The hell with it . . . Let chaos reign . . ."

It was too late. Literary journalism, which Hayes had contended was all that New Journalism ever was, would live on, but the great flowering of the sixties was over. The times that had inspired it were passing. *Esquire,* its first home, was not what it had been, and Harold Hayes, the editor, was about to become a publisher.

In an interview twenty years later, Blinder recalled, "We had decided that the magazine was on the downgrade again, and so we recommended to Arnold Gingrich that maybe it'd be a good idea, in the transition of the magazine, that Arnold become editor-in-chief or something or other, and make Harold the publisher, and let Harold select another young man to be the editor. And John Smart and I and Arnold had these discussions, and Arnold was quite willing to do this, in order to get another change of view in the editorial side of the magazine, and so he sat down with Harold and proposed this to him."

A long time had passed by the time Blinder gave this account, and memories blur the sequence of events, but one thing is clear: Blinder, in his late eighties but still smart and vigorous, and always a man with a remarkable memory, saw management in the driver's seat. What Hayes had begun as a move to consolidate power, management meant to finish by sending him off to the sidelines. Hayes may have already gotten wind of the disfavor blowing his way; perhaps that was why he talked with Melnick about going to Hollywood in the first place. He may have been on a search, not just for more money and a chance to make movies, but for a parachute.

In September, Blinder proposed moving him on to executive row as vice-president of communications, but Hayes resisted. Instead, on October 2, 1972, with the minimum six months of trial passed, the company announced the appointment of Erickson as executive editor and Hayes as editor and assistant publisher. The offer the company was making granted him the publisher's position, but only on probationary terms: he would hold it for nine months and if the company then chose he would lose it. In this interim, Gingrich would be designated founding editor or editor-in-chief, with the editor of Hayes's choice working under him.

Tom Hedley, off the scene by then, believed management never really wanted Hayes to be publisher; management wanted one of the advertising people in charge, someone—like Jerry Jontry—who could understand that the bottom line of *Esquire* was fashion advertising. Why should Hayes, antagonistic toward fashion, unsympathetic with advertising, be the company's choice to take on the role of publisher? It didn't make sense.

Whether or not Blinder, Smart, and Jontry were intent on ridding themselves of Hayes altogether, Hayes was afraid that as publisher he would lose the editorial control that Arnold Gingrich had had when he was first made publisher, back in the days when his young editors were, as Hayes put it, "reporting directly to him about any fucking comma changes." Even though Gingrich had ceded most of his authority to Hayes, he had remained active in the editorial process, reading manuscripts, offering suggestions, passing judgments. He was in a position to defend editorial decisions against other members of management. He was in that position by virtue of his status as founding editor; he had created *Esquire,* and he had been with the company for a span of four decades.

Hayes could not claim those distinctions as the basis for his authority. If he wanted the kind of editorial authority Gingrich had once had as publisher, he would have to build the authority into the title, and when he tried to do that, he said later, he became "too much of a pain in the ass" for management to abide. Yet without editorial authority, the publishing job was to him a meaningless post, and the magazine he had built and loved would be vulnerable to manipulation by the businessmen: Blinder, Smart, and Jontry. Gingrich had been, he once said, "the perfect buffer" between himself and the rest of management. "They bitched to Arnold about me and I bitched to Arnold about them. Like the enigmatic boarder in a Carson McCullers novel, he was a blind man counseling the deaf." Gingrich himself had found elements of Hayes's *Esquire* distasteful, but management had seldom intervened forcefully in editorial affairs. Management had hovered, management had made suggestions and offered criticisms. But for the most part, Blinder and Smart had honored the principle of editorial integrity—the promise made to Gingrich on his return that the businesspeople would let him run the editorial side of the magazine his way.

Yet once when management did kill an editorial feature, and Hayes was so upset that he cried, the best he got from Gingrich, he recalled, "was a manly show of ignoring my agony." Hayes had noticed that even when Gingrich disagreed with the business office, he went along with business in his affable way. Hayes had even begun to wonder "to what extent he could be counted on in a real crunch." He was not encouraged by what he was seeing in these crucial days. At one editorial meeting, Jontry proposed increasing ad pages in an upcoming issue. Management loved the idea, and editors weren't asked their opinions. As Hayes wrote in notes, "I myself had (now) been told to keep quiet at these affairs, and Arnold, who could speak up, didn't. The [dogs?] were loose and the emphasis now returned to 'service,' articles of some presumed value to advertisers."

Hayes had watched other editors go down in the last few years. Willie Morris had left *Harper's* in 1971, after only four years as its editor-in-chief, in just such a battle as this, resigning rather than accepting the owners' decision to turn his elegant vehicle of good journalism into a "specialized" publication. He had released a statement to the press: "It all boiled down to the money men and the literary men. And as always, the money men won." Most of the other editors and contributing editors at *Harper's* left with him. Before that, Clay Blair had made a grand last stand at the *Saturday Evening Post,* which he had led through a flamboyant renovation. Blair had invited "management to see things his way or accept the massive resignation of all chief editors, his foremost among them," Hayes observed. He became "one of the bravest ex-editors of our time."

Considering the course open to an editor facing powerful enemies, Hayes had favored shrewdness over bravery. Better, he thought, to outsmart the other side than to try facing it down. Yet dodge and feint though he might, he was finding it hard to stay on his feet. Gingrich himself had given him a shove in his memoir, *Nothing But People,* published in 1971. Gingrich recalled needing to "bench" himself back in the late fifties and let the younger men take control, because he was too out of touch with the times. "Now, a mere dozen years later, Harold finds himself in turn confronted by the same necessity." Gingrich made the point several times, almost as if he were sending Hayes a message.

Hayes understood very well what was happening. "What had happened to Arnold in the late fifties was happening now to me," he wrote in notes to himself after Gingrich's death.

Unlike Arnold I didn't know how to handle it however. In January 1973, the president, Abe Blinder, said, "Arise, Mr. Gingrich must surrender the title of publisher, I have appointed you, but there are some on the board who feel you may not be . . . well . . . *dependable.* So we want to nominate you for this role on a probationary basis." I told him I would let him know.

The trouble was, even if I had *wanted* to roll with it, the circumstances had now become completely changed. Arnold had so totally disenfranchised himself editorially—his role as publisher [consisting of] public relations—lunching with advertisers, etc., I saw no way to block what appeared to be an inevitable castration with me doing Arnold's job (nothing), someone else could get in there and produce the service—other than insisting I hold the title of editor as well.

I spent a weekend forming a plan, filled with brave projections of circulation and advertising programs—the crap management understood—and had it ready the following Monday.

Around 8 I showed it to Arnold, who looked it over and said easily, God, yes, sounds great. Let's see if they'll buy it.

On the following Thursday I was called into the boardroom: chairman of the board, president of the corporation, and Arnold. Only the president of the publishing division was missing. The president was [crying?].

"We have read your proposal and the vote is 4 to one against you. We have come to the end of the road with you. Why did you prepare all this? We know all that. Did you think we didn't?

"Jesus," the chairman said (they all, in crisis, talked like Arnold), "we'll have to see what we can do to keep this from being a bombshell on Madison Ave."

Arnold said nothing, sitting with his chin in his hand.

I left the room, sent a note to staff and left *Esquire.*

When the staff got back from lunch that day, Thursday, April 5, 1973, they found Hayes's memo on their desks:

Due to irreconcilable differences with this company's management, I am leaving *Esquire.* I would rather there not be any gossip about all this, if you can manage to keep it down. I have reached a settlement with the company which is just and fair. I have no great qualms about my future or yours. I can't remember a time in my history with this magazine when I have enjoyed working with any staff more than I have this one. Don Erickson has the strength and ability to keep this magazine on its present course, and I wish all of you continued good times and happiness in your work.
HH.

A company memo the same day, from Arnold Gingrich, announced:

Harold Hayes has tendered his resignation for personal reasons. Since Don Erickson has already assumed the role of executive editor, all editorial matters should be referred to him.

The staff gathered in Hayes's corner office; several editors wanted to quit. Gordon Lish spoke out against it. He thought Hayes was making unreasonable demands; they could be loyal to Hayes but not to what Hayes was doing. On Tuesday Hayes met the staff for lunch in an upstairs room at a French restaurant on 52nd Street, between Park and Madison, to explain what had happened. It was an uproarious affair—"wild, drunken hell-raising," Gordon Lish recalled, with everybody at their best:

an intense, emotional experience. Hayes wrote Gay Talese about it the next day, explaining that the staff hadn't known about "much of the pulling and tugging" that had gone on upstairs and were still on the brink of mutiny, until Hayes talked to them. ". . . I told them that if they really did respect me and our work together they wouldn't do it. Morris left a debacle behind him at *Harper's,* from which the magazine has still not recovered nor maybe ever will." Nobody quit except Peter Bogdanovich, the film columnist.

Hayes had been somewhat comforted to learn from a reporter that Gingrich had *not* voted against him after all; the vote against his proposal had actually been three to one—Blinder, Smart, and Jontry against, Gingrich for. In an almost charitable vein, Hayes wrote Talese that nobody had been "a real meanie" in all this—in fact, Blinder had been contemplating turning his president's job over to Hayes a couple of months before. Still, he said,

Blinder is, at best, insidious. At issue is the direction of the magazine—he knows it, I know it, and the staff fears it. Blinder and Jontry, by playing on Smart, have persuaded him I am an obstructionist to the growth potential of the magazine. And when Smart gets something in his mind he is loath to lose it—and so this has been the temper with respect to editorial, for a year or so, though, because editorial has evolved into a very strong arm of the company, they have been unable to do much about it. Now, as Harvard Bus. 101 would obtain, they have neutralized the problem, which is why of course Blinder and the other two would not dare challenge my editorial direction openly—the magazine is, at this moment, too successful to fuck around with. But with Don they hope to see even greater gains. So of course they are tickled to death I am *not* blowing the whistle on them but going out like a good boy, urging the staff to carry on, stay in there and fight etc., etc.

What they do not realize, and it is no solace to me, is that I am doing this really because bringing shit down on *Esquire* will destroy what I have built. It is very easy to do these days, too easy. Also, I got to hand it to the old man still (he really *does* have class)—Arnold that is—who took a bucket of shit himself thirty years ago, walked away quietly and never felt it necessary to make an issue of his own value. Don, meanwhile, an unknowing pawn throughout all this, has reacted splendidly and strongly and will no doubt soon be causing them his own style of headaches. And that is another reason, I don't want to see it blow: he deserves to see if he can make it work.

Hayes was responding to a letter he had received that morning from Talese, telling Hayes about a call he put in to Abe Blinder on Sunday. Talese had told Blinder that the call was his own idea and that Hayes was unenthusiastic about his making it: that Hayes wanted no public fuss. And having said that, he told Blinder he was depressed about Hayes's leaving *Esquire;* he told Blinder *Esquire* should give Hayes "whatever the hell" he wanted.

I told him that people of your talent do not come along every decade to magazines, or to any other kind of publishing business or any business. I told him that you were made for *Esquire;* you were not a man who could have worked at *Life,* or *Newsweek,* or *The New York Times*—you were a man of *Esquire,* just as Reston was (is) a man of *The Times.* . . . It is no disrespect for Don Erickson's talents to say, as I did to Blinder, that a man of your drive and personality does not come around all that often; and if you still wished to maintain the power of the editorial desk, did not want to be promoted into the advertising-promotion phase of non-involvement with writers and editorial decisions, that you damned well should get what you wanted; for you have given so much and have done so well, and the magazine has made money while not losing quality.

Blinder recalled that you had wanted to make more dough, had mentioned a movie company offer, other offers; and, Blinder said, the *Esquire* people on top did what they thought you wanted . . . and did not feel that filling Arnold's shoes was a step down in anybody's view of things. I know that there is a certain amount of bullshit here; I saw Mr. Blinder's words as dodging the real issue—you felt that if you were going to be the publisher, you had to have the power over the editorial matter as well as other matters, and there was no point to remaining at *Esquire* if you could not really run that magazine and control its tone. If you could not maintain control, there is no point in working in that building. Anyway, Blinder said you would have a meeting on Tuesday, and that perhaps something could be worked out this week, but he said you were a tough Marine, a hard guy, etc. (I interrupted to tell him you were a sweet gentle son of the south with malice toward none), and Blinder said more would be known this week.

Nothing was worked out.

On April 7, the *New York Times* reported a dispute over whether Hayes had quit or been fired. Hayes said he had been fired—had not Blinder said, "We're at the end of the road"? Gingrich believed Hayes had quit with a comment along the line of "That's the way the ball bounces" or "That's the way the chips fall." In its April 16 issue, *Time* magazine reported that Hayes had "suddenly quit" just months before he was to move into Arnold Gingrich's position as publisher because he refused to surrender editorial control. "Gingrich pronounced himself 'bitterly disappointed' by the resignation. 'He was my boy,' said Gingrich of his 46-year-old protege." *Newsweek* offered a longer, full-column account that began. "Arnold Gingrich, the elegant publisher of *Esquire* magazine, was in an uncharacteristic dither about an old colleague last week. 'He's like a horse who has always jumped all the hurdles suddenly refusing to jump the last one,' grumbled Gingrich."

The piece presented Hayes's departure as "a walkout," and ended with Hayes cleaning out his desk. " 'There was hope for me in this company,' he said wistfully. 'But an ambivalent situation has turned into a soap opera that we all regret.' "

Publicly cool, Hayes was devastated by what had happened. One night, Hayes went over to Lish's apartment on East 56th Street and stayed into the early morning hours. He was, Lish said, "inconsolable"—he wished he could have taken back what he had done. In notes he wrote after Arnold Gingrich's death, he said, "I was sick at heart when I left. I didn't much care what the company would say to the press. But I hadn't expected it to lie."

The staff wrote him notes of thanks and regret, which he saved. Tom Ferrell wrote,

Dear Harold,
We have drunk all your liquor.
You are a nice man, and in your way a great man, and I love you a lot, and I never doubt that what you do is wise. The wisdom of this will appear in its own time and way.
I owe you a million thanks for a million things, some small, some very big indeed. I also owe you several apologies. Take them all.
God bless you, Harold.

Byron Dobell wrote from *New York* magazine, where he had gone to work for Clay Felker,

As I told Eric Pace when he called, "I can't imagine *Esquire* without Harold Hayes—and they are out of their minds to let him go. If it's truly a matter of titles, they should let him call himself Editor and Publisher and King. Who gives a damn about titles when they've got the editor of the best national magazine in the U.S.?"

Rust Hills wrote, belatedly, on April 25, 1973, having heard a version of what happened from Lish: "All I've got to say is that the magazine was great while you were the editor, but that I always thought Esquire Inc. was a chintzy wily company that just *used* anyone who hadn't been with them in the old days in Chicago, . . ." He passed along the advice Malcolm

Cowley had given him when he quit the *Saturday Evening Post:* "do something bold."

John Sack read about Hayes's departure in *Time* and wrote, "Harold, you aren't the only editor in America who understood what I was up to; I think you're the only person, really. I wasn't writing for *Esquire* but for you."

When Hayes called Lois to tell him what had happened, he asked Lois to go on doing the covers. Lois said no, he couldn't. Hayes said he didn't want it to look like he came to Lois and asked him not to do the covers. Lois said, "Fuck them." Hayes said he had his reasons—please. Lois said he would try.

He got a call a couple of days later from Erickson, who said—as Lois recalled—"Harold says you're gonna do the covers. Gee, we're so excited."

"You're serious."

"Oh, yeah, we don't wanna lose you."

So Lois did a cover and he got a call back: they loved it, but could he come over and talk about it, " 'cause we wanna make some changes."

That was the end of Lois's arrangement with *Esquire.*

Hayes called him up and said, "Well, old buddy, you tried."

It was almost, Lois thought, as if he had known what would happen.

Hayes's old friend Pete Turner had taken Hayes on his first trip to East Africa, which would replace *Esquire* as the passion of his life. Now, he threw a big farewell party for him at his Carnegie Hall studio, with two bands, one for rock and one for smooth. Bob Sherrill missed the party, but wrote Hayes a long letter, ending on a note of reassurance. "I was about to worry about you, when I realized you are no waif and will come up with something good to do."

In the end, Hayes's decision to go quietly did not save the magazine. The following year, W. R. Simmons, the company that reported total audience figures for magazines (including pass-along readers), changed its method for figuring readership. *Esquire*'s total estimated audience collapsed from seven million to four million readers. When Rust Hills reported on the magazine's slide in an article for the November 1976 *More,* *Esquire* had lost almost half its ad lineage since Hayes's departure. There were rumors, by that time, that the magazine was going under. Whether or not it survived, surely no one could fail to notice, Hills said, "that the magazine over the last few years has been less, say, 'exciting' than those scathing, snotty, outrageous, big-read, fascinating issues of the Harold Hayes decade."

For more than a decade, Harold Hayes had behaved as if *Esquire* was his magazine: his because he created it as it was. He had fought off attempts by management to treat it as a commercial instrument. He had made his daily judgments not out of calculation of what would sell, to readers or to advertisers, but out of his own sense of what the magazine ought to be. Even, toward the end, when he tried on commercial thought, he reaffirmed his own basic idea of *Esquire.* And, at the very end, he could not give that up, merely for the sake of the office and salary of publisher. He was the son of a minister: "What shall it profit a man if he gain the whole world and lose his own soul?" He paid the price—he lost the magazine. And yet, losing Hayes, the owners found that they had lost *Esquire.*

It had been his after all.

Epilogue

WHAT ARE the chances of seeing a magazine like the sixties *Esquire* again—a magazine with that energy, that unruly take on the times? Some say impossible: the nineties are not the sixties. There is no civil rights movement, no Vietnam War. That, however, exaggerates the role of those public movements in *Esquire*'s vitality, sees *Esquire* simply as a mirror, reflecting the culture. *Esquire* was stirring up journalistic excitement before the later sixties, when the political drama was most intense. There are even those who think *Esquire* was at its best in the early and mid-sixties, the sunnier side of the sixties.

Of course *Esquire* would have been different in any other decade. But some of its finer moments occurred in timeless scenes of American life: Terry Southern's article on baton twirlers at Ole Miss, Jack Richardson on gambling, Bynum Shaw on Dr. Gatch, who took up the cause of the coastal poor. Gay Talese wrote his most moving piece, "The Loser," on a boxer who had seen better days. Diane Arbus photographed Tokyo Rose. Celebrities from the past floated through the magazine's pages like ghosts—Peter Bogdanovich's Humphrey Bogart, Rex Reed's Ava Gardner. Architects and scientists imagined a world to come. It would be possible to look at Hayes's *Esquire* not as a narrative, but as a tapestry, richly woven out of the fabric of American life, past, present, future. No one asks of a magazine that it be good reading past its time; yet the sixties *Esquire* is.

If *Esquire* owed its vitality to the sixties, then the debt was not just to the decade's political events. *Esquire* was riding the cultural energy released when high culture and mass culture crossed paths in the late fifties—a hybridization debunked by *Esquire*'s own movie critic, Dwight Macdonald. These were times when it was fun to be an intellectual—when the *New York Review of Books* would put a Molotov cocktail on its cover, and David Levine would lift Lyndon Johnson's shirt to show his scar: a map of Vietnam. These were times when it was fun to be a magazine journalist—to be Lillian Ross getting the goods on Ernest Hemingway, to be Truman Capote walking off with Marlon Brando's pride in his pocket. These were times to try journalistic souls: *The New Yorker* published James Baldwin's *The Fire Next Time,* Truman Capote's *In Cold Blood,* Jonathan Schell's reports on Vietnam—rising at least as high as *Esquire* to the moral challenge of the time.

Yes, *Esquire* owed something to the times, but the times owed something to *Esquire.* "When there was such an *Esquire,*" Gordon Lish says, "there was such a *Harper's,* there was such an *Atlantic,* there were other magazines that were hoping to rival *Esquire* in these ways." One magazine can make a difference. When editors change at the current *Esquire*—thinned down by its passage through the years—hope stirs. Every reader of serious magazines in America watched with bated breath as Tina Brown took *The New Yorker* in hand. How delicate is a magazine's personality: how difficult it is to give a magazine a second life.

Not everyone understands why magazine lovers care that good magazines survive. Why not watch television? Why not be satisfied with newspapers or books? Magazines offer something none of these media can touch: more than any other medium, magazines companionably track the times. To read a magazine over the years is to walk through life with a talkative friend.

Editors who want to make magazines in that mold are handicapped today if their magazines are advertising vehicles owned by corporations concerned about stockholder response and bottom lines. Management does not always understand that a magazine might have a limited number of friends—a natural circulation that can grow just so much and no more, given the magazine's personality. Management does not always understand that a dip in advertising revenue does not necessarily call for a shift in editorial direction. Management does not always understand the limits of market research: a magazine is not a detergent or an automobile or a remote-control toy. A magazine has a life.

Esquire, in the sixties, had a life. After thirty years, it was still a

family-controlled company (although publicly owned), still under the
wing of the first generation, and still with its founding editor on board, a
totemic figure protecting his protégé Hayes from the chilliest winds. Arnold Gingrich often seemed to the younger folk insignificant, but he was
not: his presence allowed Hayes to take risks. Hayes himself had to fight
for what he wanted, but when he fought, Gingrich was there to keep the
fights from being fatal. Ready as management was to pitch younger editors out, nobody was going to get rid of Gingrich, the man who made
Esquire.

There are still, today, magazines with comparable continuity over a
long span of time. For half a century, *The Progressive,* a political magazine
published in Madison, Wisconsin, has been passed down from editor to
editor, each editor choosing his successor, as Arnold Gingrich had hoped
to choose his. But *The Progressive* is a small, nonprofit magazine. The
model for commercial magazines—and *Esquire* was from its start a commercial magazine—has become something very different. There is not
much room in the commercial magazine world for the concept of a magazine as a living thing—the creation of a group of people who get to know it
and love it and pour their lives into its making. A magazine like that can
still survive on the margins, a magazine with a limited audience and modest production costs. A profitable magazine like the sixties *Esquire,* a
glorious, colorful mix for a reasonably big audience, would be an anomaly
now.

But it was an anomaly then, too. Hayes observed that *The New Yorker*
had been an anomaly in the thirties—a smart, sophisticated magazine in
the midst of a depression. The times may be what great editors make of
them. Surely, to imagine that the nineties are not capable of offering
material for creative journalism is to suffer a failure of imagination. If
commercial magazines fill the space between their ads with advice and
manufacture celebrities for their covers, it is certainly not because reality
has not offered higher drama.

This is the twilight of the twentieth century. There are wars and
rumors of wars. The ozone hole over the Antarctic opens and closes; new
viruses spread and kill. Computers have rewired workplaces, economies,
relationships between nations. Children kill children. History has not
ended; it moves powerfully on. But to take hold of these times would
require more than the ability to keep from being fired. It would take
something Harold Hayes had: the courage to look at what is there.

Esquire itself has been swept along by the currents of the last twenty years. A year after Arnold Gingrich died on July 9, 1976, at the age of seventy-two, Abe Blinder presided over the sale of *Esquire* to an English publishing company, Associated Newspapers, and its American partner, Clay Felker, who had just lost to Rupert Murdoch the little magazine empire he had built—*New York* magazine, the *Village Voice*, and *New West*. Less than two years later, in 1979, *Esquire* was sold again, this time to a Tennessee company owned by Phillip Moffitt, Christopher Whittle, and the Bonnier Newspaper Group of Sweden (although Moffitt later bought Whittle out), and Moffitt took the title of editor-in-chief, with first, Byron Dobell, then Lee Eisenberg as second in command. In 1987, *Esquire* underwent another transfer of ownership, this time to the Hearst Corporation, which retained Eisenberg as editor until 1991. By 1994, *Esquire* had two more editors in quick succession.

Over the years, several alumni of the sixties *Esquire* have returned to the magazine. Byron Dobell returned twice. Gordon Lish left to edit books at Alfred A. Knopf, and Rust Hills, who had been editing at another magazine, *Audience*, returned to *Esquire* as fiction editor. John Berendt came back to *Esquire* as a columnist. Bob Sherrill went to work for newspapers in North Carolina, and an essay he wrote for *Esquire*, "The Truth about Growing Old," appeared in *Best American Essays of 1993*.

Other editors made their way through other magazines. Ralph Ginzburg started a magazine, *Eros*, served eight months in prison on an obscenity conviction, then emerged to publish profitably several magazines, before he became, finally, a newspaper photographer. Jill Goldstein became editor of *Viva* and, later, an editor at the *Village Voice*. Tom Ferrell became an editor at the *New York Times Book Review*. After Byron Dobell left *Esquire* and began editing *American Heritage*, he hired Bob Brown, who also worked for John Berendt when Berendt was editor of *Lifestyle* and *New York* magazine. Clay Felker became editor of *Manhattan, inc.*, then, in 1991, editor-in-chief of *M Inc.* after *M* and *Manhattan, inc.* merged.

Some *Esquire* alumni wrote books and screenplays. Tom Hedley wrote the screenplay for *Flashdance*, among other movies. Aaron Latham wrote *Orchids for Mother* and the magazine article that was the basis for *Urban Cowboy*. Gordon Lish wrote *Dear Mr. Capote* and other fiction. Brock Brower wrote the novel *The Late Great Creature*, in which Harold

Hayes made an appearance as editor of *Esquire*. Thomas B. Morgan wrote *Snyder's Walk*, suggested by his experience covering a 1962 peace walk for *Esquire*. Rust Hills wrote his "fussy man" trilogy, republished in 1993 as *How to Do things Right: The Revelations of a Fussy Man*. John Berendt wrote a nonfiction best-seller, *Midnight in the Garden of Good and Evil*, his own contribution to literary journalism.

After *Bonnie and Clyde*, Robert Benton and David Newman wrote several screenplays together, including *Superman* and *Still of the Night*, which Benton directed. Benton won Academy Awards for best screenplay and best director for *Kramer vs. Kramer*, the New York Film Critics' Best Screenplay award for *Places in the Heart*, and critical acclaim for his 1995 film *Nobody's Fool*. After the Benton-Newman writing partnership broke up, Newman wrote several films with his wife, Leslie Newman, including the *Superman* sequels.

Jean-Paul Goude directed the parade for the French bicentennial celebration and created television commercials. Sam Antupit designed *Ms.*, which Gloria Steinem had started with Clay Felker's support; Antupit also designed *Harper's* twice and became vice-president of design at Harry N. Abrams, publisher.

Candida Donadio, George Lois, and Pete Turner kept on profitably doing what they had been doing. Sam Ferber became a publishers' consultant. Bud Lee moved to Florida to live a more normal life, and kept on taking pictures. Kitty Krupat became an organizer of publishing workers and, later, director of education for the International Ladies Garment Union.

Norman Mailer continued to write both fiction and nonfiction, publishing—among other things—a novel based on fact, *The Executioner's Song* (which won a Pulitzer Prize), and a fictional exploration of the history of the Central Intelligence Agency, *Harlot's Ghost*.

Gay Talese earned notoriety and wealth with his book on changing sexual mores in America, *Thy Neighbor's Wife*, and sold the rights to Hollywood for $2.5 million. He turned to the history of his own Italian family in *Unto the Sons*.

Tom Wolfe published several books, among them a novelistic account of the real lives of America's early astronauts, *The Right Stuff*, and a novel, *Bonfire of the Vanities*, both made into movies.

John Sack followed Company C into the Gulf War for *Esquire;* out of that assignment came a book, *Company C*. An earlier book, *An Eye for an*

Eye, an account of Jewish involvement in Communist-run prison camps in Poland at the end of World War II, propelled him once again into the center of controversy.

Garry Wills returned to academic life in 1973, first at Johns Hopkins University and later at Northwestern University in Evanston, Illinois. He wrote several books, including a political autobiography. His historical essay, *Lincoln at Gettysburg: The Words that Remade America* (1992), was awarded the Pulitzer Prize.

Michael Herr lived in London for eleven years, before he returned in 1991 to the upstate New York area where he grew up. He wrote several screenplays, including the narration for the film *Apocalypse Now,* and a novel that started out as a screenplay, *Walter Winchell.*

Laura Bergquist, who introduced Harold Hayes to Arnold Gingrich, committed suicide in 1982. After her death, Harold Hayes's secretary, Connie Wood, met the widower, Fletcher Knebel, and married him. James Baldwin died in 1987. Don Erickson, who was editor of *Esquire* for several years after Hayes left, died in 1988 of throat cancer. Jerry Jontry and John Smart died while this book was being written.

Harold Hayes and Susan Hayes were divorced, and Hayes married Judy Kessler, a producer at the *Today* show. In the 1970s, Hayes was host of a public television interview program and later went to work briefly for his friend Bob Shanks as editorial producer of *20/20.* In the early 1980s he was editorial director of CBS magazines, then moved to California to edit *California* magazine, formerly *New West,* created by Clay Felker. In the years after he left *Esquire,* Hayes wrote three books out of his love for Africa and a concern for the natural world that came out of that love—*The Last Place on Earth, Three Levels of Time,* and *The Dark Romance of Dian Fossey.* The film *Gorillas in the Mist* was based on a *Life* magazine article he wrote about Fossey before he wrote the book; the book itself was published after his death. Harold T. P. Hayes died of a brain tumor on April 5, 1989, in Los Angeles, at the age of sixty-two—sixteen years, to the day, after he left *Esquire.* Memorial services were held in Los Angeles, New York, and Wake Forest, where Provost Edwin G. Wilson, who had known Harold Hayes all his adult life, said of him:

> . . . inside, he never changed. If on the small-town campus he had been a man of the world, in New York he was still a man of North Carolina: attentive to old friends and old associations, unpretentious, boyish, even provincial. The blend of artlessness and elegance, of sincerity and penetrating perceptiveness, manners

which were both polished and natural—they were consistent in Harold from first to last. His life had unity.

And it had something more. I don't know what "lonely impulse of delight" drove Harold to what he called the "last place on earth." He said that, if he had not gone, he "might have lived out an otherwise self-absorbed life." What he discovered in Africa, he told us, was something "impenetrably mysterious" and "awesomely complex."

I agree that Serengeti and the animals who live there are "mysterious and complex" but no more so, I think, than the man who wrote those words about them. . . .

Afterword

SHARING THE MEATLOAF ON ELBA
HAROLD HAYES IN EXILE
by Tom Hedley

AROLD HAYES is wearing a defiantly East Coast suit and tie while driving a little Alfa Romeo convertible open to the California sun. He looks like a grown-up in a bump-'em car. It's 1986 in Los Angeles and lately he's been calculating the mileage between his past and his present. Sweet poison, he's thinking, that's what it is to taste your golden age too early. The experience, if you're not careful, has a way of distorting expectations; setting up a life of serial disappointment.

As he pulls up in front of the Ivy Restaurant on Robertson Avenue he remembers something a director friend once told him: "Orson Welles would've been one happy, thin man if *Citizen Kane* had been his *last* film," Peter Bogdanovich had said. "Sadly, it was his first."

As Harold makes his way through the fashionable cafe crowd—minimoguls on mobile phones, starlets starved to near-perfection—I can't help wondering what circumstance or conviction finally persuaded him to abandon his own orbit for Planet Hollywood. Maybe he was banished. If so, Elba does not become him. He seems rooted in a particular time and place; specifically those years in New York City Carol Polsgrove has so vividly evoked on these pages—the quintessential *Esquire* man smiling through the apocalypse.

Like other *Esquire* alumni I woke up one day with a view of the Pacific Ocean, writing screenplays. Harold, on the other hand, was eventually rustled west to edit *California* magazine, a periodical destined not to work because the concept was all wrong. A city magazine posing as a regional monthly, it couldn't quite focus its editorial voice or serve up successfully the meat and potatoes of the genre: service features so useful they become habit-forming.

Harold had asked me to become a contributing editor but I don't remember contributing much of anything. Unless, of course, you count these occasional lunches at the Ivy. He'd order the home-style meatloaf or the Louisiana blackened shrimp and when, inevitably, a mutual sore point came up—the slow, relentless transformation of *Esquire* as we knew it— you could see this was a disappointment he couldn't share. He'd abruptly change the subject and soon we'd be talking about Africa, an abiding passion. There were days when I thought he'd like to banish all talk of magazines.

But today wasn't one of them. Harold arrived at the table fuming. He had just come from watching a group of marketing executives perform "the demographic dance." They had dispatched him smugly with reader-ship surveys, consumer polls, all manner of articulated numbers and a two-page proposal on how to move *California* into the big time. He hand-ed me the proposal. I had to laugh. It read like a treatment for a perfume campaign.

The core of Harold's complaint went something like this: Demograph-ics are useful, even crucial. But they are only indicators. Apply them lit-erally to a magazine makeover and you place the reader where he doesn't want to be—in the editor's chair. This is not only a cop-out but at best a short-term solution.

The reader demands more than a mirror. The reader wants to be sur-prised, entertained, challenged, informed, tantalized, even seduced. This takes sophisticated editorial skills, imaginative narrative strategies. The fact is, the best editor is his own average reader; someone savvy enough to live under the skin of the times. What excites such an editor (if he or she is any good) excites the reader by definition. This is what used to be called an "editorial vision."

Harold believed a magazine was defined by the wit and power of its editorial voice. He resisted the market rule that says a magazine should seek a tight concept that subtly erases the boundaries between advertising and editorial in order to pitch directly to the lifestyle of the core demo-graphic.

"You can't run a magazine or a country with surveys," Harold grumbled over the meatloaf. And for a moment we both felt Western civilization descend to hell with a fanfare of trumpets and spreadsheets. Thank God the waiter arrived with the cabernet. Lunch, if not life, was back on course. "Well, hell," Harold said with a certain resignation, "the sun don't shine every day on the same dog's ass."

Time spent with Harold hadn't always been so convivial. He was a mentor and as it is with father-figures there were fights born of my own need to escape his influence and strike out toward an independent point of view. As they say in the Basque country, "The wolf and the dog agree at the expense of the goat—which together they eat."

As the years passed it became clear the old dog knew a hell of a lot more than I thought. In fact, it turned out he was very often *right.* A paternal truism, but nonetheless when after lunch he dropped by my office to see how my work was going, I felt an old emotion rise up—the need for the old dog's approval. I was surprised by this, by how some relationships are forever cast in stone, despite the passing of time.

My office walls were covered with color drawings, a kind of conceptual storyboard for a musical I had been working on. Harold sat and studied them for a moment. He often complained he was losing his memory. But the drawings were made by an artist whose name he immediately recognized because her father had been the French star of *An American in Paris.* More important, he picked up her central influence: the work of Jean-Paul Goude. Like many of us, Goude had been a Harold discovery. His contribution as an *Esquire* art director and illustrator was brilliant. In fact, later, he'd become something of a national treasure in France and was awarded the Legion of Honor.

The movie I was writing had been commissioned by David Geffen for Michael Jackson and Warner Brothers. When Harold asked me to tell him about Jackson I assumed, like everybody else, he was curious about the details of my meetings with "the Gloved One." Harold's eyes scanned the art on the wall as he grew more impatient with descriptions of vegetarian meals sent back because they weren't "green enough." *Who cares,* he suggested, waving me off. Save the anecdotes about the all-consuming solipsism of the American celebrity; save them for *People* or *Vanity Fair.* Who needs more Elvis or Marilyn or creatures of pop anxiety? No, the story is here *in the drawings.* And Harold is up, pacing, feeling the juice of a good idea. And here I am—an enduring dog's age later—missing the point again.

I should have known. Harold had not lost his talent to "approach all

stories about the truly famous from right field." He believed the secret of
dealing with stars was to fold them into the editorial process so that the
writer and editor had direct access. Not one to suffer publicists gladly, he
believed all middle managers must go. Good ideas aren't something
handed down through the celebrity booking system, he'd tell you. A magazine lives or dies on the authority of its voice, on the electricity of its
editorial buzz. He understood how crucial it was to interrupt the familiar
in surprising ways. He also understood that all important innovation was
formal, that it came from an expression of style at the highest level.

October 7, 1986, Neverland: that's what Harold wanted to call an
introductory piece to six pages of selected drawings; a matter-of-fact docu-
mentation of a single day in the life of Michael Jackson at his ranch near
Santa Barbara. As he was talking I remembered he'd published a similar
piece in *Esquire* about a day in the life of Mao Tse-tung. In fact, Goude
had rendered the illustration—Mao in a bath playing with a little rubber
duck.

A Day in the Life of Neverland would begin with our icon waking to a
spirulina protein shake and continue through the daily hair preparation,
visit to his personal zoo, choreographed workout, schedule of telephone
calls, the countless but presumably telling details that would reveal the
aging *infante* in his essence. The piece was to end with Jackson getting on
the phone to talk to me about his idea for the next drawing. The captions
for all drawings over three spreads would be in the words of Jackson;
describing exactly what he was after in every image, the meaning of each
dance number.

Harold, who couldn't identify a pop song for all the whistle in dixie,
remembered that Fred Astaire, a personal hero, had once described Michael Jackson as the "greatest living natural dancer." He was struck by this
assessment and assumed somewhere genius must be present. Extrapolat-
ing, he thought Jackson might also be an isolated perfectionist with a dark
side—both the beauty *and* the beast of *Neverland*. "You'll get this kind of
closet character to reveal himself," he insisted, "only if you have him
talking about his work."

"I'd have to sleep with the guy to get this story," I said incredulously.

"You have access. Keep a journal," Harold replied, as if to say, well,
Mao was no problem; what's your problem?

For a man who complained about memory loss, Harold recalled the
damnedest things. "You know, I rejected your title for the Mao piece," he

mused as I walked him back to his car. 'Easy on the Mao, Please . . .'
—that was it." And with that familiar confederate grin of his, he didn't
spare the derision. *"Just terrible."*

"You sure *I* wrote that?"

"Funny how you remember the really awful lines," he said, climbing
into his tiny Spider Veloce.

I knew I'd never find time to write *A Day in the Life of Neverland.* I'm
sure Harold knew too. By now he was used to his ideas falling on deaf ears.
If I had followed up his idea, I might have left the experience with some
sense of accomplishment. After what seemed like a time of endless frustration and empty intrigue the Michael Jackson movie was never made. I was
richer but poorer—the spiritual capital spent. Another wasp left to drown
in honey. As Harold drove off striking an inconsonant note in tinkletown,
I realized his music hadn't changed, mine had. The road between the past
and the present is marked by dubious achievements. And then he was
gone. How was I to know I'd never see him again?

Sources

L IKE MANY histories and biographies, this book relies on both documentary evidence and the memories of witnesses. Memory plays tricks. My sources knew that and were quick to acknowledge when they couldn't remember incidents, details, years; some of them told me, frankly, which among them had the most reliable memories. I did not often encounter significant inconsistencies among their accounts, and the variety of sources made cross-checking possible. I had an abundance of documents at my disposal—letters and memoranda their authors sometimes had no recollection of ever writing, although they did not doubt that they did.

In the end, I feel reasonably confident of the accuracy of my account. I have provided notes so that readers can themselves evaluate the information presented, and I have indicated in the text when accounts of events differed. I assume readers will understand that a conversation recollected thirty years later is not an exact reconstruction. I assume, further, that readers will understand that my story is not the work of an omniscient narrator, but a reconstruction created out of available evidence.

Among the many documents on which this book is based, one was especially useful in helping me understand Harold Hayes as an editor: the manuscript for a book on magazine editing that Hayes worked on for several years but never completed: "Making a Modern Magazine." He tried to keep from focusing too much on *Esquire* out of a reluctance to turn the book into a promotional ploy, but probably, too, out of a reluctance to speak too frankly of the magazine where he worked. He did speak of his *Esquire* experience in some detail in several chapters, "Building the Magazine's Personality: Importance of the Writer," "Working with a

Staff," and "Loose Words." Because the manuscript for "Making a Modern Magazine" exists only in draft, with multiple versions of chapters and varying headings and page numbers, I have not attempted to cite page numbers for this document.

Some miscellaneous advisories: I have used "Backstage" for "Backstage with *Esquire,*" the monthly column of comment about contents in the issue. All interviews referred to in the notes are interviews I conducted, unless otherwise indicated. When I have relied on information from an interview and the source is apparent in the text, I have not provided a note.

All quotations from correspondence are used by permission of the libraries where the correspondence is held and by permission of the holder of the copyright, except in a few cases in which I was unable to locate the copyright holder; in none of those few cases did publication appear to violate the "fair use" provision of the copyright law. In the interest of readability, I have regularized spelling and, occasionally, punctuation in quotations from unpublished papers.

Several reference sources have been repeatedly helpful: *Facts on File* (New York: Facts on File), *Contemporary Authors* (Detroit, London: Gale Research), and Herman Baron's *Author Index to Esquire: 1933–1973* (Metuchen, N.J.: The Scarecrow Press, 1976). Advertising revenue figures come from the Publishers Information Bureau unless otherwise indicated.

I was unable to tap one potential source of information. Near the beginning of my work on this project, I filed a Freedom of Information Act request for Federal Bureau of Investigation files on Arnold Gingrich and Harold Hayes. Because of the volume of FOIA requests, which are processed in order of receipt, my request was still unprocessed when this book went to press; my petition to expedite the request in time for publication was denied.

ARCHIVES

Collections in three major archives provided the foundation for this project:

Harold Hayes Collection, Rare Books and Manuscripts Department, Z. Smith Reynolds Library, Wake Forest University, Winston-Salem, North Carolina; cited as WF in the notes.

Esquire and Arnold Gingrich Collections in the Michigan Historical Collections, Bentley Historical Library, University of Michigan, Ann Arbor; cited as Bentley in the notes.

Gordon Lish Collection, Lilly Library, Indiana University, Bloomington.

PRIVATE PAPERS

I drew on correspondence and other papers in the private possession of John Berendt, Robert Brown, Byron Dobell, Rust Hills, Aaron Latham, David Newman, Bynum Shaw, Robert Sherrill, and Gay Talese.

INTERVIEWS

Bob Adelman, interviewed by telephone, August 26, 1994.

Sam Antupit, interviewed at his New York office, April 7, 1994.

Robert Benton, interviewed at his New York office, March 25, 1993.

John Berendt, interviewed at his New York apartment, March 20, 1992, and August 22, 1992.

Sheila Berger, interviewed at her New York home, April 7, 1994.

Gina Berriault, interviewed by telephone, April 25 and April 26, 1994.

Abe Blinder, interviewed by telephone, February 25, April 6, and May 28, 1993.

Brock Brower, interviewed at his office, Washington, D.C., January 29, 1993.

Robert Brown, interviewed at his New York apartment, March 26, 1993.

John Burks, interviewed by telephone, July 8, 1994.

Byron Dobell, interviewed at his apartment, April 8, 1994, and several times by telephone.

Candida Donadio, interviewed by telephone, December 12, 1991, and at her New York office, March 18, 1992.

Marvin Elkoff, interviewed by telephone, June 28, 1994.

Valerie Elliott, interviewed at her home near Syracuse, September 30, 1993.

Clay Felker, interviewed at his New York apartment, May 21, 1993, and several times by telephone.

Sam Ferber, interviewed by telephone, May 25, 1994.

Tom Ferrell, interviewed at his office, March 21, 1992.

Carl Fischer, interviewed by telephone, August 22, 1994.

Ralph Ginzburg, interviewed by telephone, August 7, 1994.

Jill Goldstein, interviewed at her New York apartment, March 20, 1992; in a New York coffee shop, March 26, 1993; and several times by telephone.

Susan Hayes, interviewed at her New York apartment, March 27, 1993, and subsequently several times by telephone.

Tom Hayes, interviewed at his New York apartment, March 18, 1992.

Tom Hedley, interviewed by telephone, April 4, 1994, and in a New York coffee shop, April 8, 1994.

Michael Herr, interviewed by telephone, March 29 and June 7, 1992, and in person at his home near Syracuse, September 30, 1993.

Rust Hills, interviewed by telephone, October 3, 1991, and at New Harmony, Indiana, June 17, 1993.

Kitty Krupat, interviewed at her New York apartment, March 20, 1992.

Aaron Latham, interviewed by telephone, April 12, 1994.

Bud Lee, interviewed by telephone, July 2, 1992, and in Bloomington, Indiana, October 21 and 22, 1992.

Gordon Lish, interviewed at a New York restaurant, August 21, 1992; subsequently in Bloomington, Indiana, July 19, 1994; and several times by telephone.

George Lois, interviewed at his New York office, August 21, 1992.

Martin Mayer, interviewed at Wake Forest University, Winston-Salem, North Carolina, April 10, 1992.

Bill McIlwain, interviewed by telephone, September 4, 1991, and December 12, 1993.

Jessica Mitford, interviewed by telephone, January 28, 1992.

Thomas B. Morgan, interviewed at his New York office, August 20, 1992.

David Newman, interviewed at his New York apartment, March 30, 1993.

Eleanor Perenyi, interviewed by telephone, March 1, 1994.

John Sack, interviewed at Weehauken, New Jersey, March 27, 1993, and several times subsequently by telephone.

Nora Sayre, interviewed by telephone, January 5, 1992.

Ann Zane Shanks, interviewed by telephone, July 22, 1994.

Bob Shanks, interviewed by telephone, July 26, 1994.

Bynum Shaw, interviewed at his home in Winston-Salem, North Carolina, May 31, 1991.

Robert Sherrill, interviewed at his home in Durham, North Carolina, June 1, 1991, and several times subsequently by telephone.

Gloria Steinem, interviewed by telephone, May 25, 1993, and in her New York apartment, October 3, 1993.

Gay Talese, interviewed in a limousine, New York to New Jersey, March 20, 1992, and at his New York home, May 20, 1993.

Pete Turner, interviewed at his Long Island home, October 2, 1993.

Gore Vidal, interviewed by telephone, February 10, 1993.

Dan Wakefield, interviewed at a Greenwich Village coffee shop, May 22, 1993.

Garry Wills, interviewed by telephone, July 22, 1993.

Tom Wolfe, interviewed at his New York apartment, April 7, 1994.

Connie Wood, interviewed by telephone, December 10, 1993.

Notes

Preface

Tom Wolfe never got over—"Introduction," in Gordon Lish, ed., *The Secret Life of Our Times: New Fiction from Esquire* (New York: Doubleday, 1973), p. xviii.

according to Gordon Lish—"Foreword," in Lish, ed., *The Secret Life of Our Times,* p. xv.

Part One

Suddenly it was 1960—"The New Sentimentality," *Esquire,* July 1964, p. 25.

O N E *Open the Windows*

Arbus had only lately—Patricia Bosworth describes this time in Arbus's life in *Diane Arbus* (New York: Alfred A. Knopf, 1984), Chapters 15 through 22. I am indebted to Bosworth's biography, more generally, for her characterization of Arbus.

He once proposed—Hayes to Dick Archbald, April 20, 1961 (WF); several complaint letters are on file (WF).

He found her—Hayes, "Diane Arbus: Reminiscences," lecture at the University Art Museum, California State University, Long Beach, February 1, 1985. Hayes gave a similar lecture at the Spencer Museum of Art, University of Kansas, on February 11, 1984; both lectures, delivered in connection with an exhibit of Arbus's magazine work, are sources for this section on Arbus's early work for *Esquire.* The Spencer Museum of Art and Thomas Southall, the curator who put the exhibit together, supplied me with audiotapes of both speeches.

But she was often indifferent—Interview, Shaw.

Tell me about Harold—Interview, Sherrill.

Once when he had asked: August 28, 1961, Arbus to Hayes, in Thomas W. Southall, "The Magazine Years, 1960–1971," in Doon Arbus and Marvin Israel, eds., *Diane Arbus Magazine Work* (Millerton, N.Y.: Aperture, n.d.), p. 163.

"Her vision"—Bosworth, *Diane Arbus,* p. 172.

When Hayes asked—Interview, Benton. Hayes gave Benton the credit for bringing Arbus to *Esquire* in "Editor's Notes," *Esquire,* November 1971, but Benton has a clear and specific recollection of Hayes showing him the pictures first. Bosworth also says Arbus's first contact was with Hayes, not Benton.

Her peculiar subjects—Bosworth, *Diane Arbus,* p. 172.

They had a special—"*Esquire*'s New York," rough typescript, unsigned, n.d. (WF); the file contains other, dated, memoranda on the issue by both Clay Felker and Harold Hayes. Hayes also discussed the ideas and pieces that went into the New York issue in "Diane Arbus: Reminiscences."

They had a thought—Bosworth, *Diane Arbus,* pp. 173–175; Southall, "The Magazine Years," pp. 154–156.

As her requests for help—Hayes, "Diane Arbus: Reminiscences."

The New York City Department of Correction—Samuel M. Badian to Toni Bliss, January 21, 1960 (WF).

In a polite letter—Hayes to Samuel M. Badian, January 26, 1960 (WF).

Crawford had never—A note, apparently describing a telephone message from Crawford via an intermediary, in the Arbus file (WF).

Arbus did not mind—Arbus to Benton, n.d. (WF).

Arnold Gingrich and Dave Smart—This account of the first issue, and all other information about the early *Esquire,* is based on Gingrich's memoir, *Nothing But People: The Early Days at Esquire, A Personal History, 1928–1958* (New York: Crown Publishers, 1971), and on interviews with Blinder.

"Dear Arnold"—September 23, 1954 (WF).

Harold Hayes had been born—Hayes, "Growing Roots in Winston," in the manuscript file for "Making a Modern Magazine" (WF).

start law school—Hayes, "Loose Words," in the file for "Making a Modern Magazine" (WF).

In a creative writing class—Hayes's journal (WF).

It was a "yeasty time"—Interview, Bynum Shaw.

He traveled to Raleigh—Joseph Rebello, interviews with Harold Hayes, February 16 and March 5, 1988 (my copy of transcript). Rebello dates the interviews in notes to his master's thesis at the University of Kansas, "The Role of Editorial Leadership in the Success of a Magazine: A Study of *Esquire,* 1956–1964" (1965).

His old friend—Interview, Sherrill.

The work was—H. T. P. Hayes, "Statement of Personal and Professional Background," n.d. (WF).

on the strength—"Background," prepared for application for a Nieman fellowship, n.d. (WF).

under Harris Shevelson—Joseph Rebello interview with Hayes; Hayes, "Making a Modern Magazine" (WF).

Without much of a budget—Joseph Rebello interview with Hayes.

When he wanted to use—Interview, Ann Zane Shanks.

Susan Meredith—Interview, Susan Hayes.

When Hayes arrived—The description of Hayes's early days at *Esquire* is based on Joseph Rebello's interviews with Hayes; Hayes, "Notes on the Occasion of Arnold's Death," draft (WF); and an unedited version of an article Hayes wrote for *The New Republic,* "For Arnold, with Love and Ambivalence" (WF); *The New Republic* ran an edited version, "Arnold Gingrich, *Esquire,*" September 4, 1976.

"It was the first time"—Gingrich, *Nothing But People,* p. 204.

Affable as he might be—Hayes, "Making a Modern Magazine" (WF).

Before Fred Birmingham left—Interview, Ginzburg.

Ralph Ginzburg and Clay Felker—The description of the young editors' early days at *Esquire* is based on interviews with Felker, Ginzburg, Hills, and Ferber, and on Rebello's interviews with Hayes; Rebello, "The Role of Editorial Leadership"; Hayes, "Making a Modern Magazine" (WF); Hayes, "What Every Man Needs to Know," *The New Republic,* May 26, 1979; Hayes, "A Chapel Talk," *The Wake Forest Magazine,* December 1960; Gingrich, *Nothing But People.*

Esquire would publish *Breakfast at Tiffany's—Esquire,* November 1958.

Felker fought against its publication—Felker to Gingrich, April 18, 1957 (Bentley). Asked
   about this incident thirty-five years later, Felker said he could not recall it. "I
   don't remember the piece, and I don't remember writing that memo. Those
   ideas that I expressed in there were not alien to me, but I was very volatile in
   those days."
"I thought"—Ginzburg to Gingrich, April 19, 1957 (Bentley).
Hayes asked Richard Rovere—Hayes to Rovere, February 26, 1957 (WF).
Hayes had been talking with Laura Bergquist—Bergquist to Rovere, September 15, 1959,
   Bergquist Collection, Special Collections, Mugar Library, Boston University.
As Hayes explained the idea—Hayes to Rovere, November 6, 1957 (WF).
Over the next few years—Morgan, "The Pleasures of Roy Cohn," *Esquire,* December
   1960; Buckley, "The End of Whittaker Chambers," *Esquire,* September 1962;
   Wakefield, "Dos, Which Side Are You On?" *Esquire,* April 1963; Brower, "The
   Abraham Lincoln Brigade Revisited," *Esquire,* March 1962.
"Though I wrote"—Richard Rovere, *Senator Joe McCarthy* (New York: World Publishing
   Company, 1959), pp. 236–237. Speaking at Wake Forest in 1960, Hayes told
   students he liked to think the McCarthy article helped to kill McCarthyism.
   Hayes, "A Chapel Talk," p. 5.
He would warn—Hayes, "A Chapel Talk."
Writing on his behalf—Gingrich to Louis M. Lyons, March 12, 1958 (WF).
Eager to begin—Hayes to registrar, June 12, 1958 (WF).
On a test—Harvard University Examination Book, Nov. 5 (WF).
passing on comments—Two undated letters, Hayes to Gingrich (WF).
Other interesting people—Interview, Susan Hayes.
Susan seemed—Interview, Steinem.
One spring week—Hayes to Gingrich, n.d. (WF).
Ginzburg had gotten himself fired—Interview, Ginzburg. Rebello, "The Role of Editorial
   Leadership," p. 70, gives a similar account based on an interview with Ginzburg,
   April 2, 1988. I have based the approximate time of his departure both on his
   disappearance from the masthead in January 1959 and on a memo from Ginzburg to Felker, July 3, 1958 (Bentley), in which he listed assignments he had
   been handling.
play well with the automobile industry—This was not the last time deference to the
   automobile industry affected editorial decisions. Later on, *Esquire* passed up the
   opportunity to publish an excerpt from Ralph Nader's *Unsafe at Any Speed,* an
   exposé of the auto industry, and Byron Dobell, the managing editor at that
   point, had no doubts that advertising considerations kept Hayes from even considering it. Another editor, Bob Sherrill, recalls proposing an article saying the
   automobile was obsolete; Hayes just smiled, and Sherrill understood there were
   limits to what a commercial magazine can do.
Benton was a slender—Hayes, "Robert Benton: From Out to In," *New York,* March 14,
   1977.
he tried to be a cartoonist—Interview, Benton.
Felker had the satisfying feeling—Interview, Felker.
profile of Sammy Davis, Jr.—Morgan, "What Makes Sammy Jr. Run?" *Esquire,* October
   1959, and "David Susskind: Television's Newest Spectacular," *Esquire,* August
   1960; interview, Morgan.
"It is not so much"—Hayes, "Introduction," in the file for "Making a Modern Magazine"
   (WF).

T W O *Dubious Achievements*

The dark arena—Based on Mailer, "Superman Comes to the Supermart," *Esquire*, November 1960, p. 127.

One night that spring—Peter Manso, *Mailer: His Life and Times* (New York: Penguin Books, 1985), pp. 299–300.

jazz club in the Bowery—Dan Wakefield, *New York in the Fifties* (Boston: Houghton Mifflin, 1992), p. 307.

"Like many another"—Norman Mailer, *Advertisements for Myself* (New York: G. P. Putnam's Sons, 1959), p. 17.

Commentary editor—Norman Podhoretz, "The Article as Art" (1958), in *Doings and Undoings: The Fifties and After in American Writing* (New York: Farrar, Straus & Giroux, 1964).

Yet Hayes opposed—The following section on Mailer's reporting of the Democratic Convention and the response to his article at *Esquire* is based on Hayes's "Building the Magazine's Personality," in the file for "Making a Modern Magazine"; (WF) Manso's *Mailer*, pp. 300–304; and Hilary Mills's *Mailer: A Biography* (New York: Empire Books, 1982), pp. 210–213.

Arriving at Pershing Square—Mailer, "Superman Comes to the Supermart," *Esquire*, November 1960, p. 122.

he found out when he received his check—in "A farewell to his honor," "The Sound and the Fury," *Esquire*, January 1961, p. 15; this is the letter quoted in the next paragraph.

Pete Hamill—Mills, p. 213.

Arthur Schlesinger—"The New Mood in Politics," *Esquire*, January 1960, p. 58.

"the approaching nightmare"—Mailer, "Superman," p. 127.

That fall—The quotations from Roth and Baldwin are taken from transcripts of the speeches in Rust Hills's private files.

John Cheever—This detail was supplied to me by a friend, Becky O'Malley, who was there.

Americans were passing through—"The Sophistication of America," typescript (WF).

photographer Pete Turner—Interview, Turner.

If a friend of Hayes's—Hayes to his parents, July 24, 1964 (WF); the friend, apparently, was Don Schanche.

Felker tried to leave—Felker to John Denson, July 5, 1961 (Bentley).

he held a second job—Yvonne Freund to Felker, September 1, 1961; also an ASMP release, undated; A. John Geraci to Felker, October 1, 1961 (all at Bentley).

Brock Brower—Interview, Brower.

Newman had come to *Esquire*—Interview, Newman.

"What I Did On My Summer Vacation"—Newman's personal papers.

Benton, especially—Hayes, "Robert Benton: From Out to In," *New York*, March 14, 1977. The description of their relationship is based on interviews with Newman and Benton and on Newman's remarks at Hayes's memorial service; I relied on a tape of the service given to me by Hayes McNeill.

"From the raspberry"—Harold Hayes, ed., *Smiling Through the Apocalypse: Esquire's History of the Sixties* (New York: McCall Publishing Co., 1969), p. xviii.

Rust Hills was polishing—The following stories come from an interview with Hills.

The weekend started—The story of the Michigan weekend is based on interviews with Newman and Hills, who also shared with me his correspondence for all the *Esquire* literary symposia in which he was involved. The file includes numerous letters and other items that provided useful background and chronology for this particular story; these were particularly useful: Gingrich to Allan Seager, November 1, 1961; Hills to Bamberger, November 7, 1961.

A correspondent at Iowa—K. Don Jacobusse, on October 31 (1961), to Hills.

Hayes wrote Gingrich—Hayes to Gingrich, "Re-organization," November 8, 1961 (WF); "Editorial Reorganization," November 13, 1961 (WF).

Hayes talked with—Interview, Herr; Herr to Hayes, November 13, 1961 (WF).

Hayes gave it instead to John Berendt—Interview, Berendt.

Take American women—Hayes to Acheson, December 20, 1961 (WF).

His wife, Susan—Interview, Susan Hayes.

Steinem felt sympathetic—Interview, Steinem.

Arnold Gingrich announced—Memorandum to staff, August 24, 1962 (Bentley); other items on which this section is based: Earl Wilson, in his column, "It Happened Last Night," *New York Post,* May 31, 1962, p. 14; Richard M. Mark to Gingrich and Hayes, June 4, 1962; Gingrich to Mark, June 11, 1962; Mark to Gingrich, July 2, 1962; Gingrich to Mark, July 16, 1962; Gingrich to Mrs. Florence Greenleaf, June 29, 1962 (all at the Bentley); and Dobell to Hayes, August 5, 1962 (WF); there is a further reference to Felker's departure in a memorandum from Gingrich to Hayes and Catherine MacBride (McBride), August 19, 1964 (Bentley).

On October 9, 1962—Dobell to Hayes (Talese's personal papers).

The *Times* unions—The description of Talese's reporting on Joshua Logan is based on an interview with Talese, and on the story itself, "The Soft Psyche of Joshua Logan," *Esquire,* April 1963.

rapport a good writer can have—Hayes, "Loose Words," in the file for "Making a Modern Magazine" (WF).

Looking back later—Morgan's remarks at Hayes's memorial service.

A conversation with Harvard economist—Arthur M. Schlesinger, Jr., "Foreword," in Richard Rovere, *Final Reports: Personal Reflections on Politics and History in Our Time* (Garden City, N.Y.: Doubleday, 1984).

Gore Vidal—Walter to Hayes, November 27, 1961 (Newman's personal papers).

The piece drew notice—Hayes to Rovere, May 31, 1962 (WF), also the source of the anecdote from Blinder.

In the *New York Post*—Milton Viorst, " 'The Establishment' and How It Grew," *New York Post,* July 8, 1962.

Mark Epernay, a name he got—Interview, Steinem.

His first piece—"Introducing the McLandress Dimension," *Esquire,* October 1962.

Jerry Jontry, *Esquire*'s advertising director—Jontry to Gingrich, October 2, 1962 (Bentley).

who proposed a photo story—Arbus to Hayes and Benton, n.d., "About eccentrics—" (WF); Hayes to Arbus, February 16, 1961 (WF).

Like Arbus, Terry Southern—Interviews, Newman, Sherrill; Hayes tells the story of Southern's stint as fiction editor in "How to Tell an Editor from a Writer," in the file for "Making a Modern Magazine" (WF). Southern offers another, fictionalized version, placing the episode in a later period, in "The Blood of a Wig," in *Red-Dirt Marijuana and Other Tastes* (New York: New American Library, 1967).

before the movie came out—Southern to Newman, n.d. (Newman's personal papers); Hayes to Southern, May 21, 1963 (WF); Southern to Dobell, April 29, 1963 (WF); Southern to Dobell, April 15 (1963) (Bentley).

Esquire ran a story by Gay Talese—"One Year Later, Still No Bomb," *Esquire,* May 1963; "Nine Places to Hide" appeared in January 1962.

The list prompted—Lawrence Wright, "Orphans of Jonestown," *The New Yorker,* November 22, 1993, p. 70.

Hayes knew—Interview, Berendt.

picture story on railroads—"Pavane for the Iron Horse," text by George Frazier, *Esquire,* December 1961.

About a year after Mailer left—Hayes, "Personality," in the file for "Making a Modern

Magazine" (WF); interview, Hills. Mailer's self-interview, "The First Day's Interview," appeared in *The Paris Review,* No. 26 (1961).

the letter Hills wrote—Hills to Mailer, November 28, 1961 (Bentley).

Hayes talked the idea over—Hills to Hayes, n.d. (WF); the fee *Esquire* paid comes from Charles Rembar to Hayes, August 14, 1962 (WF).

Hayes once called Hills—Hayes, "Personality," in the file for "Making a Modern Magazine" (WF).

that October week—Mailer, "The Big Bite," *Esquire,* April 1963, p. 74.

College students read *Esquire*—Mills, *Mailer,* p. 264.

He was a clear asset—Hayes, "Personality," in the file for "Making a Modern Magazine" (WF).

Something was happening—Interview, Lois, who is also the source of the account of his first meeting with Hayes and the Patterson cover. Lois has written two memoirs, both with Bill Pitts: *What's the Big Idea: How to Win with Outrageous Ideas (that Sell!)* (New York: Doubleday, 1991) and *George, Be Careful: A Greek Florist's Kid in the Roughhouse World of Advertising* (New York: Saturday Review Press, 1972). I have taken the account of the Wolfschmidt ad from *George, Be Careful,* p. 88.

he had tried to convince—"Talk by Harold Hayes, Articles Editor of *Esquire,* to *Esquire* Sales Staff on 'The Editorial Concept of Today's *Esquire,*'" typescript; also typed notes on speech and comments by sales staff that followed the speech, dated December 16, 1960 (WF).

In spring 1962—Jontry and Ferber to Gingrich, April 23, 1962 (Bentley).

Hayes described *Esquire*—Hayes, lecture on Diane Arbus at the Spencer Museum of Art, University of Kansas, February 11, 1984.

"Abe, please don't turn"—Hayes, "For Arnold, with Love and Ambivalence" (WF).

prompting Gingrich in April 1961—Gingrich to Macdonald, April 11, 1961 (Bentley). Macdonald's remarks on *Ben-Hur,* described in Chapter 5, provoked the letter.

a market research report—"*Esquire* Marketing Research: The New *Esquire* Subscriber" (Bentley).

the company itself (although not the magazine)—"Magazines: Look How Outrageous," *Time,* July 14, 1967, p. 42, reported a company loss of $431,175 in 1962. Blinder told me the magazine itself never lost money until about four years before it was sold in the seventies.

Robert Benton would recall—Benton was speaking generally of his years at *Esquire,* not 1962 in particular.

Hayes was jubilant—Hayes to Vidal, March 12, 1963 (WF).

THREE *Red Hot Center*

For weeks during the winter—"Backstage," *Esquire,* July 1963, p. 113.

"I guess everyone knows"—Undated, unsigned memorandum to Hayes (WF).

Norman Mailer cast his eye—"Norman Mailer Versus Nine Writers," *Esquire,* July 1963, pp. 63ff.

Esquire's lawyer—Lawyer's notes, signed AL, March 29, 1963 (WF).

Gay Talese was out interviewing—Talese, "Looking for Hemingway," *Esquire,* July 1963.

the *Esquire* fact-checker—Sherry Murakami, "Talese: *The Paris Review,*" April 2, 1963 (Bentley).

Humes was dismayed—Harold Humes to Talese, n.d. (Talese's personal papers).

Eleanor Perenyi—The following exchange is based on letters at WF: Perenyi to Hayes, November 1, 1962; Hayes to Perenyi, November 8, 1962; Perenyi to Hayes, November 13, 1962; Hayes to Perenyi, November 19, 1962; Hayes to Perenyi, March 26, 1963; Perenyi to Dobell, April 10, 1963; Hayes to Perenyi, April 18,

1963; Perenyi to Hayes, April 22, 1963; Hayes to Perenyi, April 25, 1963; Perenyi to Hayes, April 30, 1963.

There was one figure—The characterization of Alice Glaser and the story of her trip to India are based on interviews with Goldstein, Wakefield, Talese, and Turner; on Barry Miles, *Ginsberg* (New York: Simon and Schuster, 1989), pp. 315–316; and on the piece that resulted, "Back on the Open Road for Boys," *Esquire*, July 1963.

A young southerner—Morris, *New York Days* (Boston: Little, Brown and Company, 1993), p. 23.

George Plimpton called Talese—The description of the exchange between Plimpton and Talese is based on letters in Talese's personal papers: Plimpton to Talese, August 29, 1963; Talese to Plimpton, September 8, 1963; Plimpton to Talese, September 21, 1963; Plimpton to Talese, September 21, 1963 (but written the day after the other September 21 letter); Plimpton to Talese, n.d.

In a long letter from Italy—Plimpton to Talese, August 29, 1963.

Talese returned—Talese to Plimpton, September 8, 1963.

Hills had put the final version—Interview, Hills.

Donadio had begun her career—Interview, Donadio; also the source of Donadio's impressions of Hayes and her meeting Gingrich.

but they *could* object—Hills, "The Dirty Little Secret of Norman Podhoretz," *Esquire*, April 1968, p. 92; interview, Hills.

Burton Raffel—"Letters to the Editor," *New York Times Book Review*, October 13, 1963, p. 50.

"If Orville Prescott"—Hills, "The Structure of the American Literary Establishment," *Esquire*, July 1963, p. 41.

The *Book Review* had its revenge—Harris, "Hot Lunch Center," *New York Times Book Review*, August 4, 1963.

Rust Hills responded—"Letters to the Editor," *New York Times Book Review*, September 29, 1963, p. 34.

Critic Theodore Solotaroff—Theodore Solotaroff, *The Red Hot Vacuum and Other Pieces on the Writing of the Sixties* (New York: Atheneum, 1970), pp. 150–151.

it did not do well—Blinder to Smart, August 1, 1963; Smart to Gingrich, August 1, 1963; Gingrich to Smart, August 2, 1963 (all at Bentley).

To celebrate the issue—This account is based on interviews with Goldstein, Newman, and Dobell.

he admired the way Talese—Tom Wolfe, "The New Journalism," in *The New Journalism*, an anthology edited by Tom Wolfe and E. W. Johnson (New York: Harper and Row, 1973), p. 11; Talese, "Joe Louis: The King as a Middle-aged Man," *Esquire*, June 1962, p. 93.

Tom Wolfe got his big chance—The story behind Wolfe's customized car story is based on Hayes, "Personality," in the file for "Making a Modern Magazine" (WF); "Introduction," in Tom Wolfe, *The Kandy-Kolored Tangerine-Flake Streamline Baby* (New York: Farrar, Straus & Giroux, 1965); interview, Dobell.

"The first good look I had"—*Esquire*, November 1963, p. 114.

Hayes himself came up with—Interview, Wolfe, who told me the Cassius Clay story.

A legal adviser—Handwritten memo, signature unclear, November 8, 1963 (Bentley).

She wrote Gingrich—Lawrenson to Gingrich, March 2 (1964) (Bentley).

"Hernia, hernia"—"LAS VEGAS (What?) LAS VEGAS (Can't hear you! Too noisy) LAS VEGAS!!!!" *Esquire*, February 1964, p. 97.

One day he and Wolfe and Hayes—Interview, Sherrill; Hayes, "Personality," in the file for "Making a Modern Magazine" (WF).

He had a big following—John Baskin, who was there, described this scene to me; Baskin remembers Wolfe wearing his habitual "ice-cream suit." In "The New Journalism," *Dateline,* April 1969, Wolfe says he showed up in a green tweed suit; since he went several times, he probably wore more than one outfit.

Wolfe made several trips—Interview, Wolfe, who also told the story about the phone call from Hayes.

once when Wolfe owed—Hayes, "Personality," in the file for "Making a Modern Magazine" (WF).

but mostly (he himself has said)—Interview, Wolfe.

"In the nunnery"—Boris Pilnyak, *The Naked Year,* translated by Alec Brown (New York: Payson and Clarke, 1928), p. 58.

"Bangs mane bouffant"—"The Girl of the Year," in Wolfe, *The Kandy-Kolored Tangerine-Flake Streamline Baby,* p. 204.

A writer like Wolfe—Hayes, "Personality," in the file for "Making a Modern Magazine" (WF).

f o u r *Around the Bend*

the *New York Times* advertising columnist—Jontry to Gingrich, Hayes, Blinder, Smart, September 12, 1963; Gingrich to Smart, Blinder, Hayes, n.d.; Jontry to Gingrich, October 1, 1963 (all at the Bentley, which also has a clip of Bart's column, "In the Ad World: Culture Booming? Publishers Dubious," dated September 1963).

the company bestowed—Press release, "Hayes Named *Esquire*'s Editor, Dobell Managing Editor" (WF).

In a memorandum defining—Hayes, "For Arnold, with Love and Ambivalence," unedited manuscript for article published in *The New Republic,* September 4, 1976 (WF).

When he found some copy—Note signed, on Gingrich's notepad paper, AG (Bentley); Burroughs, "Tangier," *Esquire,* September 1964.

Once a month Hayes—Interview, Dobell.

a piece on sexual behavior—The Bard College story is based on an interview with Dobell and on correspondence in the Bentley Library, particularly Thomas Rondell to Blinder, Gingrich, Hayes, Jontry, Karp, Smart, February 5, 1964; Gingrich to Thomas Rondell, February 6, 1964; Reamer Kline to Gingrich, February 24, 1964.

For the December issue—The story of the Santa Liston cover is based on interviews with Lois and Ferber; Hayes, "The $750,000 Cover," *Adweek,* October 5, 1981; Jerry Jontry, "by George," letter to *Adweek,* August 24, 1981; Jontry to Hayes, October 22, 1981 (WF); "Thirty Years of *Esquire,*" *Newsweek,* December 16, 1963, p. 88.

Gingrich tried to explain—Gingrich to A. D. Hollingsworth, November 26, 1963 (Bentley).

In the case of "The Segs"—Interview, Fischer.

Just days after the Sonny Liston issue—Interview, Ferber, who also gave me the typescript of his presentation at that meeting. Writing to me on June 3, 1994, he said that, personally, he would have preferred a more limited, high-quality circulation. The $8.3 million figure for 1963 revenue comes from the Publishers Information Bureau, not from Ferber's speech.

Rust Hills, in his office—Interview, Hills.

Two pieces already scheduled—Hayes to Vidal, December 4, 1963 (WF); interview, Morgan; "Publisher's Page," *Esquire,* February 1964.

In the days after the assassination—Hayes to Wicker, December 8, 1963 (WF).

Wicker wrote back—Wicker to Hayes, December 22, 1963 (WF).

"The war in Vietnam"—George J. W. Goodman, "Our Man in Saigon," *Esquire,* January 1964, p. 57.

Hayes would write—Hayes, ed., *Smiling Through the Apocalypse*, p. xx.

Robert Benton and David Newman had felt—The story of "The New Sentimentality" is based on the piece itself (*Esquire*, July 1964), and on interviews with Benton and Newman, who were also the source for the story of the writing of *Bonnie and Clyde*.

Jill Goldstein had been working—Interview, Goldstein.

"We put everything we knew into that movie"—Was outlaw Bonnie based on Gloria Steinem? Benton preferred not to comment; Steinem laughed off the idea, saying, "No, he always used to say he was going to write a movie about me, but that wasn't it, it was a whole different movie."

Hayes called Sam Antupit—The story of Antupit's life at *Esquire* is based on an interview with Antupit and on Steven Heller, *"Esquire* and Its Art Directors: A Survivor's Tale," *Print*, November–December 1990.

One day that spring of 1964—Interview, Goldstein.

On March 9—March 9, 1964 (WF).

Don Erickson—Interviews, Goldstein, Dobell.

Erickson wrote down some thoughts—Erickson to Dobell, May 18, 1964 (WF).

Arnold Gingrich apparently did have reservations—Interview, Goldstein.

he had always been concerned—Gingrich, *Nothing But People*, p. 91.

Once when Gore Vidal—Interview, Brower.

Lish asked Hayes—Interview, Lish.

During the week—Interviews, Susan Hayes, Tom Hayes.

He had taken tennis lessons—Interviews, Susan Hayes, Mayer, Elkoff.

He and Susan had become friends—Interviews, Ann Zane Shanks, Bob Shanks.

In late May—"Your brother" (Hayes) to "Son" (James M. Hayes, Jr.), May 25, 1964 (WF); Hayes to folks, July 24, 1964 (WF); Hayes to Richard, September 15, 1964 (WF). The *New York Herald Tribune* article by David Hoffman, "Covering a Question of Taste," appeared on May 24, 1964, p. 35.

For the first eight months—The story of the publication of *An American Dream* is based on Hayes, "Personality" and "Ideas," in the file for "Making a Modern Magazine" (WF). Manuscripts for each installment, reflecting changes by editors and queries from the research department, are in the Mailer manuscript file of the *Esquire* collection at the Bentley Library.

but he did not like the trend—"Publisher's Page," *Esquire*, June 1963.

His years at *Esquire*—Rust Hills, "How to Retire at Forty-One," in *How to Do Things Right: The Revelations of a Fussy Man* (New York: David R. Godine, 1993), pp. 87–90.

Gingrich was surprised—Gingrich to Mrs. D. V. Klucken, January 31, 1964 (Bentley).

Hayes once left a chapter—Hayes, "Going Over to the Other Side," *New Statesman*, January 1974.

In installment seven—Mailer's comments, in response to a letter from me, were passed on by his assistant, Judith McNally.

Mailer had to meet deadlines—Brock Brower, "Norman," in *Other Loyalties: A Politics of Personality* (New York: Atheneum, 1968).

To get them all in—Manso, *Mailer*, p. 394.

After installment six—Message from Mailer to Hayes (WF).

reviews were mixed—Manso, *Mailer*, p. 403, quoting the reviews.

Newman wrote a parody—Newman's personal papers.

In August—Hayes tells the story of Mailer's report on the 1964 Republican Convention in "Personality," in the file for "Making a Modern Magazine" (WF).

When *Esquire*'s lawyers told him—Hayes, "Loose Words," in the file for "Making a Modern Magazine" (WF).

Mailer, on his part—Mailer's comment, via Judith McNally.

Mailer found him "cold"—Wakefield, *New York in the Fifties*, p. 296.

Hayes, in turn—Hayes, "Personality," in the file for "Making a Modern Magazine" (WF).
Time magazine—May 17, 1963.
Marvin Elkoff—Interview, Elkoff.
"How does a man"—"Everybody Knows His Name," *Esquire,* August 1964, p. 63.
Hayes thought—"Great Editors and Other Dinosaurs," in the file for "Making a Modern Magazine" (WF); typescript for speech "On Race," n.d. (1965), audience not identified (WF).
eventually he apologized—Baldwin to Hayes, May 5, 1966 (WF).
something he had wanted to do—Interview, Antupit.
Esquire got hold of—Interview, Sherrill.
On August 13—"Mayor Considering Delay in Endorsing Kennedy for Senate," *New York Times,* August 13, 1964, p. 15:1.
That fall, the *Columbia Journalism Review*—Penn T. Kimball, "The Non-editing of *Esquire,*" *Columbia Journalism Review,* Fall 1964, pp. 33–34.
In a memorandum dated October 27—WF.

F I V E *Editor Hayes*

As his body—Hayes, typescript for speech "On Race," n.d. (1965), audience not identified (WF).
article *Esquire* had run—William Worthy, "The Red Chinese American Negro," *Esquire,* October 1964.
"The Segs"—Reese Cleghorn, "The Segs," *Esquire,* January 1964; Gingrich reprinted the *Geneva County Reaper* editorial in his "Publisher's Page," *Esquire,* March 1964, p. 12.
in remarks—Hayes, "On Race" (WF).
On April 17—Judith Clavir Albert and Stewart Edward Albert, *The Sixties Papers: Documents of a Rebellious Decade* (New York: Praeger, 1984), p. 12. Other books that have served as factual reference works for me include John Morton Blum, *Years of Discord: American Politics and Society, 1961–1974* (New York: W. W. Norton, 1991); Gerald Howard, ed., *The Sixties* (New York: Paragon House, 1991); Todd Gitlin, *The Sixties: Years of Hope, Days of Rage* (New York: Bantam Books, 1987).
"What *do* you want?"—"Cal Kid," *Esquire,* September 1965, p. 83.
In a draft—"Memo to AG. Subject: Editorial intentions of *Esquire,*" n.d. (WF). I have dated this draft from internal cues and a study of Publishers Information Bureau figures for *Esquire* for the 1960s; this appears to be the only point at which this memorandum would have been written.
articles with attitude—James Barkley, "The Fifteen Dirtiest Plays," *Esquire,* October 1965; Alice Glaser, "The Making of the President, 1968!" *Esquire,* December 1965.
in late spring—Interview, Susan Hayes, who provided much of the subsequent account of their journey.
For three weeks—Hayes to Gingrich, Sunday, n.d. (WF; the originals of Hayes's letters from England are at the Bentley).
When an *Esquire* reporter—Marion Magid, "The Death of Hip," *Esquire,* June 1965.
It was not easy—Hayes to Gingrich, Sunday, n.d. (WF).
One night in early June—Interview, Susan Hayes; letter, Hayes to Gingrich, Sunday, n.d. (WF).
even naming him his daughter Carrie's godfather—Interview, Susan Hayes.
Years later—McNeill to Hayes, October 5, 1988 (WF).
"It's impossible"—Hayes to Gingrich, Sunday, n.d. (WF).
That afternoon at Muggeridge's—Hayes to Muggeridge, July 16, 1965 (WF).

Hayes had been back—Hayes to Muggeridge, December 29, 1965 (WF); the narrative that follows is based on Hayes's long letter to Muggeridge. I made my own call to Beacon Press, which was not able to locate for me any correspondence or information on this episode; I did find the book readily available from two Indiana libraries.

"The Care of Devils"—"Book Review of a Very Limited Edition," *Esquire*, May 1966, p. 159.

The Man Who Kept the Secrets—New York: Alfred A. Knopf, 1979, pp. 64–65 and note, p. 320.

But a couple of Republican congressmen—"Fortas Assailed and Defended in Angry Congressional Clash," *New York Times*, July 30, 1965, p. 10:7–8.

Meanwhile, in June—Michael Wreszin, *A Rebel in Defense of Tradition: The Life and Politics of Dwight Macdonald* (New York: Basic Books, 1994), p. 400.

"Tom Wolfe really"—Gingrich to Lawrenson (Bentley).

As proof that *The New Yorker*—"Lost in the Whichy Thicket," *New York*, April 18, 1965, p. 20.

written in retaliation—*The New Yorker* ran an unsigned parody of Wolfe in "Talk of the Town," March 6, 1965, pp. 32–33. The piece was attributed to Lillian Ross in John Berendt's idea memos for October 8, 1965 (Berendt's private papers), and Tom Wolfe told me it was widely attributed to Ross at the time.

Shawn even sent a telegram—Richard Kluger, *The Paper: The Life and Death of the New York Herald Tribune* (New York: Vintage Books, 1989), p. 706.

During Macdonald's years—Gingrich to Mrs. Richard Olson, October 20, 1969 (Bentley).

In an early review—"Films," *Esquire*, March 1960, pp. 52, 54.

The letters poured in—Macdonald to Gingrich, July 23 (1960) (Bentley); Macdonald to Hayes, September 30, 1964 (Bentley).

to Macdonald, he professed—Gingrich to Macdonald, July 26, 1960 (Bentley). Eight months later, though, Gingrich forbade Macdonald to comment further on the affair, unless his comments had something to do with a current film; Gingrich to Macdonald, April 11, 1961 (Bentley).

"Blast and let blast"—Macdonald to Hayes, November 12, 1965 (WF).

in the *New York Review of Books*—"The Kandy-Kolored Tangerine-Flake Streamline Baby by Thomas Wolfe," August 26, 1965. The second article appeared February 3, 1966.

He did not admire Shawn's attempt—Hayes, "Great Editors and Other Dinosaurs," in the file for "Making a Modern Magazine" (WF).

"perversely," Hayes wrote Muggeridge—February 9, 1966 (WF).

"Oh Truman"—Long, "In Cold Comfort," *Esquire*, June 1966, p. 176.

The same month—"The Personal Voice and the Impersonal Eye," *The Atlantic Monthly*, June 1966, pp. 86–90.

To Tom Wolfe—Interview, Wolfe; "The New Journalism," *Dateline*, April 1969; his theory appears in fullest form in his introduction to Wolfe and Johnson, eds., *The New Journalism*. *Esquire* ran an excerpt in December 1972, "Why They Aren't Writing the Great American Novel Anymore."

In an introduction Hayes wrote—Hayes, ed., *Smiling Through the Apocalypse*, p. xxii.

When even the *Wall Street Journal*—"Editor's Notes," *Esquire*, January 1972, p. 12.

If *Esquire* had a program—Sherrill to me, n.d. (April 1992).

A young editor who came along—Speech by Lee Eisenberg, Wake Forest University, April 9, 1992. The lines themselves are quoted from the opening page of the piece, *Esquire*, November 1970, p. 141.

When Brown read—Interview, Brown; Bergen, "What I Did Last Summer," *Esquire*, December 1965; Berriault, "The Naked Luncheon," *Esquire*, February 1966.

William F. Buckley, Jr., told—Wakefield, *New York in the Fifties*, p. 296.

A writer never knows—Interview, Hedley.

June 24, 1965, memo—WF.

When *Esquire*'s records columnist—Hayes to Mayer, October 16, 1966 (WF).

Writers would call him—Garry Wills gave a good sense of what it could be like for a writer
    to work with Hayes in "Introduction: After the Fact," in *Lead Time: A Journal-
    ist's Education* (New York: Doubleday, 1983).

"representative for the harshest"—Hayes, "Making a Modern Magazine" (WF).

"This stinks"—Memorandum, Hayes to staff, February 7, 1966 (WF).

Checking off the many things—Wolfe to Hayes, August 27, 1976 (WF).

Almost three decades later—Wakefield, *New York in the Fifties,* p. 296.

"a long and powerful relationship"—The description of their relationship is based on
    interviews with Benton and Goldstein and on the Bogdanovich correspondence
    file at Wake Forest, including especially Bogdanovich to Hayes, December 29,
    1965, and Hayes to Bogdanovich, January 17, 1966.

Hayes never let friendship—Gingrich to Lawrenson, September 27, 1973 (Bentley).

Once, later on—Humphrey to Hayes, October 13, 1972 (WF); Hayes to Humphrey,
    October 17, 1972 (WF).

Hayes rejected—"Notes on the Occasion of Arnold's Death," draft (WF).

As an editor, he was playing a role—Hayes, "Ideas," in the file for "Making a Modern
    Magazine" (WF).

Talese had quit—Interview, Talese.

profile of the *Times'*—Talese, "Mr. Bad News," *Esquire,* February 1966; Talese to Con-
    nie Wood, November 14, 1965 (WF).

Hayes had set up the job—The story of the Sinatra piece is based on a series of letters and
    cables in the WF collection: Hayes to Jim Mahoney, October 26, 1965; Talese
    to Hayes, November 6, 1965; Hayes to Mahoney, November 11, 1965; Talese to
    Hayes, November 13, 1965; Talese to Connie Wood, November 14, 1965; Hayes
    to Mahoney, November 16, 1965; Talese to Hayes, November 24 (1965).

"music to make love by"—Talese, "Frank Sinatra Has a Cold," *Esquire,* April 1966, pp.
    89–90.

In 1987, in his introduction—*Best American Essays for 1987* (New York: Ticknor &
    Fields, 1987).

Talese pursued Joe DiMaggio—Talese to Hayes, February 16, 1966 (WF); "Joe, Said
    Marilyn Monroe," *Esquire,* July 1966.

providing a detailed critique—Letters to Talese and Wolfe about the books mentioned are
    in the WF collection.

Hayes would write about Talese's rise—Hayes, "Personality," in the file for "Making a
    Modern Magazine" (WF).

He brought that outsider's stance—Interview, Talese.

Part Two

"What? Has it really been"—"Remember the Sixties," *Esquire,* August 1966.

S I X *History All Around*

In the fall of 1965—Unless otherwise indicated, the story that follows is based on inter-
    views with John Sack; on the story, "M," *Esquire,* October 1966; and on letters
    in the WF collection: Sack to Hayes, October 25, 1965; Hayes to Sack, October
    28, 1965; Sack to Hayes, November 5, 1965; Sack to Hayes, December 23, 1965;
    cable, Sack to Hayes, June 15, 1966; cable, Hayes to Sack, June 16, 1966; cable,

Sack to Hayes, June 17, 1966; cable, Hayes to Sack, June 20, 1966; Sack to Hayes, June 21, 1966; cable, Hayes to Sack, July 23, 1966; cable, Sack to Hayes, n.d. ("HELICOPTER HIT").

"A Negro specialist-four"—John Sack, "M," *Esquire,* October 1966, p. 156.

"The captains told"—"M," p. 147.

Esquire's lawyer wanted Sack—The signed permission statements are filed with the manuscript of "M" at the Bentley.

Esquire's Vietnam articles—"An Armchair Guide to Guerrilla Warfare," *Esquire,* March 1966; campus issue, *Esquire,* September 1966.

"A living breathing communist"—"When Demirgian Comes Marching Home Again. (Hurray? Hurrah?)," *Esquire,* January 1968, pp. 126–127.

Hayes wanted Ruby's story—Hayes, "Ideas," in the file for "Making a Modern Magazine" (WF).

Garry Wills was never sure—The story of Wills's and Demaris's reporting on Jack Ruby is based on an interview with Wills; "Backstage," June 1967, the source of Demaris's comments on Wills; and on the piece itself, "You All Know Me! I'm Jack Ruby!" *Esquire,* May 1967. A second installment of the story, on Ruby's trial, appeared in June 1967.

his review of James Baldwin's—Buckley to Hayes, December 7, 1966 (WF). The review was "What Color is God?" *National Review,* May 21, 1963.

"the detritus"—"The Disposal of Jack Ruby," *Esquire,* June 1967, p. 172.

"The pasteboard star"—*Esquire,* May 1967, p. 79.

"As usual, he cannot sleep"—Ibid., p. 160.

William Humphrey—Humphrey to Hayes, April 18, 1967 (WF).

Theodore Peterson—"Magazine Content: The Nude in 'Jubilee' and Other Pleasures," speech at the School of Journalism, University of Minnesota, Minneapolis, April 16, 1968, typescript (WF).

as he and Benton—Newman's personal papers.

Bob Sherrill made—The story of the demonstration and Sherrill's fight and arrest is based on interviews with Sherrill, Dobell, and Berendt. The *Wall Street Journal* mentioned the demonstration in an article a couple of years later, "Profitable Iconoclast," May 8, 1968, p. 1:1.

which *Time* found—"Magazines: Look How Outrageous!" *Time,* July 14, 1967, p. 42. The numbers that follow are from *Time,* except for the numbers in the sentence beginning "Advertising had risen"; those were supplied by the Publishers Information Bureau.

the Sunday *Times*—"WHAT THE OTHERS SAW: the year through the eyes of the world's great magazines," London *Times,* January 2, 1966.

Arnold Gingrich received—"L.I.U. Announces Polk News Prizes," *New York Times,* March 1, 1967, p. 88:1.

myth-shattering article—"The American Newspaper Is . . . ," *Esquire,* March 1967.

to provoke a newspaper company—Paul S. Denison to Gingrich, March 14, 1967 (Bentley).

When Gingrich received—"Nieman Curator Criticizes *Esquire,*" *New York Times,* March 22, 1967, p. 30:5.

He wrote to his—Sherrill to Shaw, n.d. (Shaw's personal papers).

John Berendt led—Berendt's personal papers; the *New Republic* article was entitled "Keep Off the Grass."

Gingrich balked—Hayes to Berendt, n.d. (WF).

such domestic arrangements were—Interview, Ferber.

Arthur Schlesinger—Blum, *Years of Discord,* p. 290.

Esquire had considered—Hayes, "Making a Modern Magazine" (WF).
William Worthy's report—"The American Negro Is Dead" and "Backstage," *Esquire*, November 1967.
"If there are 'villains' "—"The Black Power Establishment," *Esquire*, November 1967, p. 131.
At midnight—Worthy, "Aftermath: A Negro Reporter's Dilemmas," *Esquire*, March 1968, pp. 6off.; "Growing Dangers," quoted p. 60.
Several years later—Hayes to Evan Forgelman, May 18, 1970 (Bentley).
He had been disturbed—Speech manuscript, "On Race" (WF).
Fritz Bamberger—Bamberger to Hayes and Gingrich, undated note attached to typescript for first "Politics" column (Bentley).
Dobell had assured—Dobell to Bamberger, October 31, 1966 (Bentley).
"Esquire, of course"—"Publisher's Page," *Esquire*, January 1967, p. 6.
"apolitical to the point of indifference"—Hayes, "Notes on the Occasion of Arnold's Death," draft (WF).
In the November issue—"Publisher's Page," *Esquire*, November 1967.
"Any point of view"—Hayes, ed., *Smiling Through the Apocalypse*, p. xix.
Dwight Macdonald once—Macdonald to Hayes, August 16, 1970 (WF).
poured out his anger—"A Sense of Style," *Esquire*, November 1967, pp. 7off.
Macdonald gave—"Politics," *Esquire*, November 1967, pp. 4off.
Herb Mayes—Transcript, luncheon speech at *Esquire*, n.d. (November 1967) (WF).
When Garry Wills came up—This account of Wills's reporting for "The Second Civil War" is based on an interview with Wills; the piece itself, which appeared in *Esquire* in March 1968; Wills, "Introduction," in *Lead Time;* and Wills, *The Second Civil War: Arming for Armageddon* (New York: New American Library, 1968). Wills recalled the number of pieces he agreed to write as initially four, later three; Hayes to Wills, April 10, 1970 (WF), recalled the number as three.
When Wills set out—Wills, *The Second Civil War*, p. 16.
Wills had worked—Interview, Wills; Wills, "Introduction," in *Lead Time,* the source of the quotations.
There was a move afoot—Blum, *Years of Discord*, pp. 279–280, 289–290.
Hayes gave his secretary—Interview, Wood.
Macdonald wrote—"Politics," *Esquire*, May 1968, pp. 41ff.; Mailer's account appeared in *Harper's* in March 1968.

S E V E N *Hell-bent*

Back in May 1967—The account of Herr's reporting in Vietnam is based on interviews with Herr; "Hell Sucks," *Esquire*, August 1968; and correspondence at WF, particularly Herr to Hayes, January 7 (1967), February 5 (1967), May 4 (1967), May 18 (1967), June 1, 1967, November 15 (1967).
Considering the proposal—In a letter to Hayes dated November 15 (1967), on the brink of his departure for Vietnam, Herr said, "We've never discussed expenses on this, except to agree that there would be some, a limited amount." His agent, Donadio, would be talking to Hayes about it. On the upper right-hand corner of Herr's ideas letter, June 1, 1967, Hayes jotted "$600 expenses in Vietnam; . . . sample column—$400."
Then Herr saw the first—Herr, "Hell Sucks," p. 68.
"The very top"—Ibid., p. 110.
"desolate city"—Ibid., p. 69.
"There is a map"—Ibid., p. 66.
When the article came—Hayes to Gingrich, n.d. (WF).
The "Backstage" comments—*Esquire*, August 1968, p. 32.

In late 1967—Hayes to McGeorge Bundy, December 15, 1967 (WF).

back in January 1960—Hayes to Charles Tyroler, January 8, 1960 (WF); Hayes to Arthur Schlesinger, February 12, 1960 (WF).

when he put Vietnam—Berendt's idea lists (personal papers).

Berendt was leafing through—The account of the GI photograph is based on an interview with Berendt, who has in his possession the photograph of the headless bodies that appeared in the newspaper; he also has the following correspondence, on which this section is based: Berendt to Major General Wendell J. Coats, May 22, 1968; Coats to Berendt, May 29, 1968; Joe Carey (the photographer who supplied the prints) to Berendt, n.d.; draft of the text, "Giants," with one word cut; cut identified as the lawyer's in Don Erickson's marginal note, dated 6/28/68; Erickson to Medina (the lawyer), n.d., with note written on upper right-hand corner: "*Rush* HH wants for Nov."; Don Erickson to Harold Hayes, "Legal Report on Proposed 'Giants' feature," June 28, 1968, with Joe Carey's phone nunmber written on the bottom left-hand corner.

The year before—Smart to Gingrich, June 19, 1967 (Bentley). Deaken, "The Dark Side of L.B.J.," *Esquire*, August 1967.

When *Esquire*'s newest editor, Tom Hedley—Interview, Hedley; also "Backstage," *Esquire*, September 1968.

As soon as Garry Wills heard—The description of Wills's journey comes from an interview with Wills and from the piece itself, "Martin Luther King Is *Still on the Case!*," *Esquire*, August 1968, the source of the quotations.

Later, Todd Gitlin—Gitlin, *The Sixties*, p. 30.

Dwight Macdonald climbed—Wreszin, *A Rebel in Defense of Tradition*, p. 448.

the university called in—Albert and Albert, *The Sixties Papers*, p. 30.

Murray Kempton piece—"The Emperor's Kid Brother," *Esquire*, July 1968.

Gingrich did explain—"Publisher's Page," *Esquire*, September 1968.

"What can you do"—Wills, *Lead Time*, p. xi.

Many anti-war activists—Albert and Albert, *The Sixties Papers*, pp. 32–33.

Hayes had started out—The account of the Democratic Convention is based on John Berendt, "Hog-Wild in the Streets," in Walter Schivin, ed., *Telling It Like It Was* (New York: Signet, 1969), to which I am especially indebted; the articles in the November 1968 *Esquire:* Terry Southern, "Grooving in Chi," Jean Genet, "The Members of the Assembly," William Burroughs, "The Coming of the Purple Better One," and John Sack, "In a Pig's Eye"; the Democratic Convention files in the Wake Forest collection; and interviews with Berendt, Sack, and Fischer.

spotted the *Esquire* correspondents—Norman Mailer, *Miami and the Siege of Chicago* (New York: Donald I. Fine, 1968), p. 148.

Around lunchtime Monday—Typed notes to "Harold," unsigned, "Monday" (WF).

"You children"—Berendt, "Hog-Wild," p. 96.

"It had been a bad night"—Ibid., p. 101.

"And what of the trees"—Genet, "Members," p. 87.

Norman Mailer stood—Mailer, *Miami and the Siege of Chicago*, pp. 186–190.

"recording and playing back"—Burroughs, "Coming," p. 89.

"These are rubber people"—Berendt, "Hog-Wild," p. 104.

"to go outside and touch a tree"—Genet, "Members," p. 88.

"at the height"—Southern, "Grooving," p. 86.

He fell into a paranoid tantrum—Edmund White's account of this episode in *Genet: A Biography* (New York: Alfred A. Knopf, 1993) differs from mine. White says Genet tore up his manuscript because he was angry at Hayes for turning down an article on Vietnam that Hayes had agreed to publish. Correspondence at WF does not bear out that sequence of events. According to that correspondence,

Seaver mentioned the torn manuscript to Berendt on September 6, 1968, and did not send the translation of the Vietnam piece until September 17, 1968, by which time Genet was in London and had talked to his agent, Rosica Colin, who wrote to Hayes on September 16 without any apparent knowledge of a decision by *Esquire* not to run the Vietnam piece. Hayes turned the Vietnam piece down in a letter to her dated October 1, 1968.

Later, the FBI—Interview, Hedley.

"The thighs are very beautiful"—Genet, "Members," p. 253.

"Why when I was fourteen"—Burroughs, "Coming," p. 91.

Hayes sent—Hayes to Gingrich, "Friday"; Hayes to Gingrich, "Monday"; Hayes to Blinder, September 6, 1968 (all at WF).

the results were disappointing—Hayes to assignment editors and art department, February 27, 1969 (Bentley).

They appeared in—Daniel Walker, *Rights in Conflict* (New York: Bantam Books, 1968).

In its own way, *Esquire*—In a coda to the whole affair, Senator Eugene McCarthy showed up at *Esquire*'s thirty-fifth anniversary party on September 12, at the Algonquin Hotel, where three hundred celebrants gathered in the Rose Room. "McCarthy Brings Campaign Parable to *Esquire*'s Party," *New York Times,* September 13, 1968, p. 43:1.

In a television film—Produced for ABC in 1975; Wake Forest has the film.

In speeches he made—"Farewell to the Sixties," draft, n.d. (WF); approximate dating by reference to seeing *Easy Rider* and *Alice's Restaurant* with his twelve-year-old.

"There are manifestoes"—"Speech for Authors' League," February 20, 1968, typescript (WF). An accompanying letter, Elizabeth Janeway to Hayes, January 2, 1968, identifies the speech as being made to the Authors Guild on that date.

unless they were expressions—Interview, Hedley.

When Dan Wakefield—Hayes to Wakefield, November 27, 1968 (WF). *Esquire*'s movie critic, Wilfrid Sheed, had already reviewed *Titticut Follies* in March 1968.

The *Esquire* attitude—Hayes, "Introduction," in the file for "Making a Modern Magazine" (WF).

the issue had been briefly banned—"Post Lifts *Esquire* Ban," *New York Times,* July 18, 1968, p. 30:7.

the Magazine Publishers Association—"Advertising: Talk Aplenty on Magazine Day," *New York Times,* September 18, 1968, p. 68:3.

But the next month Hayes—October 31, 1968 (WF).

Morris went after the best writers—Willie Morris, *New York Days* (Boston: Little, Brown, 1993), p. 86.

Warren Hinckle—Warren Hinckle tells the story of *Ramparts* in *If You Have a Lemon, Make Lemonade* (New York: G. P. Putnam's Sons, 1974).

Burks had learned his trade—Interview, John Burks.

its historian Robert Draper—Robert Draper, *Rolling Stone Magazine: The Uncensored History* (New York: Doubleday, 1990), p. 6.

When Michael Herr interviewed Westmoreland—Michael Herr, *Dispatches* (New York: Avon Books, 1977), p. 233.

Edward Grossman—"Endgames," *Commentary,* May 1970, p. 98.

By 1968, Hayes himself would say—Robert Sherrill, typescript, proposal for an article on "The Esquirization of Practically Everything Periodical," n.d., "sometime in the '70s," Sherrill said in the accompanying letter to me.

"Against the aridity"—Hayes, ed., *Smiling Through the Apocalypse,* p. xv.

The Dubious Achievement Awards—"*Esquire*'s Eighth Annual Dubious Achievement Awards," *Esquire,* January 1969, p. 53.

E I G H T *Ugly beyond Belief*

Three months—Hayes described the call in "Loose Words" (in the file for "Making a Modern Magazine"), a chapter devoted to the Buckley-Vidal affair; he wrote the chapter as a magazine article, which was not published (WF). The description of the affair that follows is based on "Loose Words" and on the lengthy correspondence and depositions related to the case at Wake Forest.

During the convention—Transcript, "Excerpt from David Susskind Show—5/11/69—Gore Vidal speaking on WFB" (WF).

Vidal called Buckley—Hayes, "Loose Words," in the file for "Making a Modern Magazine" (WF).

He had once accused—Vidal to Hayes, n.d. (1963) (WF).

Back in 1964—Hayes to staff, "What's wrong," October 27, 1964 (WF).

piece on Norman Podhoretz's—"The Dirty Little Secret of Norman Podhoretz," *Esquire*, April 1968.

Esquire turned up a statement—Quoted in Hayes, "Loose Words," in the file for "Making a Modern Magazine" (WF).

"faggotry is countenanced"—Buckley, "On Experiencing Gore Vidal," *Esquire*, August 1969, p. 132.

He passed a later draft—Hayes to AG (Gingrich), n.d. (WF).

the chief of research—Interview, Krupat.

Hayes asserted—Hayes to Buckley, April 25, 1969 (WF).

on May 6, Buckley—"Buckley, in Defamation Case, Sues Esquire for $1-Million," *New York Times*, August 14, 1969, p. 55:2.

When Harvard professor—Buckley reprinted his exchange of letters with Galbraith in "Buckley v. Vidal, *Esquire*," *National Review*, October 13, 1972, pp. 1113–1115.

his lawyer sent *Esquire*—C. Dickerman Williams to Harold Medina, May 6, 1969 (WF).

Medina responded—Harold Medina to C. Dickerman Williams, May 7, 1969 (WF).

Pressed to say—Hayes quotes this exchange from the deposition in "Loose Words," in the file for "Making a Modern Magazine" (WF).

"But in a larger sense"—Vidal, "A Distasteful Encounter with William F. Buckley Jr.," *Esquire*, September 1969, p. 150.

in a long interrogation—quoted in "Loose Words," in the file for "Making a Modern Magazine" (WF), also the source of Rembar's brief to the court.

the court dismissed—"Buckley Drops Vidal Suit; Settles with Esquire," *New York Times*, September 26, 1972, p. 40:6.

The agreement, filed away—"AGREEMENT made this 18th day of August 1972," accompanied by a cover letter, Robert S. Rifkind to Harold Hayes, September 20, 1972 (WF).

Esquire was also to run—"Publisher's Page," *Esquire*, November 1972, p. 6.

Hayes felt obliged—Hayes to "Letters to the Editor," *National Review*, October 20, 1972 (WF); Buckley to Hayes, October 25, 1972 (WF).

For Hayes, Buckley's suit—Interview, Susan Hayes.

the decision to settle—"Notes on the Occasion of Arnold's Death," draft (WF).

The pieces themselves—"Endgames," *Commentary*, May 1970, pp. 98–99.

"as appropriate a conclusion"—Hayes, ed., *Smiling Through the Apocalypse*, p. xxiii.

that Hayes was worried about—Interview, Hedley.

"She had heard her husband's"—"An American Atrocity," *Esquire*, August 1969, pp. 60–61.

To Michael Herr—Interview, Herr.

"Mayhew, crazy fucker"—Herr, *Dispatches*, p. 138.

Valerie Elliott—Interview, Elliott.

The flower children were leaving—John Luce, "Haight-Ashbury Today: A Case of Termi-
  nal Euphoria," *Esquire*, July 1969.
When Nora Sayre—Sayre, "Politics," *Esquire*, December 1969.
Across the Bay—Wolfe, "The New Yellow Peril," *Esquire*, December 1969.
When Tom Hedley met—Interview, Hedley; the article, "Exclusive and Unauthorized:
  The Liberated Report of Professor X," appeared in the September 1969 issue.
Ralph J. Gleason—"Aquarius Wept," *Esquire*, August 1970.
a major renovation—Hayes to Morris Levine, October 28, 1968 (Bentley); Hayes to
  Smart, Blinder, and Gingrich, October 27, 1969 (Bentley); Hayes to J. Wettin,
  November 19, 1969 (Bentley).
The editors had approached—Erickson to staff, October 13, 1969 (Bentley).
Alice Glaser, who was withdrawing—Interview, Goldstein. The story of the "California
  Evil" issue is based on interviews with Goldstein, Hedley, Sherrill, Lee, and
  Talese, and on the issue itself, particularly Tom Burke's article, "Princess Leda's
  Castle in the Air," the source of the dialogue that begins *"What is she doing to
  the swan?" Esquire*, March 1970, p. 181.
According to MacDonald—Joe McGinniss, *Fatal Vision* (New York: Signet, 1983), pp.
  19, 43.
On February 19, 1970—"Alternatives to Student Discontent," Founder's Day address
  (WF).
there were those who thought—The Gordon Lish Collection at the Lilly Library contains
  several letters from writers to Gordon Lish casting a range of aspersions on
  Esquire.
When Hedley ran into Norman Mailer—Mailer gave essentially the same account in a
  letter to Hayes, except in his version Richard Nixon's asshole would wind up on
  Castro's forehead. He told Hayes that a philosophical divide separated him from
  Hayes. Mailer to Hayes, June 12, 1970 (WF).
Dwight Macdonald, no longer writing—Macdonald to Hayes, August 16 (1970) (WF);
  Hayes to Macdonald, n.d. (WF).
"Step Right Up Folks"—*Esquire*, August 1967; "Do Whites Make the Best Domestics?"
  Esquire, October 1970.
A lawyer for one of the subjects—L. M. Schulner to Hayes, September 9, 1970 (Bentley).
"Bad Names"—*Esquire*, July 1970; "Big Jocks," *Esquire*, April 1970.
Diana Duff Frazier—*Esquire*, July 1966.
Carolyn Cassady—Carolyn Cassady, *Off the Road, My Years with Cassady, Kerouac, and
  Ginsberg* (New York: Penguin Books, 1990), p. 425.

N I N E   *Joy Boys*

In the spring of 1970—The story of John Sack's reporting of Calley's story is based on
  interviews with Sack, on correspondence and other documents on file at WF
  and the Bentley, and on the three articles in *Esquire:* John Sack, "The Confessions of Lieutenant Calley," November 1970; "The Continuing Confessions of
  Lieutenant Calley," February 1971; "The Concluding Confessions of Lieutenant Calley," September 1971. I asked William Calley if he had any comments
  he wanted to make about the *Esquire* story; he did not.
He tried Garry Wills—Interview, Wills.
Sack had read the *New York Times*—The *Times'* first report, September 7, 1969, was a
  small item on p. 14:3. The front-page account appeared, at the bottom of the
  page, as Sack remembered it, on November 13, 1969.
Esquire usually paid for material—Interview, Goldstein, who handled payments to writers.
  The *Wall Street Journal* reported on May 8, 1968, that Esquire's "premium pay"
  was $1,500 per piece ("Profitable Iconoclast," p. 1:1).

Only twice before—Hayes to Blinder, April 30, 1970 (WF).
the transcripts cut, shaped, and slimmed—The transcripts are stored at the Boston University Mugar Library but are closed to the public for Calley's lifetime.
"I'm sorry, I'm not myself today"—This passage is included in manuscript copy attached to a research report, August 12, 1970 (Bentley), that bears the notation: *"NB* Changes in copy per JG from consultation with Calley's lawyer. See manuscript for pencil changes." JG was certainly Jill Goldstein, although later she did not remember making this particular change. John Sack also believed the cut had been made by Calley's lawyer; he did not recall Calley having any objection to it.
"Backstage" called Sirhan—"Backstage," *Esquire,* November 1970, p. 20.
The furor began—Interviews, Lish, Wood.
Newsweek featured it—"A Way to Get Rich," *Newsweek,* November 16, 1970.
Helen Lawrenson read—Lawrenson to Gingrich, November 16 (1970) (Bentley); Lawrenson to Gingrich, December 12 (1970) (Bentley).
Jerry Jontry—Jontry to Hayes, "Volkswagen," December 31, 1970 (WF); Blinder did not recall that the loss of advertising this time was lasting.
Possibly in preparation for—WF; I've linked these notes to the meeting on the basis of a reference to Hitler in a synagogue—a phrase from Jontry's memo—which also appears in the notes. It is possible the notes were made for another purpose.
When readers wrote in—"The Sound and the Fury," *Esquire,* January 1971, p. 30.
In his publisher's column—"Publisher's Page," *Esquire,* February 1971, p. 6.
Newsweek began—"Third Installment," *Newsweek,* February 1, 1971, p. 44.
Hayes drafted a letter—"Dear Sir," n.d., in two drafts (WF). The letter did not appear in *Newsweek* and Hayes kept no fair copy in his files. Sack does not remember any such agreement; in fact, he remembers continuing to press Calley's lawyer for permission to let Calley tell the Mylai part of the story before he went to trial, so the book could be published right after the trial.
Sack explained—Hayes describes the misunderstanding that surfaced with the last installment in a memorandum to Blinder and Gingrich, "Calley Memoirs," May 26, 1971 (WF).
Hayes gave it to—Interview, Latham.
To be on the safe side—Erickson to Hayes, June 10, 1971 (Bentley).
in September 1974—*Facts on File,* September 28, 1974, p. 791.
Elliott's judgment was overturned—*Facts on File,* November 20, 1975.
Esquire described Calley—"Backstage," November 1970, p. 20.
Christmas card—WF.

Part Three

T E N *Stand-up Guys*

Harold Hayes was fearless—Unless otherwise indicated, the story of Lish's life at *Esquire* is based on interviews with Lish and on the Gordon Lish Collection (including letters, memoranda, and edited manuscripts) at the Lilly Library. All papers cited in this section are from that collection unless otherwise indicated.
Hayes gave it to him—Hayes referred to Lish's letter in an undated letter to Hayes McNeill (McNeill's personal papers); Hedley said Lish got the job because he wanted it so much.
Tom Wolfe later wrote—"Introduction," in Lish, ed., *The Secret Life of Our Times,* p. xviii.
Hayes told Marine stories—Interview, Latham.
Carver expressed polite concern—Carver to Lish, "Sunday pm."

Lish sent it on to Erickson—Lish to Erickson, August 24, 1970.

The "Neighbors" that ran—The edited manuscripts are in the Gordon Lish Collection at
    the Lilly Library.

a writer he particularly liked: Lish to DE, HH, July 9, no year.

Doris Betts—Betts to Lish, June 28, 1970; Doris Betts told me she sold the story elsewhere
    when we spoke briefly on the telephone, July 25, 1994.

Paul Bowles—Bowles to Lish, May 18, 1970.

Hayes returned one story—Hayes to Lish, September 14, 1970.

Lish responded—Lish to Hayes, September 17, 1970.

Hayes himself was negotiating—The WF collection contains several letters related to
    Hayes's negotiations with Jones and Roth.

He explained to Abe—Hayes to Blinder, November 5, 1970 (WF).

"Harold," Tom Hedley said—Interview, Hedley.

Perhaps feeling—"Editor's Notes," *Esquire*, January 1971, p. 8; Lish's full memorandum,
    from which Hayes excerpted for his column, is dated October 7, 1970.

John Gardner—Gardner to Lish (December 18, 1970).

Hayes even tried to turn him—Hayes, "Editors and Money," in the file for "Making a
    Modern Magazine" (WF).

poetry was replacing—Hayes to staff, July 15, 1970 (WF); the description of poetry and
    cartoons as "space filler" is mine.

Dickey's characters—"Fiction," *Esquire*, December 1970, p. 104.

Wilfrid Sheed, *Esquire*'s movie critic—Hayes described the break in a letter dated Octo-
    ber 17, 1972, to William Humphrey (WF); Hayes responded in an undated
    letter to Sheed (WF).

Dickey wrote back cheerfully—November 19, 1970.

sent Lish a reaction—n.d.

on April 12, 1971—Steinem to Hayes (WF).

Helen Lawrenson's piece—"The Feminine Mistake," *Esquire*, January 1971.

She wrote back—Steinem to Hayes, May 21, 1971 (WF); Tom Hayes said in an interview
    that his father asked for the album back during this fracas over the profile, and
    he showed me the three albums, still in their cellophane wrappers. Hayes had
    never opened them.

"Ruth's Song (Because She Could Not Sing It)"—Gloria Steinem, *Outrageous Acts and
    Everyday Rebellions* (New York: Holt, Rinehart, and Winston, 1983).

Hayes had laid out for him—n.d. (WF).

Hayes encouraged Gore Vidal—Hayes to Vidal, March 31, 1971 (WF).

She was particularly concerned—Steinem to Judy (Jones), Friday (1971) (Bentley); jj (Judy
    Jones) to Cathie McBride, July 9, 1971 (Bentley).

"I don't mean"—Steinem to Judy (Jones), Friday (1971) (Bentley).

Steinem had lawyers send *Esquire*—E. Douglas Hamilton to Blinder, July 2, 1971.

Blair Chotzinoff—Chotzinoff to Gingrich and Hayes, July 10, 1971; Chotzinoff to Erick-
    son, July 22, 1971 (Bentley).

"She"—*Esquire*, October 1971.

Tom Morgan—Interview, Steinem.

Aaron Latham, the editor—Latham to Hayes, July 6 (Latham's personal papers).

In a speech—Typescript, n.d. (reference to Earth Day the preceding April) (WF).

article on breasts—Interview, Latham.

a spread of *Esquire* cartoons—"Sins of the Fathers," *Esquire*, July 1973, p. 122.

Craig Karpel—"October Memo," October 23, 1970 (Gordon Lish Collection, Lilly Li-
    brary).

Willie Morris thought cost him—Morris, *New York Days*, p. 356.

"Whether Mailer gets Greer"—"Publisher's Page," *Esquire*, September 1971, p. 6.

In fact, when Greer came to lunch—Interviews, Lish, Latham.

Hayes reported to the readers—"Editor's Notes," *Esquire,* September 1971, p. 12.

Back in 1968—Hayes to Blinder, Gingrich, M. Newland, March 14, 1968 (Bentley); Blinder to Hayes, October 30, 1968 (Bentley).

The year before—Interview, Goldstein, who also told me the story of the bare-breasted model; that photograph appeared in "Remember the Sixties," *Esquire,* August 1966.

Her death shook—Interview, Susan Hayes.

Hayes wrote—"Editor's Notes," *Esquire,* November 1971, p. 8.

Hayes gave a talk—"Diane Arbus: Reminiscences."

After Rust Hills left—Hills describes the experience in "How to Retire at Forty-One," in *How to Do Things Right,* pp. 157–174.

The proposal had surfaced—Erickson to Hayes, December 3, 1970 (WF); Hayes to Smart, Blinder, Gingrich, Jontry, December 3, 1970 (WF).

they learned the news—Interview, Hedley; "Esquire Shrinking Size with September Issue," *New York Times,* January 4, 1971, p. 51:4.

E L E V E N *An Uproarious Affair*

On March 13, 1972—Hayes to Gingrich, March 13, 1972 (WF). Hayes mentioned the MGM proposal to his parents in a letter of March 20, 1972 (WF).

Five years earlier—Hayes to Gingrich, January 16, 1967 (WF).

an average of $40,000—Hayes to Bob (no last name) at the Harry Walker agency, December 23, 1971 (WF).

interested in making movies—A few months later, on November 8, 1972, he floated a proposal to Blinder to form a film company that would produce nonfiction general-release movies; a Benton idea, the company would produce stylized films for a specialized audience. Hayes believed the development of home videotape players presented a promising opportunity for this kind of venture (Bentley).

Berger discovered—Berger to Hayes, December 3, 1971 (WF).

when Gingrich reached seventy—Don Erickson explained in a letter to Helen Lawrenson dated May 17, 1973 (Bentley), that although Gingrich was forced by corporate bylaw to retire from his transferrable position of publisher, he could remain on the job in the nontransferrable post of "Founding Editor."

On March 28—Hayes to Gingrich, March 28, 1972 (WF).

It was—Arnold Gingrich, "Announcement," n.d. (Latham's personal papers).

Jerry Jontry, president—Jontry to Hayes, April 22, 1971 (WF).

The *New York Times*—"Advertising: Magazines Report on 1st Half," *New York Times,* April 20, 1971, p. 71:3.

Jontry was reporting—Hayes to Gingrich, "Circulation," n.d. (March 1972) (WF).

For six years—Rust Hills, *"Esquire'*s Biggies: Capote, Talese, Wolfe, W. R. Simmons. W. R. Simmons? Right. W. R. Simmons," *More,* November 1976. Circulation figures are from Standard Rate and Data Service.

The strategy worked so long as—Interview, Ferber.

But ultimately the strategy failed—A. J. van Zuilen offers a detailed analysis of the postwar magazine economy in a published dissertation, *The Life Cycle of Magazines: A Historical Study of the Decline and Fall of the General Interest Mass Audience Magazine in the United States during the Period 1946–1972* (Uithoorn, Netherlands: Graduate Press, 1977).

Print magazine had reported—Carol Stevens, "Promotion Design at *Esquire,* Inc.," *Print,* 21 (March–April 1967), p. 46.

In March 1972—Hayes to Gingrich, "Circulation," n.d. (March 1972) (WF).

"If any icons"—*"Esquire* and Its Art Directors: A Survivor's Tale," *Print,* November–December 1990, p. 157.

He would pull back sometimes—Interview, Lois.

The month after Hayes's memo—The following section on covers is based on memoranda in the Bentley: Jontry to Smart, Blinder, Gingrich, Hayes, April 18, 1972; Hayes to Jack Shurman, February 18, 1972; Hayes to Smart, Blinder, Gingrich, Jontry, May 9, 1972; research report (JJ) to Don Erickson, May 4, 1972; Jontry to Erickson, June 5, 1972; Erickson to Jontry, June 7, 1972; Hayes to Jontry, June 7, 1972; Jontry to Smart, Blinder, Gingrich, Hayes, Erickson, Shurman, Petzel, June 8, 1972; Jontry to Erickson, June 9, 1972; Shurman to Jontry, June 9, 1972.

Smart had always wanted—Interview, Ferber.

His mood was bleak—Hayes to staff, July 13, 1972 (WF).

Clay Felker hired away—Interviews, Felker, Latham.

He wrote Hayes—Latham to Hayes, April 18, 1972 (WF).

Hayes retired his softball shirt—Hayes to staff, March 20, 1972 (Latham's personal papers).

Esquire received—Elie Abel to Harold Hayes, April 6, 1972 (WF).

Atlantic Monthly magazine column—L. E. Sissman, "Innocent Bystander," *Atlantic Monthly*, April 1973, p. 32.

They couldn't just take—Interview, Latham.

In spring 1972—Hayes to Blinder, April 4, 1972 (WF).

Hayes wrote to Mailer—Hayes to Mailer, April 19, 1972 (WF); the file also contains an earlier draft of the letter with "Dear Norman" replaced, in Hayes's writing, by "Dear Mr. Mailer."

Reflecting on the absence—Undated memo (mid-1972) (WF).

"With any luck at all"—Wolfe, "Why They Aren't Writing the Great American Novel Anymore," *Esquire*, December 1972, p. 272.

In September—Hayes to Talese, n.d. (WF). This letter is one of two private, detailed descriptions by Hayes of the events of his last days at *Esquire*. The other was a draft he titled, "Notes on the Occasion of Arnold's Death," September 4, 1976 (WF).

on October 2—Arnold Gingrich, "Esquire Editorial Promotions," October 2, 1972 (Bentley).

The offer the company was making—Hayes to Talese, n.d. (WF); interview, Blinder.

Hayes was afraid that as publisher—Hayes to Talese, n.d. (WF)

he had remained active—On January 23, 1969, Gingrich reminded Hayes who was in charge with an angry memorandum on a pictorial spread that had superimposed text on illustration, a practice that Gingrich believed insulted the written word. He asked that Hayes see it did not happen again, ever, so long as Gingrich was around. Gingrich to Hayes, January 23, 1969 (Bentley). There is plentiful evidence in the Gordon Lish Collection (Lilly Library) of Gingrich's involvement in editorial matters.

If he wanted the kind of editorial authority—Hayes to Talese, n.d. (WF).

"the perfect buffer"—"For Arnold, with Love and Ambivalence," draft (WF).

Gingrich himself had found—Martin Mayer said much of the sixties *Esquire* was distasteful to Gingrich. "A Memoir, with Arnold," draft (WF).

Yet once when management—Hayes, "Notes on the Occasion of Arnold's Death," draft (WF).

As Hayes wrote in notes—Ibid.

Willie Morris had left *Harper's*—Morris, *New York Days*, p. 356.

Before that, Clay Blair—Hayes, "Making a Modern Magazine" (WF).

Gingrich recalled—Gingrich, *Nothing But People*, p. 212.

"What had happened to Arnold"—Hayes, "Notes on the Occasion of Arnold's Death," draft (WF).

In an interview, Blinder gave his version of Hayes's departure. According to Blinder,

Gingrich had reported to Blinder and John Smart that Hayes had agreed to turn the editor's position over to Don Erickson. "And the next thing I knew, Harold came in to see me—he apparently had gone back to Arnold Gingrich—and said he did not want to do this. He'd thought about it overnight, he did not want to do this. He wanted to be not only publisher but editor as well. So Arnold Gingrich said, 'Well, that's an unusual thing, why don't you go in and talk to Abe Blinder.' So he came in to see me, and outlined exactly that viewpoint, that he wanted to be both. I said, 'We've never had the position of publisher and editor in one person—we've always felt it was proper to have a separation of the two—to have a publisher and have an editor.'

"So I said, 'We find you have made a great contribution to the magazine. We recommend that you be the publisher.' Arnold said that he would be, I think, editor emeritus, or founding editor or something like that. But that was something they had arranged.

"And he said, 'No, no I've got to be publisher and editor.'

"I said, 'Are you saying, Or else?'

"And he said, 'Or else.'

"I said, 'Well, that's your choice. It's your decision.'

"And he left.

"I didn't fire him. We didn't fire him."

When the staff got back—Interview, Lish.

"Due to irreconcilable differences"—Memorandum, April 5, 1973 (Bentley).

A company memo—Gingrich to all employees, April 5, 1973 (Bentley).

On Tuesday Hayes met the staff—Hayes to Talese, n.d. (April 11) (WF).

to learn from a reporter—Hayes, "Notes on the Occasion of Arnold's Death," draft (WF).

a letter he had received—Talese to Hayes, April 8, 1973 (WF).

On April 7—*"Esquire's* Publisher and Editor Dispute the Latter's Departure," *New York Times,* April 7, 1973, p. 31:1–2.

Time magazine—"Short Takes," *Time,* April 16, 1973, p. 53.

Newsweek offered—"Down the Up Staircase," *Newsweek,* April 23, 1973, p. 48.

Publicly cool—He may have changed his mind about going quietly. On September 5, 1976, after Gingrich's death and Hayes's piece on Gingrich appeared in *The New Republic,* Martin Mayer wrote to him, "In the days after your departure, Arnold was manning the trenches to make sure Blinder et al. didn't try to gyp you of severance pay. He felt that the things you wanted to say might jeopardize those arrangements, and he was being tough on you For Your Own Good." Elsewhere, Mayer observed that Gingrich and Hayes had given him "exactly the same account" of events leading to Hayes's departure. "A Memoir, with Arnold" (WF).

In notes he wrote—"Notes on the Occasion of Arnold's Death," draft (WF).

Tom Ferrell wrote—All the letters quoted in this section are at Wake Forest: Ferrell, April 6, 1973; Dobell, April 9, 1973; Hills, April 25, 1973; Sack, April 15, 1973.

When Hayes called Lois—Interview, Lois.

he threw a big farewell party—Interview, Susan Hayes.

Bob Sherrill missed the party—Sherrill to Hayes, n.d., postmarked May 14, 1973 (WF).

When Rust Hills reported—*More,* November 1976, p. 48.

Index